Infectious Diseases and Microbiology

nova
Medicine & Health
New York

Infectious Diseases and Microbiology

Psychological Consequences of the COVID-19 Pandemic on Children, Teenagers and Adults
Jean-Pascal Assailly, PhD (Editor)
2022. ISBN: 978-1-68507-963-5 (Softcover)
2022. ISBN: 979-8-88697-072-2 (eBook)

COVID-19 Contracting: Opportunities, Actions and Reimbursements
Eric Neudorf (Author)
2022. ISBN: 978-1-68507-710-5 (Hardcover)
2022. ISBN: 978-1-68507-733-4 (eBook)

The Aviation Industry and COVID-19
Stefan Schneider (Author)
2022. ISBN: 978-1-68507-712-9 (Hardcover)
2022. ISBN: 978-1-68507-729-7 (eBook)

Diseases Transmitted by Ticks
Hacer İşler (Editor), Metin Özdemir, MD (Editor)
2021. ISBN: 978-1-68507-359-6 (Hardcover)
2021. ISBN: 978-1-68507-383-1 (eBook)

Impacts and Implications of COVID-19: An Analytical and Empirical Study
Anand Sharma (Editor)
Prateek Agrawal (Editor)
Vishu Madaan (Editor)
Anuj Agarwal (Editor)
2021. ISBN: 978-1-53619-670-2 (Hardcover)
2021. ISBN: 978-1-68507-081-6 (eBook)

More information about this series can be found at
https://novapublishers.com/product-category/series/infectious-diseases-and-microbiology/

Vijayalakshmi Kakulapati
Editor

Data Science Applications of Post-COVID-19 Psychological Disorders

nova
Medicine & Health
New York

DOI: https://doi.org/10.52305/KRLL5890

Library of Congress Cataloging-in-Publication Data

ISBN: 979-8-88697-165-1

Published by Nova Science Publishers, Inc. † New York

Contents

Preface

Abstract

Data science has improved healthcare as new data sources and analytic techniques have become available. Data science applications are valuable technologies, which could powerfully improve health care service delivery, especially in mental illness. COVID-19's undesired psychological health repercussions, such as depression symptoms, have been widely anticipated. COVID-19 has several physical health risk factors; however, it is unknown if there are any psychological risk factors. Data science enables statistical cooperation, data analytic technique development, and data administration for psychiatric and mental health research. Although data science is not commonly employed in the mental health profession, there is hopeful evidence that it can substantially affect it. Researchers may use data science to evaluate mental diseases' consequences in the US and worldwide. When the consequences are measured and backed up by statistics, it makes a stronger argument for much-needed provisions. When the consequences are defined and validated by evidence, it provides a robust discussion for allocating critical resources to accessible psychological health diagnosis and care. Diagnostic reports, pharmaceutical sales, physicians' observations, and diagnostic testing are all examples of data. Data from health applications and monitoring tools can be used to gain valuable insights and, ultimately, break the stigma of psychiatric conditions in enhancing health care.

This book explores the concepts of data science, including ML (machine learning), DL (Deep learning), and AI (Artificial Intelligence) in psychological health care and the recent research developments focusing on pandemic healthcare systems worldwide.

The chapters in this book analyse the chances of effectively using data science (DS) in healthcare, especially in coronavirus-related issues and healthcare systems. They also present some use cases of DS in psychological problems in the catastrophic pandemic period and show its potential to improve care services delivery to overcome future challenges.

Definitions

Data science: data science is a rapidly evolving field of data analysis and application that emphasizes assembling, computing, displaying, analysing, archiving, and utilizing vast volumes of data. In the branch of psychotherapy, data science raises the potential for information gathering and processing, streamlining, and supplementing initiatives to identify neurological development. Data science technologies can allow new fields of study, including cognitive neuroscience. Scientists may help data science evaluate the consequences of psychological disorders and worldwide demographics. Once the effects are defined and substantiated by evidence, it implies a more powerful argument for allocating strategic resources to accessible psychological healthcare diagnosis and care.

Machine learning: It is being used by cognitive psychologists and physicians worldwide to support therapeutic interventions for patients. Machine learning assists in identifying a few of the leading indicators of psychiatric illness as symptoms develop. One feature is that machine learning can assist therapists in determining who is at the probability of developing a specific condition. Mental illness, distress, depressive illness, posttraumatic stress disorder (PTSD), and depressive symptoms are common in COVID patients after their recovery from illness. Because of the high incidence of psychiatric disorders and efficient psychotherapy, there has been an upsurge in investigation into how ML can improve recognition, assessment, and dealing with psychological disorders. ML approaches can create additional possibilities for understanding conscious behavioural traits, discovering psychological symptoms and comorbidities, anticipating consequences regarding disorder progression, and identifying and enhancing medications.

Artificial intelligence: In assisting diagnosing, treatments, and clinical management, AI can enhance mental health care and development. The detection of abnormalities may enable further precise, enhanced descriptions of such disorders. There's tremendous variation in the pathophysiology of mental illness, and diagnosis of abnormalities may help to improve diagnoses of such mental conditions. Using AI approaches, researchers can create appropriate pre-diagnosis methods and risk approaches to assess a person's tendency for, or the possibility of developing, mental illness. The application of artificial intelligence for behavioural psychology might give clinicians important information.

About the Pandemic

COVID-19 has generated many psychological problems, such as panic, anxiety, post-traumatic stress disorder, and other trauma and demotion disorders. Some have experienced significant, life-threatening COVID-19 sickness; some, as relatives and healthcare professionals, have observed people's sufferings; and some have understood the destruction of complications. As a result, research became more interested in detecting social and communal anxiety to assist the populace emotionally. The risk assessments implemented in response to the outbreak had varying effects on people, depending on their social context. All these people tend to be more vulnerable to frustration, depression, and post-traumatic symptoms as people are susceptible and emotional. Post-COVID-19 is causing a few people's intellectual and central nervous system difficulties to continue for a considerable length of time. Such people's psychological health has taken a long time to regain. Psychosocial stressors may be socioemotional issues first caused by the immune system's response to the infections.

Psychological Impacts

Depression can be caused by stress, rumination, and the sadness of becoming ill or spreading illness to peers and can cause uneasiness, jitteriness, numbness and panic attacks, chest pains, and respiratory complications.

Structure of the Book

Chapter 1: Introduction to Post-COVID-19 Mental Disorder & Its Consequence

The most common long-term post-COVID-19 consequence in COVID-19 patients has been recognized as psychological anguish. COVID-19 is associated with several psychological problems and illnesses, although it is uncertain if any psychological factors exist. The SARS pandemic was also related to the rise in PTSD, anxiety, and emotional discomfort among patients and caregivers. Patients with a history of psychiatric, nervous, or drug usage issues are substantially further vulnerable to SARS-CoV-2 disease and may have an advanced risk of devastating consequences, even mortality. Over the year after the catastrophic sickness, patients have continued psychiatric disruption, including severe cognitive discomfort, melancholy, and persistent PTSD distress.

Chapter 2: Contemplating the Psychological Resilience of People during the COVID Era

Mood swings are anticipated in a person's lifetime. In all circumstances, including the epidemic, the assumptions concerning emotional stability in regular duties have been investigated, established, and demonstrated. This chapter employs students, enterprises, educators, and many others to evaluate the underlying concepts of mental health and their usefulness in a range of tasks.

Chapter 3: Data Science Applications of Post-COVID-19 Mental Illness

Data science can assist us in improving solutions for psychological difficulties. Several patients attempt a variety of psychologists, therapeutic strategies, and drugs before discovering what works for them. The procedure of locating suitable treatment is especially troubling considering how long most patients have to suffer before actually obtaining any treatment and the expense and mental strain associated with attempting many choices. As a result, it is critical to determine whether or not a specific medicine is effective.

Chapter 4: Prediction of Mental Distress about COVID-19 among Higher Education Students in Odisha India

The anxiety of contamination, the epidemiological scenario, unanticipated confinement, and the deployment of virtual classrooms are all probably influencing students' emotional health throughout the COVID-19 outbreak. Five hundred forty-one undergraduates performed an internet survey in this investigation. All of these are undergraduates, KIIT Deemed to be University and BPTU Bhubaneswar, who came from all across the nation and some overseas countries. These issues were screened using a psychographic assessment, awareness, panic, worry, and emotional exhaustion scores.

Chapter 5: Post-COVID-19 Syndrome in Hospitalized Patients with COVID-19 Theoretical Learning- Insights of Patient Mental Illness

Long-term complications of coronavirus illness 2019 are persistent. Intensive care units place more emphasis on mild and severe COVID-19. The ongoing assessment of people with post-COVID conditions will be a significant challenge in characterizing and minimizing the psychosocial and therapeutic long-term consequences of COVID-19 and utilizing data science techniques to evaluate the insights of patient mental illness.

Chapter 6: Computational Intelligence Models for Stress.

The concept of computational intelligence (CI) is influenced by measurable and valuable properties of people and natural cognition. The objective of CI-based technologies is to analyse and conceptualize data from multiple types. CI is inextricably linked with the rise in available information and computational power, directly supporting elements. Complications of physical and emotional responses include undesirable tension and depression. Anxiety has both adaptive and maladaptive consequences. Coronavirus caused severe biological illness, which became an epidemic in 2020. COVID-19 wreaked havoc on public mental health. COVID-19 has triggered a countrywide lockdown. Melancholy, panic, and stressful effects were seen.

Chapter 7: Multimodality Analysis of Psychological Disorders

The COVID-19 epidemic has triggered and will continue to create tremendous emotional challenges associated with psychiatric diseases, including sadness, sleeplessness, appetite loss, anxiousness, and traumatic stress. This chapter illustrates how social dangers and epidemic pressures might have a devastating effect on psychiatric problems. Professionals, patients, and doctors should work together to develop long-term alterations of supply techniques for emotional and mental health therapy specifically aimed at reducing health care disparities.

Chapter 8: Mathematical Analysis of Mental Illness

Emotional difficulties have become more common in post-COVID-19 patients. The complex computer modeling will be built to predict the rate of increase and factors that lead to different issues, including depressive disorder, schizophrenia, binge eating, mental illness, traumatic stress, psychiatric features, etc. A comprehensive statistical analysis will be carried out to establish the significant level to recommend suitable medical instructions. This chapter includes declaring the numerous psychological diseases, identifying the psychiatric disorders after recovering from COVID with several guidelines, efforts made in mathematics, and the deep interactive analysis with the mapping of psychiatric illnesses.

Chapter 9: Elderly People's Emotional Stress

Distress is a significant psychological condition among the older, affecting the overall standard of living. Being apart from loved ones, solitude, misinformation on social media, economic hardship, and stigmatization are risk factors for older adults. To overcome, diagnose, and control such issues, it is necessary to know and investigate the emotional effect and critical parameters. Assistance services for worried persons, mobile-based, online networking & assistance communities, supporting relaxation, analysing mental repercussions, and creating and implementing appropriate remedies are among the recommended initiatives.

Chapter 10: Work from Home-Related Depression Analysis

The epidemic has left the world on its head, leading to a transformation in the workplace atmosphere of the whole working community to improve a substantial influence on the physical and psychological disorders of vast numbers of employees. The chapter focuses on examining home-related stress caused by work-from-home (WFH) on both males and females and methods to resolve this current predicament to restore humanity's average intellect.

Chapter 11: Effect of Psychological Disorder on Students' Academic Performance

Over a few years, the globe has been hit by a massive epidemic. COVID-19, a disease that began in China in December 2019, has caused a long-term epidemic around the planet. This chapter determines the impact of psychological problems on student performance.

Chapter 12: Psychological Resilience

Psychological resilience is human beings' mental or emotional ability to cope with a crisis, conflicts, problems, issues, or challenges and quickly return to normal or earlier situations. Psychological resilience gives strength to mankind and a support system to work for life's goal and overcome negativity, challenges, adversities and work through problems. The study has proposed a conceptual framework or model for being more resilient in day-to-day business, which will help individuals develop their strengths and capabilities and achieve desired goals.

Chapter 13: Challenges & Privacy Concerns related to Mental Health

So far, over 268 million cases and 5.28 million recorded fatalities have been documented, and the case burden is increasing in several nations. People with prior morbidities are more likely to suffer from acutely severe medical consequences, which can be deadly. Addressing the mental health needs of this group has emerged as a critical problem for healthcare professionals. The regional and federal governments' privacy regulation frameworks are putting pressure on processes to protect the privacy of those suffering from post-COVID-19 depressive symptomatology syndrome.

Chapter 14: Impact of Post-COVID Skin Allergies

The outbreak raises a number of concerns for care providers. Early accurate diagnosis, susceptibility categorization, effective utilisation of severe medical services, proper drugs, observation, and quick release are vital for protecting as victims as feasible. This chapter discusses several ML (machine learning) implementations and improvements for analysing facial skin concerns. The study attempts to give safe and effective professionals a strategy plan to grasp its potential and difficulties. Effective ML approaches, such as ensemble learning algorithms, are applied in this work. This chapter establishes an intelligence assessment assistance to reliably detect a specific type of hypersensitivity ailment for development.

Chapter 1

Post-COVID-19 Mental Disorder and Its Consequences

Vijayalakshmi Kakulapati[1,*], Sheri Mahender Reddy[2,†] and A. Paramasivam[3,‡]

[1]Department of IT, Sreenidhi Institute of Science and Technology, Hyderabad, India
[2]Otto-Friedrich University of Bamberg, Germany
[3]Department of Mechanical Engineer, Rajalakshmi Engineering College, Chennai, India

Abstract

The current epidemic of severe coronavirus illness has led to global medical issues. Furthermore, the ongoing and protracted post-COVID-19 or chronic COVID imposes a significant burden on health care professionals because of inadequate medical facilities. Heart disease has been identified as the most prevalent enduring post-COVID-19 consequence of coronavirus persistence. COVID-19's undesirable psychological repercussions, such as anxiety and depression, have been generally anticipated but have yet to be fully assessed. COVID-19 has several physiological conditions and diseases. However, it is unknown whether there are possible psychological causes. The severe acute respiratory pandemic was also related to a rise in PTSD, tension, and emotional anguish among victims and doctors. In the context of certain

*Corresponding Author's Email: vldms@yahoo.com.
†Corresponding Author's Email: mahendersheri@gmail.com.
‡Corresponding Author's Email: paramasivam.a@rajalakshmi.edu.in.

In: Data Science Applications of Post-COVID-19 Psychological Disorders
Editor: Vijayalakshmi Kakulapati
ISBN: 979-8-88697-165-1

occurrences, the effects might be rapid and then last for a significant period. COVID-19 may induce severe psychological issues like disorientation, restlessness, and dementia. Patients who have had psychological, cognitive, or medication abuse issues are significantly more susceptible to SARS-CoV-2 infection and may have a higher risk of devastating outcomes, even fatality. During one year post-acute, victims of the devastating disease have ongoing psychological disturbance, with considerable psychological distress, sadness, and chronic posttraumatic depression. Most people with symptomatic respiratory failure have neuropsychological problems, such as poor concentration, cognition, remembering, and intellectual information processing. This chapter addressed the post-COVID psychological issues and their consequences.

Keywords: post COVID, consequence, psychological, stress, anxiety, disorder, mental, survivor, PTSD, risk, factor, complication

Introduction

While most patients with COVID-19 recover in a few weeks, a few develop post-COVID symptoms. These issues are several emerging, reoccurring, or continuous medical difficulties that have occurred four or even more weeks since being infected with the pathogen that causes COVID-19. Even patients who did not exhibit COVID-19 indications in the days following infection can develop post-COVID problems. Such post-COVID symptoms might be protracted COVID, lengthy COVID sequelae, or persistent COVID. Experts worldwide are trying to learn more about the short-term and long-term health effects of COVID-19, as well as who gets these symptoms [1].

The long-term impacts of COVID-19 last for at least two weeks [2]. This change has been described primarily in patients with acute and catastrophic illnesses, but it may also occur in those with minor ailments that do not require treatment [3]. Unfortunately, it is unknown whether gender, ethnicity, age, origin, pre-existing medical complications, infectious load, or the course of COVID-19 influence the likelihood of long-term consequences [4].

After recovering from COVID-19, patients can have many complications. Post-COVID-19 causes respiratory, psychological, circulatory, skin rashes, sensory nerve, and kidney and cardiovascular system problems, increasing the likelihood of long-term, life-threatening health problems. Nevertheless, the infection can affect the host for three months following diagnosis. It could lead to significant changes in certain people, who receive a subsequent tangible result even after they have recovered, although it does not necessarily suggest that the infection remains communicable [5].

Some typical indications and consequences of post-COVID problems could include [6]:

- Muscle aches, ligament pain, or headaches
- increased glucose levels
- Flu
- Tiredness, feelings of exhaustion, or drowsiness
- Impaired sense of smell
- Chest discomfort or hypotension
- Chest tightness or pain in the chest
- Mellitus :
- muscle pain
- A lack of attention, poor decision-making, or cognitive confusion
- Sleeplessness, stress disorder, or sadness
- lightheadedness
- rashes on skin

Problems can be complicated by incorporating physical or psychological behavior. The consequences of epidemics might last many years, affecting every community. The COVID-19 epidemic was quickly documented, analogous to post-traumatic stress disorder (PTSD) [7]. Therefore, individuals who had affected coronavirus and recovered are more probable to create PTSD symptoms [8]. Several PTSD and depression effects were cited by COVID-19 sufferers [9]. One of the most common problems in PSTD includes stressful experiences, sleeplessness, nervousness, restlessness, cognitive problems, exhaustion, and emotionally painful recollections [10].

Background

Psychological disorders affect approximately a million individuals worldwide. The COVID-19 epidemic has dramatically raised emotional stress due to the ongoing physical and emotional health danger. Additionally, feelings of loneliness resulting from being isolated have significantly contributed to stress. Throughout this epidemic, data show a significant increase in the number of people affected by cognitive impairments.

The virus has an effect on neurogenic and brain neuroinflammation, which causes long-term neuromuscular issues, intellectual incapacity, and emotional distress [11–15]. An analysis of SARS2 and the Middle East respiratory syndrome (MERS) observed numerous long-term symptoms that impact systems of the body, such as tiredness, significantly reduced functional fitness, joint pain, suicidal behavior, nervousness, PTSD, and insomnia [16]. Psychological therapy must be intended to improve individual cognition at multiple stages. Consequently, how important is it to evaluate PSTD's physical and psychological repercussions that influence life expectancy [17] in terms of strengthening intervention systems to assist patients and families in planning effective treatment programs?

A pandemic causes emotional distress to non-patients, caretakers, and medical practitioners because of its infectious potency, the ambiguity of aspects and clinical outcome, and legal restrictions caused by social, interpersonal, and emotional disorders, as well as parental, financial, and other domains. Unconfirmed reports, a lot of news in the media worldwide, significant changes in everyday life and routines, fear, intolerance, ignorance, a feeling of being alone, and sadness all add to the stress [18].

Severe COVID-19 disease can be life-threatening. People have observed peers' disease and misery as relatives and hospital employees; people who have observed the fatal injury or uncertainty of the death of loved ones or acquaintances due to infection; and individuals who have suffered severe vulnerability to affective facts [19]. During the intense phase of the illness, confusion is prevalent among people who require treatment due to COVID-19. The evidence on protracted psychological consequences in this patient population is still incomplete. This may be equivalent to an earlier coronavirus pandemic.

One year after discharge, victims of acute illness have prolonged mental and emotional dysfunction with considerable feelings of anxiety, sadness, and PSTD. Most individuals with SARS had neuropsychological deterioration, such as reduced focus, cognition, and intellectual response time [20]. Elderly sufferers may have difficulty continuing normal living functions or returning to employment. Victims may have muscular vulnerabilities and constant inflammation. Psychologically, such people may struggle with focus and consciousness [21]. According to the WHO, females are disproportionately more likely than males to experience psychological problems. One in every five females intends to leave their respective occupations or limit their working responsibilities, with many citing exhaustion and family obligations as primary motivators. Before the epidemic, more females observed increased psychological symptoms than males [22–24].

Depression, PTSD, and mental disabilities are far more common in ICU COVID-19 high-risk patients than in patients who received regular treatment [25]. Additionally, experiences of stiffness, exhaustion, and irregular heartbeat after COVID-19 were significant indicators of PTSD [26]. Mortality, terror, intrusive medicine, anguish, insanity, disconnectedness, weariness, joint pain, cognitive disorders, and insomnia can all affect them [27]. There was a statistically significant link between developing cognitive problems and panic, sadness, PTSD, and agitation [28].

On the other hand, neurocognitive impairments were connected to an elevated risk of incurring mental impairment. As a consequence, the incidence of depression has risen. Whenever psychological aspects are included, this can significantly increase psychotic issues [29] and, in rare cases, possibly mortality [30]. This became crucial in analyzing the psychosocial rehabilitation method for post-COVID-19 sufferers and indications to improve preemptive family support components that respond to anxiety.

Usage of Data Science in Healthcare Systems

A computer program progressively supports physicians in everyday activities, such as effective decision-making. The majority of intelligence predictive challenges are performed by applying machine learning methodologies. Therefore, the analytical ability of machine learning apps is inadequate. Even though it is correct, a learned machine learning system never describes the "how" of executed recommendations. Data sciences have enormous promise; merging analytics and AI will benefit health services. Data science is the application of various techniques, tools, and techniques to analyze valuable knowledge from well-designed data gathered. This type of "deterministic issue" is challenging to solve, particularly in the health care system, because clinicians do not desire to make people's lives assessments without an accurate description of how the technology originated its observations.

Data science should be used in clinical psychologists' assessment, treatment, and prevention. This might necessitate a shift from different perceptions and toward scientific proof study employing data science. The key benefit is much less variation in psychological disorder diagnostics and treatment. Portable monitoring systems will allow therapists to collect data within the therapeutic workplace by analyzing and supervising activities, behavior, and other relevant factors throughout the day [31, 32, 33].

Applications

- Investigators may use data science to evaluate the consequences of psychological diseases over time on humans.
- Patients say that disaster counselling communications use an algorithm to find people at high risk for depression, anxiety, or loss of consciousness.
- The recorded information assists in therapist learning and panic psychologists can refer individuals to the specialist advice they may require.
- Suicidal thoughts can be anticipated by examining patient records, resulting in a significant reduction in mortality risk.
- The classification model was developed to combine data from hospitalizations, such as maturity level, gender, postal code, prescription, and diagnostic information, to estimate the chance of every person's life being driven to suicide. Accessibility to such information can survive.
- Organizations and insurance providers can utilize chatbots to identify patients battling drug and alcohol addiction, distress, or anxiety.
- By using machine learning techniques, it is possible to find differences in how well people take their medications based on how they behave digitally and how much psychological distress they feel.
- The Ginger.io app helps doctors and nurses keep track of their patient's progress, spot signs of distress, and develop personalized care suggestions.
- Data Science and Machine Learning techniques can help with many initiatives, from identifying suicidal behavior alert messages in youngsters to advising that therapies will be effective for certain people [33, 34, 35, 36, 37].

Post COVID Complications and Their Consequences

Patients recovered from COVID-19 disease may struggle with a few comparable clinical manifestations for several weeks after being discharged from the clinic, including weariness, muscle pain, coughing, dry cough, breathing difficulties, and other symptoms. Consequences reported in patients include adverse effects on the lungs, organs, and cardiovascular and the emergence of a black fungus infection termed Mucor mycosis. Psychological health consequences from isolation, poor economic situations, and a lack of access to treatment may exacerbate conditions.

After recovery from COVID-19, patients experience distress among hospitalized, non-hospitalized caregivers and medical professionals accruing to the unpredictability of symptoms and severity and government prohibitions. Gossip, a deluge of facts and social media, variations in ordinary life and routines, financial turmoil, intolerance, stigma, a sense of isolation, and regret add to the panic.

The psychological tendency to express concern, worry, and dread of becoming ill or contaminating people can express uneasiness, jitteriness, loss of coordination and arrhythmias, breathlessness, and throat irritation. In severe circumstances, patients may experience sadness, characterized by feelings of sadness, weariness, hopelessness, sleepiness, hunger, and a progressive decrease in productivity levels. Elderly individuals are much more fragile, and they require extra attention.

Becoming conscious, admitting, and understanding that someone has mental illnesses seems essential in treatment. Communicating with a therapist, keeping regular and better health, eating nutritious food, preventing smoking and narcotics, and experimenting with new hobbies such as playing, listening to music, reading, drawing, and performing can all assist with anxiousness. Limiting or prohibiting access to online entertainment is beneficial [38].

Most COVID-19 victims are symptomless; most have minor issues resolved independently. Someone should look at the existing situation favorably, believing that the odds of contracting an illness are minimal. Simple precautions such as face mask use, isolation, and good hygiene are sufficient to avoid contamination.

Inhaling toxins, caffeine, and corrosive materials in vaporizer juice adversely affects the respiratory system and reduce resistance. The consequences of smoking include a harmful influence on the mind, which causes cognitive problems and poor knowledge acquisition in those who smoke.

Post COVID-19 Psychological Impacts

Anxiety has become a frequently observed psychological wellness sign. One in three patients experienced a combination of sadness and worry after being discharged from the clinic. Insomnia and neurological problems were also indicated as psychological problems. In COVID-19 cases, there was a significant drop in cognitive indicators, such as recognizing things right away and understanding what they mean [39, 40, 41, 42, 43, 44, 45].

The consequence of multiple COVID-19-related catastrophic stress and the impacts are minor extreme forms of stress. Due to the epidemic, several people have experienced PTSD (posttraumatic stress disorder).

Lack of PPE (personal protective equipment), concerns about virus exposure, exhaustion, mortality despite efforts to recover patients, and hard predictions about which victims will receive fewer resources are all sources of stress. However, researchers studied PTSS (post-traumatic stress symptoms), fear, sadness, and other disorders in the general population [46].

Consequences

The epidemic has harmed public mental health, resulting in psychological crises [47]. Throughout the COVID-19 epidemic, infected people displayed various symptoms of cognitive trauma, including emotions, sadness, and anxiety; mood changes; impatience; sleeplessness; cognitive impairment; PSTD; and hostility [48]. Persistent publicity may also create anxiety, according to investigations [49]. Nonetheless, in the existing environment, correctly predicting the mental and cognitive implications of COVID-19 is difficult. A pandemic may affect the quality of life of people at multiple levels of the community, ranging from contaminated patients and clinicians to relatives, kids, educators, and patients with psychiatric illness, due to the infectivity of the disease, the percentage of transmission, and the eventual resultant fatality rate [50].

Perplexity or Strange Attitude

The epidemic may cause neurological anguish and impede cortex activity, affecting cognitive performance. Nevertheless, such impairments were only observed in individuals who reported post-COVID signs. Furthermore, some nerve disorders, such as disorientation, have been linked to migraines and fatigue [51].

Patients experiencing schizophrenia may have a distorted perception of life, which frequently influences their behavior, causing them to operate in unusual ways. Monitoring a person's behavior can be affected by mental disorders or illnesses. Humans affected by schizophrenia may exhibit unusual habits [52].

Sleep Disorder

Insomnia, particularly drowsiness, was a common psychological condition following COVID-19 or reported, including severe and symptomatic phases of the infection. Lack of sleep affects psychological and meta-cognitive control, leading to irritation and cognitive issues [54]. During the advanced stages of an illness, cognitive and emotional pressure can activate biological processes that drive the development of pro-inflammatory cytokines that can interact with metabolic disorders and activities connected to sleep [53].

Addiction to Substances

A drug consumption disorder is a neurological dysfunction that impacts a patient's cognition and behavior. It can lead to incapacity to manage drugs, including authorized or illicit medicines, liquor, or prescriptions. Addiction seems to be the most severe consequence of drug misuse, with effects ranging from mild to chronic. Certain medications may initially alleviate specific effects of psychological diseases and exacerbate the clinical symptoms.

Self-Destructive Attitude

Suicidal thoughts and behavior are likely to arise in patients experiencing post-COVID disorder due to signs of psychological, cognitive, and metabolic disorders and inflammation damage to the nervous system. Variations in suicidal behaviour continued for various socioeconomic categories in the first year of the epidemic. Suicidal thoughts are more likely in patients who have experienced financial, relational, increasing drug use, or COVID-19 infection assaults [55].

Anxiousness

It can also be found in various mental conditions, such as severe anxiety, anxiety attacks, and nightmares. Although all such diseases are unique, they share the suffering and dysfunction associated with worry and dread. Panic is a typical reaction to risk or psychological stress. Panic disorder causes anxiety and contributes to the importance of the quality role. The sympathetic nervous system reacts when confronted with a potentially harmful scenario [56].

Mood Swings or Depression

Older people are more insecure and require extra attention. Symptoms of depression, such as melancholy, are classified as such. It's associated with increased anxiety, frustration, grief, or rage, interrupting one's daily activities. Patients who consistently feel down or desperate, on the other hand, may be suffering from mental health issues [57]. Youngsters may also be concerned about schooling or jobs, money, their capacity to participate in critical communal and socioeconomic events and hobbies, or other aspects of life [58]. The number of hours spent in isolation is crucial in post-COVID melancholy.

Post-COVID Stress Disorder

Post-COVID Stress Disorder (PCSD) is a psychological health condition that affects people who survived COVID-19. It is comparable to PTSD. Migraine, nervousness, sleeplessness, tiredness, irritation, and poor concentration are indications of PTSD. Patients who've already healed from COVID-19 are more prone to develop PTSD, including extreme fears of re-infection, mortality, and the loss of family, as well as dreams about the epidemic. These impacts might be induced by recognition of clinics and the epidemic, epidemic reporting, or anything related to the pandemic. People with post-traumatic stress disorder (PTSD) will strive to avoid anything to do with the outbreak, such as going to the doctor for any reason [59].

A Poor Understanding of Contagion

Inadequate awareness is most likely the leading cause of fear and uncertainty, especially during the initial phases of an epidemic, reflecting the importance of information. Rapidly alleviated with increasing, an appropriate measure may be the quick and efficient publishing of credible experimental findings in a general context. Individuals with inadequate public health awareness cannot comprehend the gravity of the epidemic and the precautions that must be taken to avoid getting the disease. Whereas most individuals are emotionally responsible, a small percentage of people neglect preventative measures and interaction due to the absence of knowledge and perception of COVID-19 [60]. Consequently, it is critical that the general population, particularly the aged, be familiar with and knowledgeable about COVID-19.

Subconscious

The subconscious results are from perceptions about oneself and the aspects associated with such emotions. Consequently, the ideas lead to tension, frustration, and melancholy. The method of constructing a judgment or coming to a judgment is presented. People can become persistent as they interpret and support dysfunctional attitudes. As a result, they may be intended to shield people from anguish, frustration, and humiliation [61].

Social Problems

The financial sector is estimated to harm the mental health of its employees, increasing suicidal behavior and alcohol-related fatalities. Raising liquor prices and limiting distribution reduces the significant impact on human health and improves patient outcomes. Efficient labor services intended to assist the public in keeping or regaining employment mitigate the financial crisis's psychological effects. Financial assistance initiatives will aid in reducing the deficit, while affordable and effective inpatient care will assist people at risk and avoid psychological health consequences [62].

False News

Social Networking allows individuals to stay interconnected even when they are physically isolated. The daily reports on mortalities and intensifying case statistics can be distressing, specifically for persons susceptible to psychological complications or who are currently taking prescriptions for psychiatric diseases. In a study on misleading information, deception and propaganda are frequently employed [63]. A few are using the aspects to categorize between consciously distributed incorrect information. They subconsciously mislead people about misconceptions as the "inappropriate information exchange of misleading info" and falsehoods as the "conscious conception and exchange of info recognized to be completely bogus" [64].

Rumours have been defined as neither "posting inaccurate facts intending to be inaccurate nor having a common objective in transmitting incorrect news." In contrast, propaganda has been defined as "trying to influence and deceiving persons purposely to accomplish different goals" [65]. Simultaneously, many people use incorrect terminology [66], whereas others define misrepresentation as false news or propaganda that is purposefully false information [67]. The concept of disinformation refers to false or incomplete data, irrespective of consent.

Inflexibility

Resilience is a significant intellectual capability that relates to a person's psychological, behavioral, and interpersonal (or alignment) in instances of transition, innovation, and ambiguity. The capacity to modify somebody's thoughts to adapt to fluctuating, unfamiliar, diverse, and unpredictable conditions are associated with behavioral compliance. The capability to modify the kind, amount, and intensity of attitude or activity to traverse fluctuating, unfamiliar, unpredictable, and ambiguous contexts is referred to as social cognition. Feelings' modulation is accompanied by the capacity to change one's customary or prevalent emotions when engaging with altering, unexpected, unpredictable, and ambiguous conditions [68].

Security of Family

Teaming migrant kids with their families is essential to addressing the impacts of the trauma they have encountered. The fight will undoubtedly continue, but kids are probably significantly more likely to have committed and caring women who give birth and protect them. The percentage of families also reported improved home relations, such as spending more quality family time together, feeling connected, displaying affection, and noticing adaptability in children. Families associated with improvements are in unfavorable and good contact with their kids as part of the COVID-19 epidemic, probably due to more possibilities for parents.

Additionally, a higher majority of parents concerned about their kids' economic well-being due to the epidemic probably spend more personal time with them, displaying additional attention and compassion and recognizing persistence in the children. A more significant percentage of families concerned about the kids' psychological difficulties mentioned giving them greater unconditional love. Parents may collectively participate in more talks and initiatives [69–70]. A recent study found that even though parents have more responsibilities because of the epidemic, they also have more chances to make new friends.

Discussion

The epidemic is spreading over the globe, and it is producing increasing anxiety and distress. These are reasonable and acceptable emotions given the changeable and unpredictable position everybody is experiencing. The question confronting us seems to be how we handle and respond to the problematic scenarios happening so quickly in our broader society. Therefore, we may use the incredible qualities of toughness and collaboration that we, thankfully, also possess as humans. Being diagnosed as susceptible to COVID-19 and being informed may be exceedingly scary and frightening for aged people, including those with pre-existing medical problems. Panic, worry, and anger may all significantly affect such people.

Its consequences can be especially tough for elderly adults facing intellectual impairment or dementia. Furthermore, some elderly adults may be interpersonally lonely and unhappy, which can exacerbate psychological problems. Females after recovery from COVID-19 were likewise shown to be more likely to experience feelings of disturbance than their male counterparts. People who survived COVID-19 and experienced emotional suffering had greater cyclothymiacs and depressed mental emotions and more significant aspects of loss of impulsive management and inability of coherence.

Conclusion

The cognitive effects of the COVID-19 outbreak might endure for a few generations after the epidemic. Even during the post-pandemic period, the frequency of common mental health disorders and fatality is predicted to rise. Individuals' psychosocial issues may worsen due to COVID-19, lowering their well-being.

References

[1] https://www.cdc.gov/coronavirus/2019-ncov/long-term-effects/index.html.

[2] Tenforde, M. W. et al. Symptom duration and risk factors for delayed return to usual health among outpatients with COVID-19 in a multistate health care systems network—United States, March-June 2020. *Morb. Mortal Wkly Rep.* 69, 993–998.

[3] Townsend, L. et al. Persistent poor health post-COVID-19 is not associated with respiratory complications or initial disease severity. *Ann. Am. Thorac. Soc.*

[4] Gemelli Against, C. P. A. C. S. G. Post-COVID-19 global health strategies: The need for an interdisciplinary approach. *Aging Clin. Exp. Res.* 32, 1613–1620.

[5] https://www.pacehospital.com/post-covid-complications-long-term-effects-of-coronavirus-after-recovery.

[6] Raker E. J., Lowe S. R., Arcaya M. C., Johnson S. T., Rhodes J., Waters M. C. Twelve years later: The long-term mental health consequences of Hurricane Katrina. *Soc Sci Med.* (2019) 242 :112610. DOI : 10.1016/j.socscimed.2019.112610.

[7] Liu, N., Zhang, F., Wei, C., Jia, Y., Shang, Z., Sun, L., Wu, L., Sun, Z., Zhou, Y., Wang, Y., & Liu, W. Prevalence and predictors of PTSS during COVID-19 outbreak in China hardest-hit areas: gender differences matter. *Psychiatry Res.* (2020) 287 :112921. DOI : 10.1016/j.psychres.2020.112921.

[8] Xiao S., Luo D., Xiao Y. Survivors of COVID-19 are at high risk of posttraumatic stress disorder. *Glob Health Res Policy.* (2020) 5 :29. DOI : 10.1186/s41256-020-00155-2.

[9] Vindegaard N, Benros ME. *COVID-19 pandemic and mental health* consequences: a systematic review of the current evidence. *Brain Behav Immun.* (2020) 89 :531–42. DOI : 10.1016/j.bbi.2020.05.048.

[10] Rogers, J. P., Chesney, E., Oliver, D., Pollak, T. A., McGuire, P., Fusar-Poli, P., Zandi, M. S., Lewis, G., & David, A. S. Psychiatric and neuropsychiatric presentations associated with severe coronavirus infections : à systematic review and meta-analysis with comparison to the COVID-19 pandemic. *Lancet Psychiatry.* (2020) 7 :611–27. DOI : 10.1016/S2215-0366(20)30203-0.

[11] Wu, Y., Xu, X., Chen, Z., Duan, J., Hashimoto, K., Yang, L., Liu, C., & Yang, C. Nervous system involvement after infection with COVID-19 and other coronaviruses *J. Brain. Behav.,* 87 (2020), pp. 18-22.

[12] Ellul, M. A., Benjamin, L., Singh, B., Lant, S., Michael, B. D., Easton, A., Kneen, R., Defres, S., Sejvar, J., & Solomon, T. Neurological associations of COVID-19, *Lancet Neurol.* (2020), 10.1016/S1474-4422(20)30221-0.

[13] Wostyn P. COVID-19 and chronic fatigue syndrome: Is the worst yet to come? *J. Med. Hypotheses.* 146:110469. https://DOI.org/10.1016/j.mehy.2020.110469.

[14] Komaroff, A. L., L. Bateman Will COVID-19 lead to myalgic Encephalomyelitis/ chronic fatigue syndrome? *J. Front. Med.*, 7 (2021), p. 1132.

[15] Disser, N. P., De Micheli, A. J., Schonk, M. M., Konnaris, M. A., Piacentini, A. N., Edon, D. L., Toresdahl, B. G., Rodeo, S. A., Casey, E. K., & Mendias, C. L. Musculoskeletal consequences of COVID-19 *J. Bone Joint Surg. Am.,* 102 (2020), pp. 1197-1204.

[16] Ahmed, H., Patel, K., Greenwood, D., Halpin, S., Lewthwaite, P., Salawu, A., Eyre, L., Breen, A., O'Connor, R., Jones, A., & Sivan, M. Long-term clinical outcomes in survivors of severe acute respiratory syndrome (SARS) and the Middle East respiratory syndrome (MERS) coronavirus outbreaks after hospitalization or ICU admission: a systematic review and meta-analysis *J. Rehabil. Med.*, 52 (2020), pp. 1-11.

[17] Steiner, W. A., L. Ryser, E. Huber, D. Uebelhart, A. Aeschlimann, G. Stucki Use of the ICF model as a clinical problem-solving tool in physical therapy and rehabilitation medicine *J. Phys. Ther.*, 82 (2002), pp. 1098-1107, 10.1093/ptj/ 82.11. 1098.

[18] https://www.narayanahealth.org/blog/psychological-problems-associated-with-covid-19.

[19] https://www.psychiatrictimes.com/view/post-covid-stress-disorder-emerging-consequence- global-pandemic.

[20] Rogers J. P., Chesney E., Oliver D., Pollack T. A., McGuire P., Fusar-Poli P., Zandi M. S., Lewis G., David A. S. Psychiatric and neuropsychiatric presentations of severe coronavirus infections: a systematic review and meta-analysis with comparison to the COVID-19 pandemic. *Lancet Psychiatry.* 2020; 7:611–627.

[21] https://www.medpagetoday.com/infectiousdisease/covid19/86556.

[22] https://www.kff.org/coronavirus-covid-19/issue-brief/the-implications-of-covid-19-for-mental-health-and-substance-use/.

[23] Wu, Y., Xu, X., Chen, Z., Duan, J., Hashimoto, K., Yang, L., Liu, C., & Yang, C. Nervous system involvement after infection with COVID-19 and other coronaviruses, *J. Brain. Behav.* 87 (2020) 18–22.

[24] Halpin, S. J., McIvor, C., Whyatt, G., Adams, A., Harvey, O., McLean, L., Walshaw, C., Kemp, S., Corrado, J., Singh, R., Collins, T., O'Connor, R. J., & Sivan, M. Post-discharge symptoms and rehabilitation needs in survivors of COVID-19 infection: a cross-sectional evaluation, *J. Med. Virol.* 93 (2021) 1013–1022, https://DOI.org/10.1002/jmv.26368.

[25] Singleton, N., G. J. S. O. Lewis, Better or Worse: A Longitudinal Study of the Mental Health of Adults Living in Private Households in Great Britain: *Report Based on Surveys Carried Out by the Office for National Statistics in 2000 and 2001 for the Department of Health and the Scottish Executive Health Department,* 2003.

[26] Liu, D., Baumeister, R. F., Veilleux, J. C., Chen, C., Liu, W., Yue, Y., & Zhang, S. Risk factors associated with mental illness in hospital discharged patients infected with COVID-19 in Wuhan, China, *J. Psychiatr. Res.* 292 (2020) 113297, https://DOI.org/10.1016/j.psychres.2020.113297.

[27] D. Wade, R. Hardy, D. Howell, M. Mythen, Identifying clinical and acute psychological risk factors for PTSD after critical care: a systematic review, Minerva Anestesiol. 79 (2013) 944–963, https://DOI.org/10.1177/216770261 4553230.

[28] Méndez, R., Balanzá-Martínez, V., Luperdi, S. C., Estrada, I., Latorre, A., González-Jiménez, P., Feced, L., Bouzas, L., Yépez, K., Ferrando, A., Hervás, D., Zaldívar, E., Reyes, S., Berk, M., & Menéndez, R. Short-term neuropsychiatric outcomes and quality of Life in COVID-19 survivors, *medRxiv.* (2020), https://DOI.org/10.1111/joim.13262.

[29] Yuan, B., Li, W., Liu, H., Cai, X., Song, S., Zhao, J., Hu, X., Li, Z., Chen, Y., Zhang, K., Liu, Z., Peng, J., Wang, C., Wang, J., & An, Y. Correlation between immune response and self-reported depression during convalescence from COVID-19, *Brain Behav. Immun.* 88 (2020) 39–43, https://DOI.org/10. 1016/j.bbi.2020.05.062.

[30] Hatch, R., D. Young, V. Barber, J. Griffiths, D. A. Harrison, Watkinson PJCc. Anxiety, depression and posttraumatic stress disorder after critical illness: a UK-wide prospective cohort study, *Crit. Care* 22 (2018) 310, 10.1186/s13054-018-2223-6.

[31] https://www.oxfordbibliographies.com/view/document/obo-9780199828340/obo-9780199828340-0259.xml.

[32] https://towardsdatascience.com/data-science-in-mental-health-ccd09ba2148a.

[33] https://www.discoverdatascience.org/social-good/mental-health/.

[34] Ndiaye, B. M., L. Tending, D. Seck, *Analysis of the COVID-19 pandemic by SIR model and machine learning technics for forecasting.* Xiv:2004.01574. URL http://arxiv.org/abs/2004.01574.

[35] Mohri, M., Rostamizadeh, A., and Talwalkar, A. (2012). *Foundations of Machine Learning.* Cambridge, MA: The MIT Press.

[36] Karaarslan E, Konacaklı E. Decentralized solutions for data collection and privacy in healthcare. Artificial intelligence for data-driven medical diagnosis. In *De Gruyter* (in press).

[37] Karaarslan, E., E. Adiguzel, Blockchain based dns and pki solutions, *IEEE Commun. Stand. Mag.* 2 (3) (2018) 52e57.

[38] https://www.narayanahealth.org/blog/psychological-problems-associated-with-covid-19/.

[39] Arab-Zozani, M., F. Hashemi, H. Safari, M. Yousefi, H. Ameri Health-related quality of life and its associated factors in COVID-19 patients *Osong Public Health Res. Perspect.*, 11 (2020), pp. 296-302, 10.24171/j.phrp.

[40] Daher, A., P. Balfanz, C. Cornelissen, A. Müller, I. Bergs, N. Marx, *Muller-Wieland, D., Hartmann, B., Dreher, M., Muller, T.* Follow up of patients with severe coronavirus disease 2019 (COVID-19): Pulmonary and extrapulmonary disease sequelae *Respir Med.*, 174 (2020), pp. 106-112.

[41] Garrigues, E., Janvier, P., Kherabi, Y., Le Bot, A., Hamon, A., Gouze, H., Doucet, L., Berkani, S., Oliosi, E., Mallart, E., Corre, F., Zarrouk, V., Moyer, J.-D., Galy, A., Honsel, V., Fantin, B., & Nguyen, Y. Post-discharge persistent symptoms and health-related quality of life after hospitalization for COVID-19. *J. Inf. Security.*, 81 (2020), pp. e4-e6.

[42] Xiong, Q., Xu, M., Li, J., Liu, Y., Zhang, J., Xu, Y., & Dong, W. Clinical sequelae of COVID-19 survivors in Wuhan, China: a single-Centre longitudinal study *Clin. Microbiol. Infect.*, 27 (2021), pp. 89-95.

[43] Halpin, S. J., McIvor, C., Whyatt, G., Adams, A., Harvey, O., McLean, L., Walshaw, C., Kemp, S., Corrado, J., Singh, R., Collins, T., O'Connor, R. J., & Sivan, M. Post-discharge symptoms and rehabilitation needs in survivors of COVID-19 infection: a cross-sectional evaluation *J. Med. Virol.*, 93 (2021), pp. 1013-1022, 10.1002/jmv. 26368.

[44] Méndez, R., Balanzá-Martínez, V., Luperdi, S. C., Estrada, I., Latorre, A., González-Jiménez, P., Feced, L., Bouzas, L., Yépez, K., Ferrando, A., Hervás, D., Zaldívar, E., Reyes, S., Berk, M., & Menéndez, R. Short-term neuropsychiatric outcomes and quality of Life in COVID-19 *survivors Journal of Internal Medicine.* (2020), 10.1111/joim.13262.

[45] De Lorenzo, R., Conte, C., Lanzani, C., Benedetti, F., Roveri, L., Mazza, M. G., Brioni, E., Giacalone, G., Canti, V., Sofia, V., D'Amico, M., Di Napoli, D., Ambrosio, A., Scarpellini, P., Castagna, A., Landoni, G., Zangrillo, A., Bosi, E., Tresoldi, M., Ciceri, F., Rovere-Querini, P. Residual clinical damage after COVID-19: a retrospective and prospective observational cohort study. *PLoS One*, 15 (2020), Article e0239570, 10.1371/journal.

[46] https://www.psychiatrictimes.com/view/post-covid-stress-disorder-emerging-consequence-global-pandemic.

[47] Xiang Y. T., Yang Y., Li W., Zhang L., Zhang Q., Cheung T., Ng, C. H. Timely mental health care for the 2019 novel coronavirus outbreak is urgently needed. *Lancet Psychiatry*. 2020;7(3):228–9.

[48] Brooks, S. K., Webster, R. K., Smith, L. E., Woodland, L., Wessely, S., Greenberg, N., & Rubin, G. J. The psychological impact of quarantine and how to reduce it: a rapid review of the evidence. *Lancet*. 2020. 14;395(10227):912–20.

[49] Neria Y., Sullivan G. M. Understanding the mental health effects of indirect exposure to mass trauma through the media. *JAMA*. 2011;306(12):1374–5.

[50] Ryu S., Chun B. C., Epidemiology of K. S. An interim review of the epidemiological characteristics' of 2019 novel coronavirus. *Epidemiol Health*. 2020;42: e2020006.

[51] https://timesofindia.indiatimes.com/life-style/health-fitness/health-news/coronavirus-symptoms-the-most-unusual-side-effects-people-report-after-covid-diagnosis-according-to-nhs/photostory/78268656.cms?picid=78268802.
[52] https://www.medicinenet.com/unusual_behavior/symptoms.html.
[53] Hao, F., Tam, W., Hu, X., Tan, W., Jiang, L., Jiang, X., Zhang, L., Zhao, X., Zou, Y., Hu, Y., Luo, X., McIntyre, R. S., Quek, T., Tran, B. X., Zhang, Z., Pham, H. Q., Ho, C. S. H., & Ho, R. C. M. A quantitative and qualitative study on the neuropsychiatric sequelae of acutely ill COVID-19 inpatients in isolation facilities *J. Transl. Psychiatry.*, 10 (1) (2020), pp. 1-14, 10.1038/s41398-020-01039-2.
[54] McNally, R. J., D. J. Robinaugh, G. W. Wu, L. Wang, M. K. Deserno, D. Borsboom Mental disorders as causal systems: a network approach to posttraumatic stress disorder *Clin. Psychol. Sci.*, 3 (2015), pp. 836-849, 10.1177/ 2167702614553230.
[55] https://www.nimh.nih.gov/health/topics/substance-use-and-mental-health.
[56] https://www.msdmanuals.com/home/mental-health-disorders/anxiety-and-stress-related-disorders/overview-of-anxiety-disorders.
[57] Valencia Higuera and Kimberly Holland Everything you want to know about depression Updated on February 11, 2020, available at http://www.goosexx.com/health/depression.
[58] Canadian Mental Health Association, BC Division COVID 19 and Anxiety available at https://www.heretohelp.bc.ca/infosheet/covid-19-and-anxiety.
[59] https://www.india.com/health/post-covid-stress-disorder-signs-treatment-and-everything-you-need-to-know-5103917.
[60] Daoust, J. F. Elderly people and responses to COVID-19 in 27 countries. *PLoS ONE* 15, e0235590. https://DOI.org/10.1371/journal.pone.0235590 (2020).
[61] Phaedonos P., Anastassiou-Hadjicharalambous X. (2011) Self-Judgment. In: Goldstein S., Naglieri J. A. (eds) *Encyclopedia of Child Behaviour and Development.* Springer, Boston, MA. https://DOI.org/10.1007/978-0-387-79061-9_2549.
[62] https://www.euro.who.int/__data/assets/pdf_file/0008/134999/e94837.pdf.
[63] Farkas, J., Schou, J. Fake News as a Floating Signifier: Hegemony, Antagonism and the Politics of Falsehood. *Javn. Public* 2018, *25*, 298–314.
[64] Wardle, C. *Information Disorder: The Essential Glossary*; Shorenstein Center on Media, Politics, and Public Policy, Harvard Kennedy School: Harvard, MA, USA, 2018.
[65] Benkler, Y.; Faris, R.; Roberts, H. *Network Propaganda: Manipulation, Disinformation, and Radicalization in American Politics*; Oxford University Press: Oxford, UK, 2018; ISBN 0-19-092364-4.
[66] Floridi, L. Brave. Net. World: The Internet as a Disinformation Superhighway? *Electron. Libr.* 1996, *14*, 509–514].
[67] Keshavarz, H. How Credible Is Information on the Web: Reflections on Misinformation and Disinformation? *Infopreneurship J.* 2014, *1*, 1–17].
[68] Martin, A. J. (2017). Adaptability - What it is and what it is not. *American Psychologist*, *72*, 696-698. http://dx.DOI.org/10.1037/amp0000163.

[69] Johnson K. *Parenting during COVID-19: a new frontier*. Canadian Paediatric Society; 2020.

[70] Ye J. Pediatric mental and behavioral health in the period of quarantine and social distancing with COVID-19. *JMIR Pediatr Parent* 2020;3: e19867. DOI:10.2196/19867pmid: http://www.ncbi.nlm.nih.gov/pubmed/32634105.

Chapter 2

Contemplating the Post-COVID Psychological Disorders in a Selective Sample Using DASS-21 and the WHO-5 Well-Being Index

G. Yogapriya[1,*], G. Vijay Krishna[1] and C. V. Subramanian[2]

[1]School of Environment Architecture and Design, SRMIST, Ramapuram, India

[2]Faculty of Architecture and Planning, PMIST, Thanjavur, India

Abstract

Background: Earlier this year, the virus COVID-19 was detected for the first time and has since spread worldwide, causing widespread illness and death. A rise in emotional and psychological challenges worldwide has resulted from the disease's direct and indirect effects on individuals and families. It is usual for people to experience worry, tension, and other emotional responses during times of instability. Additional stress can increase symptoms in those already who have a mental illness.

Methods: A survey is conducted on selective samples like students-teachers, COVID and non-COVID patients, small-medium scale entrepreneurs. A measurement scale of the WHO-5 Well-Being Index and The Depression, Anxiety, and Stress Scale-21 items (DASS-21) were taken in the questionnaire survey. When it comes to post-COVID mental diseases, data science is usually used to investigate the prevalence of these disorders, with a particular emphasis on their worry and

*Corresponding Author's Email: yogaprig@srmist.edu.in.

In: Data Science Applications of Post-COVID-19 Psychological Disorders
Editor: Vijayalakshmi Kakulapati
ISBN: 979-8-88697-165-1

melancholy. WHO-5 well-being index and the DASS-21 have their score calculations carried out in this study.

Results: Among the 154 respondents of 77 males and 77 females, the WHO-well-being index has shown an average score of 55 among the sample selected. The male displayed a high score of 100 in 1.94%, and female respondents have reached 92 only. The Happiness index doesn't depend on the infection also. The DASS-21 shows a severity score, more in COVID affected persons than the non-affected ones. The students (COVID), Teachers (COVID), Medium Entrepreneurs (COVID) have shown the value of ≥60% in Depression and Stress. The anxiety value is comparatively less in both cases.

Keywords: anxiety, COVID, COVID patient, DASS-21, depression, happiness index, infection, mental diseases, mental illness, WHO-5, wellbeing index, post COVID, psychological disorders, questionnaires surveys, stress

Introduction

Our world is now suffering a worldwide pandemic disaster. By the 16th of December in 2021, the World Health Organization had documented more than 273 million cases worldwide. Unfortunately, the coronavirus was responsible for infecting over 5.3 million people [1]. The increase in cases and deaths has been documented, impacting people of all socio-economic backgrounds. As soon as the SARS virus was discovered in Wuhan in December 2019, many people watching television or reading about it in the news had no idea that it would soon knock on their door and infect them with the disease. The virus is still spreading. Even though it has been experimented with, vaccines are in their tracks. New ideas on how the virus spreads in an environment offered to explain why the virus is still spreading. In several nations, a state of emergency has been proclaimed, and social isolation is widely seen as a critical technique for slowing the spread of the virus.

In addition to cholera, malaria, and swine flu, all of these illnesses are ones that individuals of today's age are likely to be acquainted with [2]. However, the COVID pandemic has left an indelible mark on people's thoughts, and there is still a great deal of worry, tension, and anxiety linked with it [3].

The sense of fear that pervades society despite the government's decision to lift the lockdown here and there does not decrease. Anxiety may be expressed in several ways depending on the scenario. Learning and teaching have moved online, and educational institutions are still trying to find a way to include both conventional and online methods in their curriculum [4].

System interfaces such as Zoom, Cisco, and Google Meet have been simplified to meet the education on track. If the current state of things continues, all sides are afraid of what might happen [5]. People are preoccupied with questions such as whether or not we are under lockdown, whether or not we have a new variant, and whether or not we are in excellent health. It is also up for contention whether or not someone dies or is admitted to the hospital when the day-to-day schedule cannot be followed. Since its inception, the epidemic has caused widespread suffering, mental anguish, and fear among the general public.

According to peer-reviewed research, post-pandemic mental health concerns will likely rise because of an emotional epidemic curve [6, 7]. Anxiety levels vary among patients who have recovered from COVID. Post-COVID, people were more worried about their health, even if it was only a slight ailment. Alternatively, they may be at home recuperating or in serious condition at the hospital. They developed mental toughness as a consequence of their previous experiences. Their emotions were far more critical when it came to the second one. These people are entirely unaware of how their stress levels have risen with the number of sick days they were in. There is a lot of self-reflection about what happened, how it may happen again, and how their circumstances could be better controlled in the future.

Small businesses and entrepreneurs have recently faced threats to their interdependence livelihoods and mental health due to a scarcity of financial resources. Populations that have been found to be disproportionately affected have been identified [8]. Even while it's generally known that entrepreneurs are quick on their feet, this has not always been the case in the business world. In addition to various causes such as uncertainty and health worries, entrepreneurs' poor mental health was aggravated by a lack of social support and aid. According to recent research findings, entrepreneurs may overcome difficulties and cope in the wake of the pandemic's setbacks, uncertainties, and tensions.

Depending on the dose received, the body may exhibit a range of symptoms after being exposed to COVID-19. Post-traumatic stress disorder and anxiety disorders are two additional prevalent mental health problems in conjunction with depression and suicidal ideation [9]. Treatment, services, and social support that are not maintained over time can lead to relapse, aggravated even more by a lack of access to therapeutic resources. Several people have committed suicide due to the neuropsychiatric symptoms and socio-economic implications of COVID-19 exposure, which have been documented. COVID-19 is also accountable for other crimes such as stigmatization, racism, and hate crimes. Diversity is encouraged and welcome among all types of marginalized groups, including racial and ethnic minorities; immigrants; refugees; LGBTQ individuals; and those who have been marginalized due to their sexual orientation or gender identity [10].

Analytical Framework

Literature Review

As a result of the current economic crisis and the widespread usage of lockdowns, it is projected that the number of suicides and mental diseases linked to suicide will climb dramatically. It is expected that the number of Canadians unemployed is likely to rise by 1.6% in 2020 and 1.2% in 2021. First and foremost, increased unemployment rates resulted in more than 418 suicides between 2020 and 2021. An increase of 14.0% in 2020 and a 13.6% increase in 2021 are expected, with an additional 2114 suicides in the 2020-2021-time period [11, 12]. The same trend may be observed in several countries, including the United States, Pakistan, India, France, Germany, and Italy. According to three different research examinations, higher psychological distress was observed in the general public, people suffering from mental illnesses, and healthcare workers all at some point [13, 14].

These challenges point to the crucial need for additional public mental health and policy support during this challenging time, which should be prioritized. Many risk factors have been discovered as being connected with depressive symptoms in the COVID-19 pandemic, and they are currently being investigated in further depth to determine their significance. According to this study's findings, women are more prone than men to have depressive symptoms [15, 16].

Urban dwellers, those with a poor self-rated health rating, and those who have recently divorced or been bereaved are more prone to experience depression-like symptoms, as is being single or divorced, or widowed. In addition, people who have a history of mental stress or medical issues are more likely to have depression-like symptoms. Individuals exposed to COVID-19 are more prone to experience depressive symptoms due to news stories shared on social media.

Several risk variables have been discovered as being connected with depressive symptoms in the period, and they are currently being investigated in greater detail. Individuals who were married reported higher feelings of anxiety when compared to those who were not married, according to one study, which was conducted on this topic [17]. An abundance of risk factors has been identified as being associated with depressive symptoms in the COVID-19 pandemic, and they are currently being studied more thoroughly.

Extending the quarantine time raised the likelihood of developing anxiety-related side effects resulting from the procedure. According to one study, the intuitive assumption is that earlier exposure to COVID-positive persons or items would increase anxiety symptoms. This has been confirmed to be true in one study [18]. Individuals who were divorced or bereaved experienced more feelings of stress, according to the findings, than participants who were single or married, according to the results [19].

According to the data, an alarming 40.4% of the young people in the research on the impact of COVID-19 on adolescents' mental health showed susceptibility to mental illness [20]. At COVID-19, 230 medical staff members from an infectious disease tertiary referral center were asked to participate in a survey to determine the prevalence of anxiety and stress disorders among those working in the field of infectious diseases. According to the study's findings, researchers observed a high frequency of anxiety and stress problems among medical staff [21].

Methods

Questionnaire Tool

The World Health Organization defines health as "a condition of complete physical, mental, and social well-being." It does not just imply that one will not become ill or suffer from a handicap. This is the definition that has been in use since 1948. People's subjective well-being, as a result, is a significant component of how they evaluate the overall quality of their life.

Positive emotions such as contentment, satisfaction, and happiness are included in this category, along with negative emotions such as depression and anxiety. There are various reasons why well-being is a standard outcome measure across diverse groups of people (for example, people in the hospital versus those in the hospital), including the following: (e.g., pre-post treatment or comparisons of different treatment conditions). It is one of the most widely used methods to determine overall well-being in patients and non-patients. The WHO-5 allows us to analyze general health over a period using five questions.

People are asked to score their feelings about each of the five statements over the last two weeks using a Likert scale with a maximum of six points. The scale ranges from 0 to 5, with 0 denoting "no time" and five representing "always" as the starting point. Pleasant mood (good spirits, relaxation), vitality (being active and waking up fresh and invigorated), and general interest are all factors that contribute to a person's subjective quality of life, according to the World Health Organization (having a public interest in things). The higher one's score, the better one's health, and the app are accessible in various languages to accommodate different cultures (Table 1).

Table 1. WHO-5 Well-Being Index [22]

	Between the period Jan 2020-Dec 2021	Every time	The majority of the time	Almost half of the time	In less than half of the cases	Now and then	At no point in time
1	I've been feeling upbeat and optimistic.	5	4	3	2	1	0
2	I've been feeling peaceful and relaxed.	5	4	3	2	1	0
3	I've been feeling energized and active.	5	4	3	2	1	0
4	I felt rejuvenated and refreshed when I awoke.	5	4	3	2	1	0
5	My daily existence has been full of things that pique my curiosity.	5	4	3	2	1	0

The listed value, as per Table 2, showcases a collection of three self-report scales used to assess the different components of depression, anxiety, and stress that a person may be experiencing. The findings of these tests are used to determine how people are feeling about various issues such as depression, anxiety, and stress. In total, there are three DASS-21 scales, each of which contains seven items that are further broken into subscales that have identical content to the major scale.

Table 2. Items Depression Anxiety and Stress Scale-21 with their respective constructs

Item	Question	Construct
1	It was so hard for me to calm down	Stress
2	Felt Dryness in my mouth	Anxiety
3	Not able to experience feelings of positivity	Depression
4	Having some breathing difficulties (such as wheezing and breathlessness without having made any physical effort)	Anxiety
5	Feeling to initiate and to do activities	Depression
6	Deliberated to embellish when reacting to circumstances	Stress
7	Felt unstable (for example, in my hands)	Anxiety
8	Sensed nervousness in me	Stress
9	Things that could have made me panic and look silly made me nervous.	Anxiety
10	Sensed I had no wanting towards anything	Depression
11	Sensing restless	Stress
12	Hard to relax	Stress
13	Sensed having no motivation and felt depressed.	Depression
14	Not happy with the things that kept me from doing what I had been doing.	Stress
15	Sensed that being panic	Anxiety
16	Sensed unenthusiastic about all things around	Depression
17	Felt like I was worthless as a person	Depression
18	Sensed being over sensitive/emotional	Stress
19	Even though I hadn't engaged in any strenuous physical activity, I was aware that my heartbeat had shifted	Anxiety
20	Felt afraid without reason	Anxiety
21	Felt my life is meaningless	Depression

When using the depression scale technique to analyze depression symptoms such as dysphoria and despair, it is essential to include anhedonia, lethargy, and other factors. All variables are assessed on a five-point scale: sympathetic stimulation, skeletal muscle effects, anxiety symptoms, and the individual's assessment of their anxiety levels.

A variety of degrees of chronic, non-specific arousal in people may be measured using the stress scale, which can be found here. This scale, among other things, assesses the capacity to relax, the amount of anxiety, the ability to become angry, the level of irritability, and the level of impatience in a person. The scores for depression, anxiety, and stress are calculated by summing up the values from each category relevant to the situation. In addition to being based on dimensional thinking rather than category thinking, this tool effectively assesses mental health. Initially, researchers hypothesized that the differences between average people and people suffering from a medical disease in terms of sadness, anxiety, and stress mainly differed in degree rather than actual differences in severity [22].

DASS-21 - Survey in Malaysia

The COVID-19 pandemic has had a devastating impact on people's mental health worldwide. In previous studies, programs and interventions that use social networks are beneficial for improving mental health. Even though there is a pressing need for more research in low and middle-income countries, most current evidence comes from high-income regions, which is problematic. A study is conducted to describe the potential value of a hybrid health carnival in promoting mental health and increasing access to screening services.

A mental health carnival was held in Malaysia to commemorate World Mental Health Day, with the theme "Mind Your Mental Health" as the focus (Cakna Kesihatan Mental). Participants had the opportunity to interact face-to-face and participate in virtual activities during the carnival. A free online therapy session was made available to groups identified as high risk during the screening process. There was also a pre- and post-assessment to determine the program's impact on participants' knowledge, which was done through social media metrics.

Five hundred fifteen people showed up to take part in the carnival! (78.8 percent virtual participants). According to social media metrics, more than 5,585 people saw all of the event's Facebook activities during the day. A statistically significant increase in mean knowledge scores was observed (p 0.05). This digital approach will continue to evolve as a new frontier for high-risk populations and anyone seeking mental health support and treatment in any setting. Figure 1 gives the idea of analysis.

A Survey Conducted in Tamil Nadu in DASS 21 and WHO-5 Well-Being Indexes

Mental health condition from Jan 2021 to Dec 2021 - Survey is conducted. As part of the study's selection process, the two survey questionnaires. It has been floated among a sample of both COVID and non-COVID patients representing a variety of demographics, including students, teachers, small- and medium-sized businesses in google form. The survey is conducted to understand the psychological disorders of the sample population in the mentioned period, especially after the first and second wave of COVID and make them understand their mental health symptoms. Participants in this survey must do so, as stated explicitly in the description.

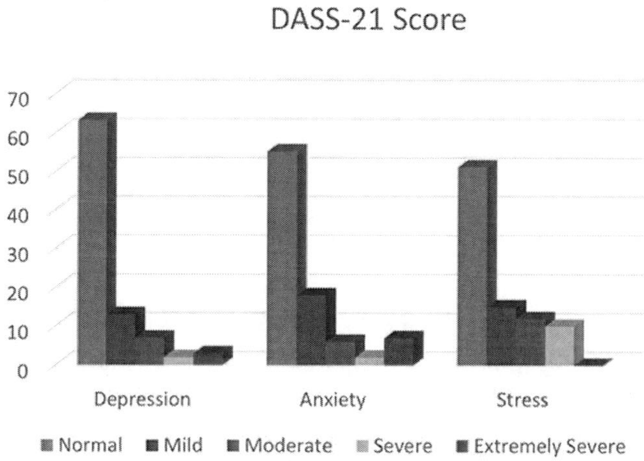

Source: Mat Ruzlin et al., 2021.

Figure 1. Bar graph of DASS-21 scores according to severity among participants attending mental health screening [31].

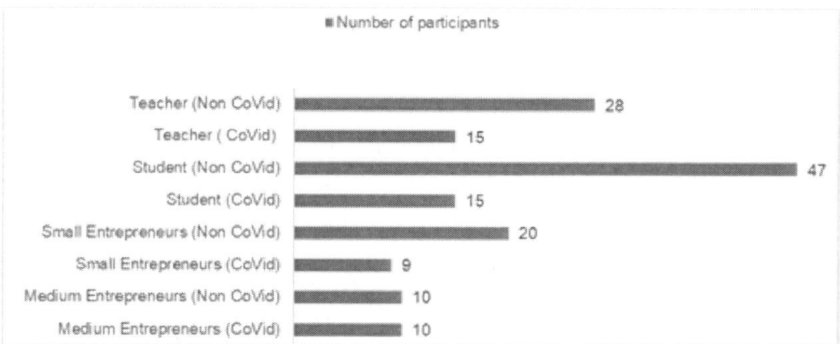

Figure 2. Number of respondents.

The respondents are mainly from Tamil Nadu, India. The gathering will bring together more than 154 people, including 77 men and 77 women. The graph depicts the number of samples selected from the broader group of samples. Students in the non-COVID category show the most significant interest in completing the Google form. In contrast, small entrepreneurs in the COVID category show the slightest interest in completing the form (Figure 2).

Results and Analysis

WHO-5 Well-Being Index

The WHO-5 well-being index categorizes people's levels of well-being based on their answers to the five questions mentioned. For the final score, which spans from 0 to 100, it is essential to multiply the raw score by four, with 0 indicating the poorest possible well-being and 100 representing the best possible well-being. A favorable attitude about one's well-being is characterized by a score greater than 50 on the questionnaire. As seen in Table 3, the average female score is around 53.5, and the average male score is roughly 54.2 for the gender-specific category. The median for both males and females is 52, and the mode is 44, which implies less than 50% of the population. According to the data in the table, the well-being index is at the center scale for males and females. In this study, evidence suggests that a score of 50 or below (the cut-off score) reflects a sad mood, but not necessarily depression itself. This indicates that both males and females are in a bad temper during COVID administration. When the scoring value is taken in category value of Non-COVID and COVID samples among the selective participants, we couldn't see much scoring value difference among both the category and the median of 44 and mode value of 52 in most of the classes as shown in Table 4.

Table 3. WHO-5 Well Being Index score in gender base

Gender	Average	Median	Mode	SD
Female	53.50649351	52	44	19.17139
Male	54.02666667	52	44	19.22669

Among the 154 samples, no female respondent has reached the score of 100, and 1.94%, as shown in Table 5, the male respondent has achieved the maximum score of best well-being. A person of 55 years old has performed the best well-being index shows that aged person tries to keep the happiness and pursuit of happiness in a better way than the younger ones and the pandemic doesn't impact him much as shown in Table 6.

The selective sample with COVID affected or without COVID has shown the well-being index score less than 60 showcases that the people are not happy between the period of Jan 2019 to Dec 2021. One is the other way; they want to survive in the period, not bothering on being Happy. The Male category has reached the maximum score of 100 and 25. Female has achieved a score of 92 and the least score of 22. The results can be taken so that females have less well-being index than males irrespective of the COVID conditions, as shown in Table 6.

Table 4. Score in category base

Category	Number of participants	Average	Median	Mode	SD
Medium Entrepreneurs (COVID)	10	55.86957	44	52	18.54139
Medium Entrepreneurs (Non COVID)	10	55.2233	44	52	17.6596
Small Entrepreneurs (COVID)	9	54.85149	44	52	17.17646
Small Entrepreneurs (Non COVID)	20	56.11538	44	52	18.1853
Student (COVID)	15	53.97468	60	52	18.55137
Student (Non COVID)	47	51.96429	44	48	18.28302
Teacher (COVID)	15	56	44	52	17.90047
Teacher (Non COVID)	28	56.04301	44	52	18.48924

Table 5. Maximum score

Gender	Age	Category	Score
Male	21	Student (Non COVID)	100
	25	Student (Non COVID)	100
	55	Medium Entrepreneurs (COVID)	100

Table 6. WHO-5 Well Being Index score range based on gender and age

Gender	Age	Score
Male	20-55	100-25
Female	20-47	92-22
COVID	55-22	100-22
Non COVID	56-20	92-20

DASS-21

Lovibond's original 42-item DASS was shortened to a 21-item version [23] adjusted again. Research on reliability and validity is done, and the severity scale scoring is given in Table 7. This has been published worldwide, all of which demonstrates that it is a well-established instrument for measuring symptoms of depression, anxiety, and stress in both clinical and non-clinical samples of adults [24-29]. It is calculated by entering the D, A, and S scores according to questions 1 to 21 in the appropriate fields. To sum the scores for each of the D, A, and S subscales and the total of each subscale, it is necessary to multiply each by two.

Table 7. Subscale - 21 items

	DASS21-D	DASS21-A	DASS21-S
Normal	0-9	0-7	0-14
Mild	10-13	8-9	15-18
Moderate	14-20	10-14	19-25
Severe	21-27	15-19	26-33
Extreme Severe	28+	20+	34+

According to standard severity labeling, the following cut-off scores should be used as guidelines: (ranging from average to severely Severe). The higher the score, the more often the person reports experiencing the symptoms. The Cronbach's alphas for depression, anxiety, and stress were 0.94, 0.87, and 0.91, respectively, when the subscales were used as a basis.

There are several limitations to this significant scale. It is very homogeneous (primarily cognitive and emotional symptoms) and does not capture all clinical criteria for major depressive disorder. These include sleeping problems, changes in appetite and weight, fatigue, and psychomotor slowness and agitation, among other things [30].

As shown in Table 8, the mild DASS-21 subscale is either less than or equal to zero in all categories. This demonstrates the evidence that stress, depression, and anxiety are classified as severe, moderate, or extremely severe in the sample under consideration (see Figure 1). The number of COVID affected people is higher than that of non-affected people. As shown in Table 9, the severity of depression is less severe in non-COVID samples and more severe in COVID-affected instances. As illustrated in Figure 3, the Anxiety scale is significantly lower in all cases when compared to the Depression and Stress scales overall.

Table 8. Subscale in the respondents

	Severity	SE (COVID)	SE (Non COVID)	STU (COVID)	STU (Non COVID)	TE (COVID)	TE (Non COVID)	ME (Non COVID)	ME (COVID)
		%	%	%	%	%	%	%	%
D	Normal	56	55	9	27	13	36	50	40
	Mild	22	0	0	0	0	11	30	0
	Moderate	0	30	13	40	0	18	0	0
	Severe	11	10	43	20	40	14	0	0
	Extreme Severe	11	5	36	13	47	21	20	60
A	Normal	33	55	13	7	7	14	40	40
	Mild	22	0	0	0	0	0	0	0
	Moderate	22	20	19	33	33	25	40	0
	Severe	0	10	26	27	27	32	0	0
	Extreme Severe	33	15	43	33	27	29	20	60
S	Normal	33	50	11	20	7	14	40	30
	Mild	33	0	0	0	0	0	0	0
	Moderate	22	25	21	33	33	25	40	0
	Severe	0	10	23	27	27	29	0	0
	Extreme Severe	22	15	45	20	33	29	20	70

Table 9. Severity subscale in the respondents

		SE (COVID)	SE (Non COVID)	STU (COVID)	STU (Non COVID)	TE (COVID)	TE (Non COVID)	ME (COVID)	ME (Non COVID)
DASS21-D	Severity	22	15	79	33	87	35	60	20
DASS21-A	Severity	33	15	43	33	27	29	60	20
DASS21-S	Severity	22	25	68	47	60	58	70	20

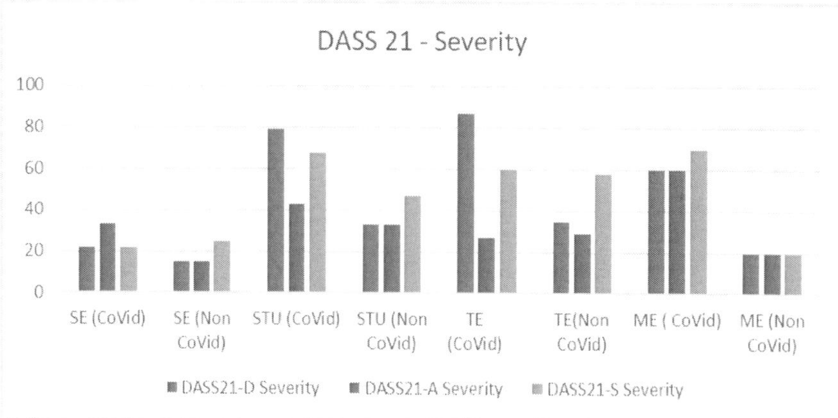

Figure 3. Severity subscales.

Conclusion

The virus COVID-19 was discovered for the first time and has since spread worldwide, causing widespread illness and death. A survey is conducted on respondents such as students, teachers, COVID and non-COVID patients, small- and medium-sized business owners, and other interested parties. Only 92 percent of female respondents received a high score, whereas male respondents received a high score of 1.94 percent of total respondents.

The evidence of the severity score is more substantial in COVID affected individuals than in non-affected individuals. Participants in the WHO well-being index and the DASS-21 have reported a greater awareness of their health and well-being. No one believes that there is a long-term solution to this problem, and no one understands what it means to be completely satisfied all of the time. A straightforward questionnaire is used to collect information about current well-being from participants.

Participants in the survey are not informed of the responses until after the survey has been administered. One of the primary goals of the research is to increase general public awareness and understanding of the well-being index. Because many infection mutations cause a pandemic, the survey results may be used in the future to assess the level of scale diversity present in disease transmission. Through the use of the DASS-21 questionnaire, researchers can further contribute to developing the ability to distinguish between depression, anxiety, and stress. Most of the time, people report feeling stressed regardless of physically presenting themselves.

Because the current generation is experiencing this for the first time, this poll describes the situation in question. We do not take any further action due to the survey's results because the information contained in the results, including the scope, scale, and subscale values, is used solely for non-clinical purposes.

References

[1] Piret, J. and Boivin, G., 2022. *Pandemics Throughout History.*

[2] Salari, N., Hosseinian-Far, A., Jalali, R., Vaisi-Raygani, A., Rasoulpoor, S., Mohammadi, M., Rasoulpoor, S. and Khaledi-Paveh, B., 2020. Prevalence of stress, anxiety, depression among the general population during the COVID-19 pandemic: a systematic review and meta-analysis. *Globalization and Health*, 16(1).

[3] Who. int. 2022. *Weekly epidemiological update on COVID-19 - 21 December 2021.* [Online] Available at: <https://www.who.int/publications/m/item/weekly-epidemiological-update-on-COVID-19---21-december-2021> [Accessed 18 January 2022].

[4] Dhawan, S., 2020. Online Learning: A Panacea in the Time of COVID-19 Crisis. *Journal of Educational Technology Systems*, 49(1), pp. 5-22.

[5] Mertens, G., Gerritsen, L., Duijndam, S., Salemink, E. and Engelhard, I., 2020. Fear of the coronavirus (COVID-19): Predictors in an online study conducted in March 2020. *Journal of Anxiety Disorders*, 74, p. 102258.

[6] KFF. 2022. *KFF Health Tracking Poll - December 2020: COVID-19 and Biden's Health Care Agenda - Methodology*. [online] Available at: <https://www.kff.org/report-section/kff-health-tracking-poll-december-2020-COVID-19-and-bidens-health-care-agenda-methodology/> [Accessed 18 January 2022].

[7] KFF. 2022. *The Implications of COVID-19 for Mental Health and Substance Use.* [online] Available at: <https://www.kff.org/coronavirus-COVID-19/issue-brief/the-implications-of-COVID-19-for-mental-health-and-substance-use/> [Accessed 18 January 2022].

[8] Statista. 2022. *Topic: COVID-19 and mental health*. [online] Available at: <https://www.statista.com/topics/7106/COVID-19-and-mental-health> [Accessed 18 January 2022].

[9] Hossain, M., Tasnim, S., Sultana, A., Faizah, F., Mazumder, H., Zou, L., McKyer, E., Ahmed, H. and Ma, P., 2020. Epidemiology of mental health problems in COVID-19: a review. *F1000Research*, 9, p. 636.

[10] Ransing, R., Adiukwu, F., Pereira-Sanchez, V., et al., 2020. Mental Health Interventions during the COVID-19 Pandemic: A Conceptual Framework by Early Career Psychiatrists. *Asian Journal of Psychiatry*, 51, p. 102085.

[11] Ren, F. and Guo, R., 2020. Public Mental Health In Post-COVID-19 ERA. *Psychiatria Danubina*, 32(2), pp. 251-255.

[12] McIntyre, R. and Lee, Y., 2020. Projected increases in suicide in Canada as a consequence of COVID-19. *Psychiatry Research*, 290, p. 113104.

[13] Mamun, M. and Ullah, I., 2020. COVID-19 suicides in Pakistan, dying off not COVID-19 fear but poverty? - The forthcoming economic challenges for a developing country. *Brain, Behavior, and Immunity*, 87, pp. 163-166.

[14] Thakur, V. and Jain, A., 2020. COVID 2019-suicides: A global psychological pandemic. *Brain, Behavior, and Immunity*, 88, pp. 952-953.

[15] Hao, F. et al., "Do psychiatric patients experience more psychiatric symptoms during COVID-19 pandemic and lockdown? A case-control study with service and research implications for immune psychiatry." *Brain* (2020): 106.

[16] Tan, W. et al., 2020. Is returning to work during the COVID-19 pandemic stressful? A study on immediate mental health status and psychoneuroimmunity prevention measures of the Chinese workforce. *Brain, Behavior, and Immunity*, 87, pp. 84-92.

[17] Gao, J., Zheng, P., Jia, Y., Chen, H., Mao, Y., Chen, S., Wang, Y., Fu, H., & Dai, J. 2020. Mental health problems and social media exposure during COVID-19 outbreak. *PLOS ONE*, 15(4), p. e0231924.

[18] Moghanibashi-Mansourieh, A., 2020. Assessing the anxiety level of the general Iranian population during the COVID-19 outbreak. *Asian Journal of Psychiatry*, 51, p. 102076.

[19] Lei et al., 2020. Comparison of Prevalence and Associated Factors of Anxiety and Depression Among People Affected by versus People Unaffected by Quarantine During the COVID-19 Epidemic in Southwestern China. *Medical Science Monitor*, 26.

[20] Liang, L., Ren, H., Cao, R., Hu, Y., Qin, Z., Li, C., & Mei, S., 2020. The Effect of COVID-19 on Youth Mental Health. *Psychiatric Quarterly*, 91(3), pp. 841-852.

[21] Huang, J. & Han, M. & Luo, T. & Ren, A. & Zhou, X. 2020. Mental health survey of 230 medical staff in a tertiary infectious disease hospital for COVID-19. Zhonghua Lao dong wei sheng zhi ye bing za zhi = Zhonghua laodong weisheng zhiyebing zazhi = *Chinese journal of industrial hygiene and occupational diseases*. 38. E001. 10.3760/CMA.j.cn121094-20200219-00063.

[22] Mirza, W., Mirza, A. M., Saleem, M. S., Chacko, P. P., Ali, M., Tarar, M. N., Babar, A., Freiwald, J., & Talitskiy, K. 2018. Well-being Assessment of Medical Professionals in Progressive Levels of Training: Derived from the WHO-5 Well-being Index. *Cureus*.

[23] Lovibond, S. H., Lovibond, P. F., 1995. *Manual for the Depression Anxiety Stress Scales*. 2nd edition. Sydney: Psychology Foundation of Australia.

[24] Antony, M. M. et al., 1998. Psychometric properties of the 42-item and 21-item versions of the depression anxiety stress scales in clinical groups and a community sample. *Psychological Assessment*; 10: 176-181.

[25] Sinclair, S. J. et al., 2012. Psychometric evaluation and normative data for the depression, anxiety, and stress scales-21 (DASS-21) in a non-clinical sample of U. S. adults. *Eval. Health Prof.;* 35: 259-279.

[26] Henry, J. D., Crawford, J. R., 2015. The short-form version of the Depression anxiety stress scales (DASS-21): construct validity and normative data in a large non-clinical sample. *Br. J. Clin. Psychol.*; 44: 227-239.

[27] Bottesi, G., et al., 2015. The Italian version of the Depression anxiety stress scales-21: factor structure and psychometric properties on community and clinical samples. *Compr. Psychiatry* 2015; 60: 170-181.

[28] Tonsing, K. N., 2014. Psychometric properties and validation of Nepali version of the Depression Anxiety Stress Scales (DASS-21). *Asian J. Psychiatr.* 2014; 8: 63-66.

[29] Vasconcelos-Raposo, J., Fernandes, H. M., Teixeira, C. M. 2013. Factor structure and reliability of the depression, anxiety, and stress scales in a large Portuguese community sample. *Span. J. Psychol.* 2013; 16: 10.

[30] Weiss, R. B., Aderka, I. M., Lee, J., Beard, C., Björgvinsson, T. 2015. A comparison of three brief depression measures in an acute psychiatric population: CES-D-10, QIDS-SR, and DASS-21-DEP. *Journal of Psychopathology and Behavioral Assessment*. 2015; 37:217-230. doi: 10.1007/s10862-014-9461-y.

[31] Mat Ruzlin, A., Chen, X., Yunus, R., Samsudin, E., Selamat, M. and Ismail, Z., 2021. Promoting Mental Health During the COVID-19 Pandemic: A Hybrid, Innovative Approach in Malaysia. *Frontiers in Public Health*, 9.

Chapter 3

Data Science Applications of Post-COVID-19 Mental Illness

Ch. Vijaya Bhaskar[1,*], D. S. R. Murthy[2], M. Nagaraju[1] and Sheri Mahender Reddy[3]

[1]Sreenidhi Institute of Science and Technology, Yamnampet, Ghatkesar, Hyderabad, Telangana, India
[2]Anurag University, Hyderabad, Telangana, India
[3]Otto-Friedrich University of Bamberg, Germany

Abstract

As innovative solutions and analysis methodologies became accessible, data science gained a more vital role in health. Data science can assist us in improving solutions for psychological difficulties. Several patients attempt a variety of psychologists, therapeutic strategies, and drugs before discovering what works for people. Locating suitable treatment is especially troubling considering how long most patients have to suffer before receiving treatment and the expense and mental strain of attempting many choices. As a result, it is critical to determine whether or not a specific medicine is effective. Healthcare data science has been expanding rapidly, but using objectives to analyse and address psychiatric problems has regressed the rest of the community. Psychological wellness is well adapted for data science strategies: the impact of psychological illness is enormous, primarily neglected, and remains unclear, generating immense promise for computation investigation and therapies. This chapter discussed various data science applications of post-COVID-19 psychological effects and consequences.

*Corresponding Author's Email: vijayabhaskar.ch@gmail.com.

In: Data Science Applications of Post-COVID-19 Psychological Disorders
Editor: Vijayalakshmi Kakulapati
ISBN: 979-8-88697-165-1

Keywords: data science, affective, mental, treatment, patient, psychology, physician, strategy, drug, strain

Introduction

The internal health catastrophe has surfaced because of this of the COVID-19 outbreak. As of June 2020, the US Centers for Disease Control and Prevention (CDC) approximated that over a third of Americans experienced anxiety or depressive disorders [1]. Youthful householder rates are past doubly as high, despite the truth that the frequency of internal health enterprises has increased considerably in the recent decade [2, 3]. Over 60 people who progressed from eighteen to 24 were sad or anxious, and a one-fourth had pondered self-murder in the previous month.

These numbers demonstrate that depression rates have risen significantly from roughly 11% of most grown-ups in 2019 [4] to almost 25% among university students before the epidemic. The increase in depression has corresponded with substantial disruptions in daily life, such as stay-at-home orders, grounds closures, and interpersonal distancing measures, which have altered how people live, work, research, and interact. The person's mental health is assessed utilizing a high grade of affective disease, producing substantial depressive disorders and many anxiety disorders.

Psychological disorders include nervousness attacks, depressive illnesses, and mood disorders, in addition to personality problems. Many mobile apps, intelligent devices, for example, smartwatches, and innovative groups can end up being employed to provide cell phone emotional health therapy. Personal psychiatry may also assist in predicting bipolar disorder and improving diagnosis in addition to treatment. Most intelligent techniques don't seem due to a lack of resources, especially in developing places. Within Pakistan, for illustration, the mental well-being system receives 0% of the government's health budget. There is usually a requirement for a cheap approach to diagnosing depression within Pakistan. Everybody can know about this [5].

Data science can assist us in correctly designing and applying solutions for psychiatric problems. Several patients attempt a variety of professionals, therapeutic strategies, and drugs before discovering what performs better for them. This lengthy process of locating suitable care is especially troubling depending on the prolonged majority of people waiting to obtain any treatment and the expense and emotional trauma connected with attempting many choices. It is essential to judge whether or not someone's specific therapy is effective [6].

Big data from human mobility, contact tracing, medical image resolution, virology, drug verification, bioinformatics, and electronic recording, as well as technical literature, are now widely available thanks to ever-increasing processing power and data science strategies in medicine and public health [7] Because of these advancements, the tremendous passion of teachers and practitioners, and the urgent requirement for data-driven insights, information science has performed a crucial function in understanding and dealing with the continuing coronavirus disease 2019 (COVID-19) epidemic [8].

One of data science's most exciting challenges is adapting developing technologies to produce new phenotypic and biometric characteristics that can be connected to current datasets. Various sensors, including wearable and Smartphone apps, may enable current, fine-grained monitoring of various parameters, such as sleep, mood, vital indicators fluctuation [9–10], and alcohol intake [11] These methods may reinforce scientific treatment and guideline research in locations such as circadian rhythms in psychological diseases [12].

Phenotypic data can be extracted using data mining techniques on social media and health records [13]. Ultimately, record linking to social and informative data repositories creates a genuinely comprehensive repository both in health and sickness, an integrative model of psychological processes [14]. Even worse than the pandemic may lie underneath it in terms of death rates, morbidity, and social barriers. It might be emphasized that most of the literature on the psychological effects of COVID-19 is much more retroactive than predictive. Thinking about what occurred may be less significant than analyzing what we have learned, what humans must do immediately, and what we often don't realize. Because of the fixation on syndrome phenotypes [15], investigators have learned slightly to nothing regarding the perception of intellectual illness—in this instance. Schizophrenia is connected with a highly contagious epidemic. When authors dwell upon these traditional neurobiological possibilities [16], they continue to produce more heat transfer than illumination, failing to reach definitive interpretations or effective treatments.

This chapter discusses the significance of post-COVID-19 psychiatric illness issues using data science. The context of the issue is described in the second section. Section 3 discusses relevant work in psychological wellness and the most recent data investigations. The fourth section discusses several sorts of psychological illnesses and data science applications. The fifth portion covers the proposed topic's importance, and the sixth section emphasizes the conclusion statements, which are accompanied by future enhancements.

Background

Anxiousness, sleep difficulties, misery, suicide, PTSD (post-traumatic stress disorders), and anxiousness attacks are all instances of emotional health issues [17]. New-onset mental health issues: due to COVID-19-related stress, anxiety, and loneliness; everlasting neuropsychiatric symptoms or disorders (e.g., severe ischemic stroke, pain, dizziness, ataxia, delirium, and seizures) of COVID-19 infection thanks to hard cytokine storms; enduring neuro-psychiatric symptoms or disorders (e.g., acute ischemic cerebrovascular event, headache, dizziness, ataxia, delirium, and seizures), degeneration of pre-existing Psychological disorder is caused by a deficiency of treatment resources, disruption of solutions, service supply, and support [18] Suicides: therefore, of COVID-19's neuropsychiatric indications and socioeconomic implications [19] - Other concerns: Racism, prejudice, and racial discrimination associated with COVID-19

Medical professionals, persons with pre-existing psychological conditions; class iv workers; pregnancies; disabled people and degenerative diseases; migrants; refugees; migrants; refugees; and queer community are minority groups [20] Uncertainty, lack of counseling services due to education or employment shutdown, scholastic absence, psychiatric comorbidity, anxieties, discrimination, prolonged loneliness, insecurity, long working hours, fatigue, interacting directly with ongoing instances, and suffering economic difficulties are all possible causes [21].

Data science can assist us in understanding and improving psychological problems.

- Who is suffering from severe depression?
- What indications and signs are essential investigative evidence?
- What factors influence somebody else's desire to engage in and remain in diagnosis?
- What are the characteristics of psychiatric disorders in diverse demographics?

Data science can effectively address these issues and is becoming ever more prevalent and at least more accessible. Fitness tracker information can be utilized to recognize physiological indicators related to the disorder. Online communities and internet interaction provide perspective into the behavioural effects of psychiatric well-being. Physician and therapeutic relationship documents are progressively being analyzed using machine learning and natural, and neuroimaging may be perfect for diagnosing computer vision.

Data science can benefit from understanding and executing therapies for psychological issues. Several patients attempt a variety of counselling, treatment strategies, and drugs before identifying anything that suits them. This lengthy procedure to locate suitable treatment is especially troublesome depending on how long most people have to spend until obtaining any therapy and the expense and cognitive stress involved with many choices [22].

Medical science can potentially deliver an infinite number of decision-support and self-monitoring capabilities if personal psychologists and the domain work together to steer innovative technology ahead. Instead of proactively adopting the techniques obtained by technicians, such improvements will probably collapse to incorporate with our whole turmoil healthcare system for many factors that enhance genetic variation, and cognitive science has battled to continue improving patients' lives. Collaboration of data scientists and psychologists is critical with this subsequent stage in the field's philosophical evolution [23].

- Significant actions in data science have happened since the epidemic: As per Strategy Analytics, 75% of organizational insight, information, and data scientists have worked incredibly long hours since the epidemic, so this tendency is anticipated to remain.
- The tendency towards working from home will persist, lowering the need to provide specialists to move and widening firms' talented workforce.
- Increased demand for localized and reconfiguration production processes, resulting in a requirement for more intelligent data capabilities.
- Advancements in Machine learning and artificial intelligence effectively storm financial crises (even eliminate the necessity of social distancing rules).

As organizations accumulate these competencies, new possibilities for data scientists and analytical experts will emerge. Data scientists will face a significantly altered situation in the following weeks as we transition to a post-COVID scenario [24].

Related Works

Comments concerning the global food crisis are being taken out of the preserved database for targeted keywords [25]. The collection is trained to utilize two supervised and unsupervised methods of learning: NB (Nave Bayes) and KNN (K nearest neighbour). Cloud technology is the best method for storing big volumes of large amounts of data. HDFS features for independent analysis and a massive data repository have been developed [26]. MongoDB is a massive data engine for studying global mental and behavioural health information [27]. Describes a method of implementing the big data technology 'MongoDB' for evaluating facts linked to global psychological therapies. The information is subsequently examined utilizing evolutionary algorithms for various psychiatric conditions before being placed in MongoDB for ultimate data extraction.'

Predictive modelling has also been used to identify illness throughout epidemics. Electronic datasets were evaluated [28] based on community behavior patterns, news reporting elements, and specialist tendencies of search-related illness epidemics. They discovered significant characteristics influencing trained and layman searching behaviours in healthcare professionals and patients and signals for focused messaging during catastrophes and epidemics. A disaster response team suggested [29] employing an IoT-based mobile network of wearable technology known as body area networks (BANs). The gadget is built using "intelligence architecture," a concept that aids information processing and decisions obtained from the sensors' data. Anxiousness, sadness, and sleeplessness are shared among 60% of clinicians, caregivers, and hospital interns during the COVID-19 epidemic [30] and are expected to last for multiple decades. Later, HCP performed in respiratory therapy during the SARS pandemic in 2003 showed prolonged and considerably higher aspects of perceived health problems such as tension, sadness, and PTSD symptoms [31].

One year after discharge, victims of severe illness have persistent psychiatric dysfunction with considerable stress, sadness, and PTSD. A significant proportion of individuals with symptomatic respiratory failure had neuropsychological dysfunction, such as reduced concentration, focus, remembering, and intellectual response time. Individuals with acute respiratory syndrome (SARS) and extended ventilators had significantly poorer quality of life following release from the critical care unit when contrasted to hospitalizations for other causes [32].

The feedback to the COVID-19 epidemic may be equivalent to environmental catastrophes and other devastating occurrences affecting a society [33], resulting in long-term misery in the afflicted populace [34]. The health consequences of catastrophes can last up to 12 years in only one out of six people in the afflicted community [35]. The psychiatric effect of the COVID-19 epidemic was quickly recorded; in most communities, it is comparable to PTSD symptoms in the community [36]. People who acquired COVID-19 and recovered are also more susceptible to developing PTSD symptoms [37]. Several PTSD and depression signs were described by epidemic patients [38]. According to a hypothesis, the much more common problems in the post-illness phase include a feeling of loneliness, sleeplessness, stress, agitation, cognitive problems, exhaustion, and unpleasant experiences [39].

Solving emerging difficulties using suitable actions may be difficult in several nations, especially those with limited capabilities. As a result, substantial efforts should be made to avoid psychiatric disorders and provide facilities for early recognition of psychiatric difficulties. Following the COVID-19 emergency, these psychological well-being service diagnoses and therapy methods can be categorized as general, selected, or recommended [40].

Nervousness (15.7 percent), melancholy (10.6 percent), and tension (5.2 percent) were determined to be relatively low in India compared to other countries [41]. Furthermore, over half of the medical professionals who reported such concerns lost consciousness from mild to extremely serious. Furthermore, 67 respondents experienced bodily ailments, particularly migraine, tiredness, fear, and sleeplessness, indicating bodily manifestations of discomfort. However, during the COVID-19 emergency service, army public healthcare employees from the UK were evaluated for the consequences of poor protective equipment on patients' psychological disorders. Those who already lacked appropriate tools were more likely to suffer from prevalent psychiatric illnesses (2.49 percent), PTSD (2.99 percent), worse healthcare (2.09 percent), and emotional disturbances (1.69 percent) [42].

Few investigations of mental and emotional complications among admitted patients with COVID-19 have already been documented, and much more show up. Research on inpatient but asymptomatic individuals indicated that PTSS was prevalent (96.2 percent) [43]. A document study of 841 COVID-19 inpatients discovered that more than 50% of the 841 patients had a neuropsychiatric condition. Imprecise cognitive signs, as well as abnormalities of cognition (19.6 percent), were detected, primarily in older adults or those with acute COVID-19 illness; peripheral neuropathy (3.1 percent); dysautonomia (2.5 percent); and other less related signs. Neurocognitive complaints such as sleeplessness, anxiousness, sadness, and schizophrenia were observed by 19.9 percent of such individuals, although they were not linked with depressive disorders [44].

Various respiratory distress infections have been used in several investigations to derive conclusions. A contextual of lengthy treatment outcomes for older adults of SARS and Middle East Respiratory Syndrome (MERS) in the emergency ward (ICU) demonstrated PTSD occurrence in 39%, loneliness in 33%, and anxiousness in 30% over and above six months after contamination, and also chronic obstructive lung disease and physical performance [45]. Italian specialists also found that patients of COVID-19 may experience comparable results [46].

Acute respiratory distress syndrome (ARDS) in COVID-19 ICU patients is possible, with a 25 percent chance of recovery. Like MERS and SARS victims, recipients of ARDS may have lasting exhaustion and poor activity intolerance, discomfort and weakening, neurodegenerative consequences, and the psychosocial repercussions of prolonged ICU hospitalizations. Inactivity, absence from relatives, extended medication, health complications and survivability, and later job insecurity were concerns [47]. The researchers emphasized identifying PTSD and other psychiatric disorders and providing early and aggressive interdisciplinary counselling that should persist after discharge.

Data Science Application of Post-COVID 19 Mental Illness

The science of evaluating fundamental data in massive datasets to make conclusions is known as data science. These findings are based on data collected within these collections. Data science is a multidisciplinary subject that employs analytical techniques and algorithms to obtain insights from the aggregation and analysis of data by applying meaningful conclusions throughout various applications. Data science is more of a set of skills for teaching robots to assist organizations in better decisions. While projecting demands, a corporation must recognize that it will only get more competent or innovative. The problem is figuring out how to integrate it into existing corporate procedures. Several decision-makers do not consider what will produce the strategy work after this year. The current COVID-19 scenario has made it difficult for enterprises to function by their initial strategic goals.

There have been many efforts to improve the benefits that Data Science may bring to psychological wellness. Data scientists are using algorithms to analyze massive information with the aim of diverse variables that would effectively target sources, indicators, and signs of psychiatric conditions and choose the most appropriate therapies. Scientists can uncover prophylactic ways to battle psychosomatic illnesses while pinpointing the origins. Nevertheless, the techniques utilized to carry out these activities are still being developed and will not be extensively utilized.

In theory, data science is a tremendously successful method of technology that may assist both people and corporations in combating this epidemic. Nevertheless, one must exercise caution and ensure that the technologies' professionals are as active and updated regularly. Because the conditions change so quickly, data scientists and business analytics executives must guarantee that they will immediately react [48].

Diagnosis

Some of the issues for psychological disorders are the absence of definite testing, classification, and reliance on experimentation approaches. Furthermore, conflicting signs or idiosyncratic variances can frequently result in postponed or inaccurate identification. On the other hand, Data Science can transform circumstances. By examining vast quantities of data, researchers can identify trends that otherwise would have been buried and difficult to notice. Origins, indicators, and indications can be recognized and connected to obtain a more solid and actual diagnosis.

Depression

It is common for people to develop multiple trials before finding a depression that performs for them. Big data might put a stop to this examination holistic approach to health. According to studies, mood disorders, including lack of enthusiasm, reduced activity, and inability to make judgments, indicated a lower result for antipsychotic drugs. This information might greatly enhance whether sufferers are assigned to therapies. Ml algorithms were also utilized to construct an application to forecasting that intervention would perform effectively for somebody by using vast quantities of information and allowing people struggling with melancholy to provide data about themselves and monitor the effects.

Applications

- Data Science allows investigators to quantify the consequences of psychological conditions on worldwide demographics, both past and future. Whenever the consequences are defined and backed by evidence, it makes a powerful argument for allocating strategic assets to behavioural well-being diagnosis and care accessible.
- Suicidal thoughts and depressive disorders are predicted using Natural Language Processing (NLP) approaches. Throughout the phrases they express, emergency counselling communications utilize algorithms to detect users at significant risk for adverse outcomes or consciousness.
- The acquired data enables counsellor instruction, and crisis counsellors can refer identified high clients to the patient supervision they may require.
- Suicidal thoughts can be anticipated by examining Patient Data, which lowers mortality rates dramatically.
- A predictive model developed at Vanderbilt University Medical Centre in Nashville combines hospitalization information, such as time of life, sex, postcode, prescription, and diagnosis histories, to forecast a person's chance of committing suicide. Sensitive data has the potential to aid and reduce mortality rates.
- Studies show that combining a mobile phone with an intelligence watching individual behavioural responses might be an appropriate diagnosis.
- Penn Medicine scientists used classification techniques to calculate the magnitude and form of neural systems in kids, resulting in a better diagnosis and more customized therapy for behavioural disorders.
- Imaging techniques have been proven in investigations to anticipate antidepressant therapeutic results in severe depression.

- ML tools are being designed to distinguish between those who regulate their psychotic symptoms independently or with the assistance of healthcare experts and require more protective treatment from therapists. It has the potential to assist deliver more sophisticated treatment and alleviate the scarcity of qualified people.
- A recent study revealed that learning algorithms might uncover trends in integrated care with worldwide web behavioural therapy for psychological morbidity.
- People are typically afraid to divulge concerns to a psychiatrist they've never met earlier and relax their defences using Intelligence technologies. This, together with decreased expenses, aids AI technologies in diagnostics, faster therapy, and successful healthcare consequences.
- Organizations and insurance providers may utilize Chatbots to target employees dealing with drug dependence, melancholy, or anxiousness and give access to efficient and premium assistance.
- AI can offer pre-emptive review in circumstances where people are becoming sad or nervous following obtaining poor diagnostic testing for a significant medical ailment, and
- It can assist in the generation of appropriate therapeutic strategies.
- The Ginger.io software assists professionals in tracking patient improvement, identifying moments of emergency, and developing tailored treatment plans by comparing previous evaluations and legitimate data obtained utilizing Smartphone.
- Appropriate care and individualized treatment strategies can make psychological wellness therapies increasingly affordable and effective.
- Massive data have also been analyzed to determine the association between childhood trauma and schizophrenia and psychological disorder.
- Artificial intelligence techniques investigate how parental interactions and social networking affect teen psychological wellness and whether they are crucial to someone's well-being.
- It can aid in discovering linkages underlying neurological diseases, improve preventative care for teenagers, and break the trend of multigenerational deprivation.
- Understanding suicide warning signs in youngsters, recommending which therapies will work for particular people, and using genetics to

inform schizophrenia treatments and extend the lives of those affected by schizophrenia are all topics that Data Science and Machine Learning techniques may assist.
- Data Science and ML techniques can help with various initiatives, including recognizing suicidal behavior warnings in kids, endorsing which therapies will work in which individuals, and recognizing genetic factors to advise psychiatric disorders treatments and increase life expectancy for those affected by schizophrenia.
- When used correctly, Data Science has the potential to help us discover potential risks for psychiatric disorders, get patients the best therapy for patients, measure how well individuals progress, and even examine how we may avoid psychological issues [49].

Several advantages of incorporating data science into business enterprises include:

- It reduces the chance of components not being delivered and stored on time.
- It examines transportation, inventory levels, weather changes, marketplace insufficiency, and several other factors that might affect a whole procedure in logistics.
- By utilizing the analysis process, the company can assess client demands, behavior, and industry growth. The research results are vital in determining which items are in the market demand.
- Organizations may effectively manage assets and regulate spending using projections and correctly developed inferences.

Healthcare Industry

The decision support system in the medical is a critical data science instance. The forecasting model examines historical information, analyzes it, discovers patterns, and makes estimates depending on such advancements. Because the threat of visiting a clinic enhances an individual's experience risk due to the increased likelihood of the COVID-19 pathogen being prevalent in medical centers with COVID-19 inpatient units, everybody intends to use the virtual world in the health care system to investigate better public services and drug carriers. This is how data science in medicine may benefit medical facilities:

- Obtain many connections and relationships of disorders among the consumers of healthcare blogs.
- Enhance patient safety via personalization and maintaining records.
- Increase performance of the supply chain and pharmacy procurement for greater patient accessibility.
- Anticipate worsening diagnosis and treatment, give prevention measures via videos and interactive training while using online resources to begin therapeutic as soon as possible.

Data Science in Psychiatry

The epidemic significantly influences people's quality of life, and we'll all across the universe.

1) The epidemic influences the frequency of emotional problems and psychological disorders
2) The outbreak influences the incidence of suicidal behavior
3) The probability of COVID-19 infection, catastrophic disease, and mortality in patients with psychological illnesses
4) The coronavirus influences psychiatric care
5) The efficacy of COVID-19-adapted psychotherapies in preventing or reducing mental issues and maintaining rehabilitation.

Crises Text Line

The number of texters needing emergency assistance far outnumbers the number of possible caregivers. Whereas this circumstance isn't acceptable for anybody looking for free support, the Crisis Text Line recognizes that sure victims want aid already more immediately than the others. The business developed a learning algorithms method for identifying phrases and emoticons that signal a more significant negative impact, enabling them to advance the more dangerous group to the top of the queue. The methods utilize data via text exchanges that result in an effective recovery (i.e., the utilization of rescue services), which is a novel and crucial form of information. Suicidal thoughts and deaths are callous to predict, and the research lacks an efficient testing method and other helpful forecasting techniques. Maintaining the capability to forecast these occurrences in textual communication behavior, on the other hand, offers a considerable capability to mitigate this diagnosis deficiency in a larger sense.

Ellie, the 3-D Chat Bot

Ellie is not intended to replace medical therapy but to serve as a "records collector" to better the diagnosis. Whenever an affected person interacts with Ellie, information is recorded on the pace of communication, the duration they hesitate while getting answers, and the mobility and positioning of 66 distinct spots on their face. This procedure has revealed that people with PTSD contact the heads on spikes and arms disproportionately more often than those without PTSD, a therapeutic hint that would have gone unnoticed absent Ellie's intensive data analysis. In addition, Ellie recognized more PTSD indicators in research with sick people than in the conventional Post-Deployment Health Assessment given to service members [50].

Quartet Health

It is a psychological wellness software firm established in New York City dedicated to improving the effectiveness and usability of psychiatric care through a four-pronged, comprehensive strategy. The Quartet makes every effort to assist registered users and one of the processes. Providing physicians would not get news on their customers' experiences with mental health treatment; however, Quartet integrates recommending physicians and psychological physicians to guarantee interaction among these critical parties. Quartet also offers further assistance to people in need thru the team of "Care Navigators."

COVIDiSTRESS

The adverse effects of vast loneliness, home detention, and relevant data activity are known as 'cabin fever throughout a virus.' Shuttering schools and universities and requesting individuals to sequester themselves in their residences will likely trigger psychological and pragmatic anxiety unconnected to the dread of getting the disease. Adherence to clinical practice guidelines has been proven to decline as a result of severe stress but also as a result of modest daily demands, including occupational stress or domestic chores. The scientists launched the COVIDiSTRESS open scientific cooperation to assist health officials and decision-makers organize informed responses. The dataset can assist academics and policymakers in identifying subtle differences in mental and behavioural risk variables in the perspective of the COVID-19 [51].

Risks in Education Sector

Post-The COVID-19 catastrophe, universities worldwide went to virtual meetings and other digital solutions to continue operating. Such virtual educational experiences emphasized the global challenges to online educational acceptance and learning. The education industry is increasingly using specific technology and data science to anticipate system throughput and performance.

In the educational sector, the critical efforts have been taken to provide effective educational systems and devices:

- Effective electronic devices or technology utilization significantly improves within and without the class.
- Innovative applications of data generated or acquired in professional learning environments are to customize knowledge and enhance academic learning analytics based on instructional and administrative education data, research and evaluation, and policy design.
- Personalization of instructing of Intelligence inference and educational policy
- Big data education data analysis and novel methods personalize and improve a person's learning programs using individual data obtained from Online browsing, online communities, and interconnected gadgets and devices.

COVID-19 disproportionately impacts graduate pupils due to worry about educational excellence, prospective professions, and social interactions. Before the epidemic, adolescents worldwide were experiencing increased worry, negative emotional states, a lack of emotional and psychological difficulties, drug addiction, and suicidal behavior [52]. Students require extra facilities and assistance to manage the condition's psychiatric consequences.

Female students, entirely non-Asian, in good condition, or who met someone afflicted with COVID-19 had a more significant emotional effect. Aged 18 to 24 years old, working eight or even more hrs per day on computers, and having somebody affected were all significant potential elements of antibiotic therapy. Teenagers of the above socioeconomic classes who probably spent 2 hrs outside or less than 8hrs on digital devices have been less inclined to feel adverse effects [53].

Occupational stress, emotional and social misunderstanding, insufficient training, and career uncertainty have long put pressure on the education sector. This pressure may influence teachers' wellness, leading to a rise in sick leave, delay, and poor work performance. Furthermore, protecting one's psychological state is critical because instructor interaction can be stressful for students.

E-Commerce Industry

People are shopping electronically in the post-pandemic period, and artificial intelligence on online media provides experiences akin to an authentic experience. Digital marketers instantly customize their digital marketing depending on the demographic descriptions of visitors. Changing website designs and modifying featured items, among other aspects, is a systematic strategy to get even more customers to buy digitally. Many internet sites that don't offer anything have tailored advertisements.

Further, with the development of the COVID-19 epidemic and the increasing significance of e-commerce, research in buying behavior is becoming increasingly important. The authors evaluate the correlations between the components and the intensity of the effect. Online purchases are boosted in the wake of the epidemic. The analysis found what modifications in online consumer purchase decisions are frequent during the epidemic [54].

Numerous cognitive aspects influence consumer buying behavior [55]:

- Greater levels of anxiousness and COVID-related fear might reflect trends, enhancing the urge to purchase needs.
- Increasingly stressful situations would allow customers to preserve cash or might enhance the urge to buy cash on essentials

- More significant amounts of depression are connected, including a surge in the desire to acquire both needs and non-necessities.
- Increased consciousness tactics would be connected with a greater demand for purchasing, particularly for non-necessities.
- A more excellent overall economy would be connected with a rise in the price of both needy and non-necessities.

Image Processing and Computer Vision

Healthcare and medicine, when combined, constitute a potential arena for leveraging technological advances. Because of breakthroughs in data science, the healthcare system is rising continuously. It aids in various ways, one of which is the interpretation of diagnostic imaging. This is one of the fascinating research fields in computer vision [50].

Data Science aids in detecting digitized images to identify flaws in the nervous system and assist clinicians in developing an efficient therapeutic approach. Such diagnostic image examinations included X-rays, ultrasounds, MRI (Magnetic Resonance Imaging), CT scans, etc. The appropriate examination of such images provides vital information for physicians to give effective therapy to victims.

Patients afflicted with the coronavirus COVID-19 develop psychological disorders that last or tend weeks post pathogens. Roughly 60% positively identified for mental consequences, including at least one of the categories tested (PTSD, misery, nervousness, restlessness, and obsessive-compulsive symptomatology) [56]. After transmission, roughly 40% of individuals experienced severe despair and distress. After three months of follow-up in a Chinese investigation, tension, sadness, and sleep disturbances were found in multiple other patient populations [57].

Predictive Analytics in Psychological Effects

The predictive and prescriptive method founded on Data Science generates forecasts about the patient's prognosis. This also assists in developing plans for the most proper medication for the patients. As a result, prescriptive analytics is a valuable technology that significantly contributes to the health sector.

The following are the significant advantages of data analytics in health care services:

- It assists in the treatment of acute and chronic disorders.
- It effectively analyses pharmacological distribution requirements.
- It forecasts the condition of the patient and recommends prevention methods.
- It allows for speedier healthcare information recording.
- It aids in the effective use of physicians and other services for the advantage of the most outstanding group of patients.
- It forecasts a victim's significant medical catastrophes.

Developing Drugs

It has gotten much more accessible with numerous Data Science tools in medicine. Records from billions of testing's may be handled in years, if not months. It aids in determining the efficacy of medicine using data processing. As a result, an effective vaccination or treatment can be released in less than one year. All of these are accomplished through Data Science and Machine Learning. These have changed the pharmaceutical company's technology production areas.

Genomics Data Science

Data Science technology in medicine and genetics has simplified the process. Using diverse Information Sciences and Big Data techniques, researchers can investigate genomes with less effort and dedication. Such techniques let investigators must identify genetic risk abnormalities and the medicine that better reacts to a certain kind of genome.

Remote Supervision

The apps created utilizing online guidance are an excellent illustration of Data Science in action. Data Scientists have created complete systems that provide patients with individualized interactions. Data Science-based healthcare apps enable patients to discover diseases by evaluating signs. The person only has to register their complaints, and the program will anticipate the diagnosis and prognosis. This will recommend protection, medicine, and therapy based on the patient's health status.

Discussion

Recently, there has been a surge in interest and exploratory research into the possible uses of ML for psychological disorders. The analysis summarizes data science applications in psychological wellness, highlighting contemporary trends and changes. The strategic pathway of development for ML technologies that are effective and adaptable for psychological medicine was determined by addressing current approaches and future phases of ML advances. Patients with depressive symptoms are usually stigmatized and publicly excluded by the family. They may outperform in educational institutions and employment. Therefore, individuals lose accessibility to social facilities, resulting in inadequate living conditions. Financial stress is a significant and sometimes intangible expression that leads to a state of poverty and poor wellness. The large majority of people impacted come from low- and middle-income communities.

Researchers observed no influence of isolation on emotional problems in older adults who had previously healed from COVID-19 contamination and were untreated, as judged by relationship status. It contradicts the conclusion that residing solo was an independent state of psychological discomfort in an elderly group of community people. This finding could be understood by the impact of COVID-19–related imposed confinement, which may counteract the impact of isolation on emotional exhaustion.

Data science is combined with scientific innovations, which can evaluate behavioural traits over a period. Then at the macro scale, better, healthier, and psychologically ill individuals can lead to significant inventions about observable traits allocation of healthy and unhealthy behaviour, which clinical diagnosis schemes have struggled to identify. For example, evidence collected by Cell phones and wearable technologies provides an inaccessible source of genuine conscience neurobiological facts rather than depending on primitive ontologies that manage to grasp the rich diversification of clinical findings. Such evidence provides a conceivably more precise, reliable, and diagnostically accurate objective for biological, cellular, and cognitive science psychological science to corresponding clinical manifestations with an underlying theme.

Data Science approaches can reveal therapeutically significant hidden data in massive datasets, assisting decision making. Data from clinics, pharmaceuticals, patient records, cellular phones, and online searches provide a massive set of data that may be used for therapeutic reasons, including identification, diagnostics, therapy, and further studies.

Conclusion

Data science is a fast-expanding discipline with several beneficial approaches to psychological healthcare investigation, most of which we have highlighted in this View. As crucially, it provides the intention of making genuine complexities analysis revitalized. H hope that the significant advances in treatment interventions that we are starting to witness will provide practical advantages to persons experiencing the psychological disorder.

Future Enhancement

In the future, psychiatric healthcare data science will have an enormous capacity to promote advanced investigation and significant advances in treatment and therapies. With the increase in data science and the introduction of numerous computation technologies, the healthcare system continues to be a prominent developer of data-driven services for a better quality of life and personalized services to its customers. Data scientists may generate helpful insights into improving the capabilities of healthcare and biopharmaceutical companies by analyzing a wide variety of medical data, including economic, therapeutic, R&D, management, and relevant data.

References

[1] Czeisler MÉ. et al., Mental health, substance use, and suicidal ideation during the COVID-19 pandemic—the United States, June 24–30, 2020.*Morb. Mortal. Wkly. Rep.*, 69, 1049 (2020).

[2] Twenge JM, Cooper AB, Joiner TE, Duffy ME, Binau SG. Age, period, and cohort trends in mood disorder indicators and suicide-related outcomes in a nationally representative dataset, 2005–2017. *J. Abnorm. Psychol.* 128, 185 (2019).

[3] National Center for Health Statistics, "Early release of selected mental health estimates" (National Center for Health Statistics, 2019).
[4] American College Health Association, "National college health assessment" (American College Health Association, 2018).
[5] Ayesha Kamran Ulhaq, Amira Khattak, Noreen Jamil, M. Asif Naeem, Farhaan Mirza, "Data Analytics in Mental Healthcare," *Scientific Programming*, vol. 2020, Article ID 2024160, 9 pages, 2020. https://doi.org/10.1155/2020/2024160.
[6] https://towardsdatascience.com/data-science-in-mental-health-ccd09ba2148a.
[7] Topol EJ. 2019 High-performance medicine: the convergence of human and artificial intelligence. *Nat. Med.*, 25, 44–56. (Doi:10.1038/s41591-018-0300-7).
[8] Who coronavirus (COVID-19) dashboard. https://COVID19.who.int/.
[9] Bidargaddi N. et al. Digital footprints: facilitating large-scale environmental psychiatric research in naturalistic settings through data from everyday technologies. *Mol. Psychiatry*, 22, 164–169 (2017).
[10] Khan Y, Ostfeld AE, Lochner CM, Pierre A, Arias, AC. Monitoring vital signs with flexible and wearable medical devices. *Adv. Mater.*, 28, 4373–4395 (2016).
[11] Selvam AP, Muthu Kumar S, Kamakoti, V, Prasad, S. A wearable biochemical sensor for monitoring alcohol consumption lifestyle through ethyl glucuronide (EtG) detection in human sweat. *Sci. Rep.*, 6, 23111 (2016).
[12] Bradley AJ. et al. Sleep and circadian rhythm disturbance in bipolar disorder. *Psychol. Med.*, 47, 1678–1689 (2017).
[13] Knight A, Bidargaddi N. Commonly available activity tracker apps and wearables as a mental health outcome indicator: a prospective observational cohort study among young adults with psychological distress. *J. Afect. Disord.*, 236, 31–36 (2018).
[14] McIntosh AM. et al. Data science for mental health: a UK perspective on a global challenge. *Lancet Psychiatry*, 3, 993–998 (2016).
[15] Jauhar S, Johnstone M, McKenna PJ. Schizophrenia. *Lancet*, 2022, 399, 473-86. doi:10.1016/S0140-6736(21)01730-X pmid:35093231.
[16] Rogers JP, David AS. A longer look at COVID-19 and neuropsychiatric outcomes. *Lancet Psychiatry*, 2021, 8, 351-2. doi:10.1016/S2215-0366(21)00120-6 pmid: 33836149.
[17] Ren F-F, Guo R-J, Department of Neurology, Dongfang Hospital, Beijing University of Chinese Medicine, Beijing, China. Public mental health in POST-COVID-19 era. *Psychiatr Danub*, 2020, 32, 251.
[18] Spoorthy MS, Pratapa SK, Mahant S. Mental health problems healthcare workers face due to the COVID-19 pandemic-A review. *Asian J Psychiatr*, 2020, 51, 102119.
[19] Ransing R, Ramalho R, de Filippis R. et al. Infectious disease outbreak related stigma and discrimination during the COVID-19 pandemic: drivers, facilitators, manifestations, and outcomes across the world. *Brain Behav Immun*, 2020, 89, 555–8.
[20] Cabarkapa S, Nadjidai SE, Murgier J. et al. The psychological impact of COVID-19 and other viral epidemics on frontline healthcare workers and ways to address it: a rapid systematic review. *Brain Behav Immun Health*, 2020, 8, 100144.

[21] Das N. Psychiatrist in the post-COVID-19 era - Are we prepared? *Asian J Psychiatr*, 2020, 51, 102082.

[22] https://towardsdatascience.com/data-science-in-mental-health-ccd09ba2148a.

[23] Torous, John & Baker, Justin. (2015). Why Psychiatry Needs Data Science, and Data Science Needs Psychiatry: Connecting with Technology. *JAMA psychiatry.*, 73. 1-2. 10.1001/jamapsychiatry.2015.2622.

[24] https://www.simplilearn.com/data-science-work-after-COVID-19-article.

[25] Goyal, S. "Sentimental analysis of Twitter data using text mining and hybrid classification approach," *International Journal of Advance Research, Ideas and Innovations in Technology*, vol. 2, no. 5, pp. 2454–132X, 2016.

[26] Kumar M, Bala, A. "Analysing Twitter sentiments through big data," in *Proceedings of the 2016 3rd International Conference on Computing for Sustainable Global Development (INDIACom)*, pp. 2628–2631, New Delhi, India, March 2016.

[27] Dhaka P, Johari R. "Big data application: study and archival of mental health data, using MongoDB," in *Proceedings of the 2016 International Conference on Electrical, Electronics, and Optimization Techniques (ICEEOT)*, pp. 3228–3232, Chennai, India, March 2016.

[28] Kostkova P, Fowler D, Wiseman S, Weinberg JR. (2013) Major infection events over 5 years: how is media coverage influencing online information needs of health care professionals and the public? *J Med Int Research*, 15(7), e107.

[29] Rathore MM, Ahmad A, Paul A, Wan J, Zhang D. (2016) Real-time medical emergency response system: exploiting IoT and big data for public health. *J Med Syst*, 40(12), 283.

[30] Que J, Shi L, Deng J, Liu J, Zhang L, Wu S, Gong Y, Huang W, Yuan K, Yan W, Sun Y, Ran M, Bao Y, Lu L. Psychological Impact of the COVID-19 pandemic on healthcare workers: a cross-sectional study in China. *Gen Psychiatr.*, 2020, 33(3).

[31] McAlonan GM, Lee AM, Cheung V, Cheung C, Tsang KWT, Sham PC, Chua SE, Wong JGWS. Immediate and sustained psychological impact of an emerging infectious disease outbreak on health care workers. *Can. J. Psychiatry.*, 2007, 52, 241–247.

[32] Rogers JP, Chesney E, Oliver D, Pollack TA, McGuire P, Fusar-Poli P, Zandi MS, Lewis G, David AS. Psychiatric and neuropsychiatric presentations of severe coronavirus infections: a systematic review and meta-analysis with comparison to the COVID-19 pandemic. *Lancet Psychiatry.*, 2020, 7, 611–627.

[33] Momoi M, Murakami M, Horikoshi N, Maeda M. Dealing with Community Mental Health post the Fukushima disaster: lessons learnt for the COVID-19 pandemic. *QJM.*, (2020), hcaa213. DOI: 10.1093/qjmed/hcaa213.

[34] North CS, Pfeffer Baum B. Mental health response to community disasters: a systematic review. *JAMA.*, (2013), 310, 507–18. DOI: 10.1001/jama.2013.107799.

[35] Raker EJ, Lowe SR, Arcaya MC, Johnson ST, Rhodes J, Waters MC. Twelve years later: The long-term mental health consequences of Hurricane Katrina. *Soc Sci Med.*, (2019), 242, 112610. DOI: 10.1016/j.socscimed.2019.112610

[36] Liu N, Zhang F, Wei C, Jia Y, Shang Z, Sun L. et al. Prevalence and predictors of PTSS during COVID-19 outbreak in China hardest-hit areas: gender differences

matter. *Psychiatry Res.*, (2020), 287, 112921. DOI: 10.1016/j.psychres.2020. 1129 21

[37] Xiao S, Luo D, Xiao Y. Survivors of COVID-19 are at high risk of post-traumatic stress disorder. *Glob Health Res Policy.*, (2020), 5, 29. DOI: 10.1186/s41256-020-00155-2.

[38] Vindegaard N, Benros ME. COVID-19 pandemic and mental health consequences: a systematic review of the current evidence. *Brain Behav Immun.*, (2020), 89, 531–42. DOI: 10.1016/j.bbi.2020.05.048

[39] Rogers JP, Chesney E, Oliver D, Pollak TA, McGuire P, Fusar-Poli P. et al. Psychiatric and neuropsychiatric presentations associated with severe coronavirus infections: a systematic review and meta-analysis compared to the COVID-19 pandemic. *Lancet Psychiatry.*, (2020), 7, 611–27. DOI: 10.1016/S2215-0366(20) 30203-0.

[40] Sher L. The impact of the COVID-19 pandemic on suicide rates. *QJM: An International Journal of Medicine*, 2020: hcaa202.

[41] Chew NWS, Lee GKH, Tan BYQ. et al. A multinational, multicentre study on the psychological outcomes and associated physical symptoms amongst healthcare workers during COVID-19 outbreak. *Brain Behav Immun.*, 2020, 88, 559-565.

[42] Simms A, Fear NT, Greenberg N. The impact of having inadequate safety equipment on mental health. *Occupational Medicine.*, 2020, 70(4), 278-281.

[43] Bo HX, Li W, Yang Y, et al. post-traumatic stress symptoms and attitude toward crisis mental health services among clinically stable patients with COVID-19 in China. *Psychol Med.*, 2020, 27, 1-2.

[44] Romero-Sánchez CM, Díaz-Maroto I, Fernández-Díaz E. et al. Neurologic manifestations in hospitalized patients with COVID-19: The ALBACOVID registry. *Neurology.*, 2020, 95(8), e1060-e1070.

[45] Ahmed H, Patel K, Greenwood DC. et al. Long-term clinical outcomes in survivors of severe acute respiratory syndrome and Middle East respiratory syndrome coronavirus outbreaks after hospitalization or ICU admission: A systematic review and meta-analysis. *J Rehabil Med.*, 2020, 52(5), jrm00053.

[46] Vittori A, Lerman J, Cascella M. et al. COVID-19 Pandemic acute respiratory distress syndrome survivors: pain after the storm? *Anesth Analg.*, 2020 Jul, 131(1), 117-119.

[47] Javelot H, Weiner L. Panique et pandémie: revue de la littérature sur les liens entre le trouble panique et l'épidémie à SARS-CoV-2 [Panic and pandemic: Review of the literature on the links between panic disorder and the SARS-CoV-2 epidemic] *Encephale*. 2020 Jun, 46(3S), S93-S98.

[48] https://www.expresscomputer.in/guest-blogs/data-science-to-revamp-the-businesses-post-COVID-19-era/82576/.

[49] https://medium.com/analytics-vidhya/role-of-data-science-in-improving-mental-health - care-1eb91d37a4e5.

[50] https://intellipaat.com/blog/data-science-applications-in-healthcare.

[51] Yamada, Y, Ćepulić, DB, Coll-Martín, T. et al. COVIDiSTRESS Global Survey dataset on psychological and behavioral consequences of the COVID-19 outbreak. *Sci Data*, 8, 3 (2021). https://doi.org/10.1038/s41597-020-00784-9.

[52] Holm-Hadulla RM, Koutsoukou-Argyraki A. Mental health of students in a globalized world: Prevalence of complaints and disorders, methods and effectivity of counseling, the structure of mental health services for students. *Mental Health & Prevention*. Elsevier, 2015, 3, 1–4.

[53] Browning MHEM, Larson LR, Sharaievska I, Rigolon A, McAnirlin O, Mullenbach L. et al. (2021) Psychological impacts from COVID-19 among university students: Risk factors across seven states in the United States. *PLoS ONE*, 16(1), e0245327.

[54] Gu, S, Slusarczyk, B, ´ Hajizada, S, Kovalyova, I, Sakhbieva, A. Impact of the COVID-19 Pandemic on Online Consumer Purchasing Behavior. *J. Theor. Appl. Electron. Commer. Res.*, 2021, 16, 2263–2281.

[55] Di Crosta A, Ceccato I, Marchetti D, La Malva P, Maiella R, Cannito L. et al. (2021) Psychological factors and consumer behavior during the COVID-19 pandemic. *PLoS ONE*, 16(8), e0256095. https://doi.org/10.1371/ journal.pone.0256095.

[56] Mazza MG. et al. Anxiety and depression in COVID-19 survivors: role of inflammatory and clinical predictors. *Brain Behav. Immun.*, 89, 594–600 (2020).

[57] Huang, C. et al. 6-month consequences of COVID-19 in patients discharged from hospital: a cohort study. *Lancet*, 397, 220–232 (2021).

Chapter 4

Prediction of Mental Distress about COVID-19 among Higher Education Students in Odisha, India

Kamakhya Narain Singh[1,*], Jibendu Kumar Mantri[1], Vijayalakshmi Kakulapati[2] and Chinmay Misra[3]

[1]Department of Computer Science & Applications, North Odisha University, Baripada, Odisha, India
[2]Sreenidhi Institute of Science and Technology, Yamnampet, Ghatkesar, Hyderabad, India
[3]School of Computer Applications, KIIT Deemed University, Bhubaneswar, Odisha, India

Abstract

COVID pandemic and the subsequent recent emergence of its different variants have posed significant challenges for continuing everyday lifestyle, including any educational institute's campus life. In contrast, educational institutes conduct classes, exams, placement, and other co-curricular activities online, offline, and hybrid modes. Because of this, we have achieved a web-based survey on students about their mental health and other related issues such as anxiety, worry, disturbance, fear of infection, and mental anguish caused by COVID-19 in university undergraduates. 1100 pupils completed a digital survey in this cross-sectional study. All these are college graduates from various universities in Bhubaneswar, India, and other universities in Odisha. COVID-19 awareness, nervousness, tension, panic, and mental illness in the past

[*]Corresponding Author's Email: kamakhya.vphcu@gmail.com.

In: Data Science Applications of Post-COVID-19 Psychological Disorders
Editor: Vijayalakshmi Kakulapati
ISBN: 979-8-88697-165-1

were used to screen the psychological distress. This paper reviews the current scenario of COVID-19 concerning psychological distress and related issues. Students' mental health can be affected by using the development of RST (rough set theory) principles.

Keywords: COVID-19, rule base, psychological distress, rough set theory

Introduction

COVID pandemic and subsequent recent emergences of its different variants have posed significant challenges for continuing a normal lifestyle on all fronts, including any educational institute's campus life. 2020 and 2021 will be known as one of the most turbulent years of the century. Millions died across the globe; hundreds of thousands perished in India due to COVID-19. The pandemic triggered the worst economic crisis since 1930. Major economies lost at least 4 percent of their GDP in 2020 and 2021. Due to that, government revenue declined. In addition, it led to employment loss, low salaries, and demand fall. Since 2020, the pandemic has disrupted every sector, especially tourism, aviation, manufacturing, and academic and health services. Health services have stretched the global health system beyond its limits. It made it difficult for people to pay for healthcare. Due to the pandemic, millions were pushed into extreme poverty; many in the middle class were forced below the poverty line because of healthcare payments. The pandemic hit worst on more vulnerable groups like those in the informal sector and daily wage laborers.

While educational institutions conduct classes, examinations, placement, and other co-curricular activities online, offline, and in hybrid modes, various tools and applications are used to conduct academic training virtually, such as zoom, Google meet, Microsoft edge and Skype, etc. But, sometimes, students suffer due to a lack of infrastructure, resources, and poor connectivity. Students want to attend offline classes but are disturbed, afraid, and psychologically distressed by the commencement of COVID-19 variants [1].

We have conducted a web-based survey on students about their mental health and other co-related issues such as anxiety, worry, disturbance, and fear of infection. Students at a university are experiencing mental distress due to COVID-19. In this cross-sectional study, 1100 students completed an online survey. All these are participants from KIIT Deemed to be universities worldwide, including Biju Patnayak technical university, Bhubaneswar, and other universities from Odisha. These issues of the COVID-19 awareness, anxiety, tension, panic, mental problems in the past and emotional exhaustion scores were used.

The World Health Organization has been providing rolling updates on the COVID-19 outbreak. However, this time of crisis generates psychological concerns throughout the population. It has released self-help guidelines on mental health [2]. Likewise, Indian helplines take initiatives to bring down mental health concerns due to COVID-19 through its helpline SAMHSA [3].

Any pandemic brings anxiety, fears, mental illness, and psychological distress [4]. Due to unexpected long periods of lockdown, Students often feel worried, stressed, and some other psychological issues due to their apprehension of the Coronavirus and the rapid adoption of online teaching [5]. Students need alternative ways to adapt and adjust the mechanism to avoid the fear, anxiety, and mental and physical distress from this situation [6]. COVID-19 is misunderstood by students who consume news and spend substantial time on social networks despite media and social media's best efforts to correct this misinformation [7]. The author studied students with sufficient awareness about a pandemic that refused to wear masks [9]. Students are worried and nervous because of a lack of understanding about COVID-19 or a misperception regarding disease infection [8].

However, data is Nt available about the mental condition of students during this global pandemic outbreak. Hence, there is a need to prepare data for research and study the cognitive behavior of students with respect to knowledge about pandemics, nervousness, panic, worry, and psychosomatic pain among students during this pandemic. This paper reviews the current scenario of Coronavirus concerning emotional anguish and related issues among students. Subsequently, generating the rules and preparing knowledge base to find students' psychological distress using association rules and the RST concept. The other sections are structured as Section 2 elaborates on the existing works; Section 3 explains the framework and methodology proposed. Section 4 describes the analysis of the result. Sections 5 and 6 contain the conclusion and future enhancement work, respectively, and in the last section, acknowledgment is followed by the conflict of interest.

Related Work

In literature study, many related studies deal with a survey done on university students based on various parameters to observe the students' psychological distress and co-related issues. We have also reviewed the papers which used the RST concept and other Soft Computing (SC), ML, AI, and DL algorithms for prediction, classification, clustering, and recommendation. [10] analyzed and validated the coronavirus risk predictions based on SGB (stochastic gradient boosting) and RC (recursive feature) reduction. The authors developed a method [11] based on soft, rough set models that help make decisions in any future real-life problem. Authors have applied their proposed model on coronavirus symptoms to identify the COVID-19 patients. A system prototype [12] introduced the CSCP system to predict the correlation among diseases in the same patient. The proposed prototype extracts symptoms from patients' electronic health reports (EHR) and transforms the signs into a data warehouse using association rules to find associated diseases. The method presented uses the relationship to find the frequency of illness-infected patients in a specific area at a particular time [13]. The authors identified the number of diseases that occurred month-wise throughout a year and the number of patients infected by disease at various geographical locations.

An intelligent system [14] was proposed using clinicians' and patients' association rules mining techniques. The proposed intelligent diagnostic system helps classify the diseases based on categorical, quantitative, Boolean clinical data and multimedia data in images of various scan reports. The author has applied this system to diabetic data and got a favorable result. An analytical framework [15] was presented as an analytical framework to recommend the medicine needed by the patients. The authors used the association rules technique to map the association between disease and medication recommended by the doctor. The framework includes three parts. The first part involves collecting data based on prescriptions. The second part consists of making a cluster of the top 10 diseases using a k-mean algorithm. The third part finds an association between medication and medicine needed by the patient.

Using rough set theory [16], proposed a rule to identify the COVID-19 disease. Authors have presented an exciting idea to minimize the symptoms to predict the COVID-19 patients and help clinicians and health workers decide more accurately based on symptoms supplied to rule. This idea saves time and money and allows policymakers to prepare policies and guidelines. A framework was presented [17] that offers a cost-effective treatment for COVID-19 suspected patients using the RST concept. The proposed framework considers a three-way multi-class decision instead of a three-way decision. The cost feature is indispensable and applicable for similar types of real-life problems. Subsequently, a test case using COVID19 symptoms is illustrated using this proposed framework. In [18], that generated a rule base that helps decide using reduct and core features of the RST concept. Authors have presented an analytical approach to selecting indispensable attributes, removing dispensable or redundant attributes, and validating the accuracy of selected features.

An analysis of the ongoing Omicron COVID-19 impacts on Globe [19] was presented. The author has given statistics about the effects of Omicron in the United States, Italy, South Africa, France, the United Kingdom, and India. After that, it was compared with the Delta variation on a daily, weekly, and monthly basis in India to an active case, recovery case, hospitalization rate, and mortality rate. A cohort study on an examination of the inpatient admission results percentage of infectious diseases caused by the Delta mutation in England from March 29 to May 23, 2021, compared the hospitalization output of long-suffering patients with the delta variant and the hospitalization output of patients with the alpha variant [20]. Additionally, it estimated the possibility of a patient infected with a delta variant admitted in emergency care with a patient infected with an alpha variant admitted in emergency care with and without vaccination. COVID-19 variants of distress and interest rising in India through the map were analysed in [21]. Authors have studied variant B.1.617 and interest B.1.618 transmission in India with case fatality ratio, recovered, suspected cases, every day reported cases per billion, and mortality percentage in terms of daily, the weekly, and monthly basis on respective age groups such as 20-35, 35-50, 50-75 and 75-100 in between Mar 2021 to June 2021. The researchers did a sequencing assessment based on a seven-day rolling estimate of the portion of total sequences of disease transmission of variants and various interest variants in Indian states from January 2021 to April 2021 among developed countries that have fully vaccinated. In [22], classified multiple outbreaks of the pandemic in Delhi from April 2020 to July 2021 using a BaYian algorithm to consider transmission and mortality for weekly, suspected cases, and infected rates. The proposed model also analyzed the high fatalities rate in May 2021 and replaced the B.1.1.7 with the highly contagious B.1.617.2. Subsequently, the Authors measured the correlation and differentiated the properties of the B.1.1.7, B.1.617.1, and B.1.617.2 lineage and observed the resistance is reduced to some extent inpatient by preceding infection. The vaccine effectiveness in patients contaminated with delta variants [23] was analysed. Using a test-negative case-control design, they evaluated it with patients contaminated with an alpha variant. Subsequently, authors have also compared the vaccination status of patients contaminated with either delta variant or alpha variant and patient-reported symptoms but had a negative report with the first dose, second dose, unvaccinated, and type of vaccination. Authors found a high level of effectiveness against delta variant for those who took both doses and slightly lower against alpha variant compared to delta variant. Similarly, the absolute difference was around 13% to 20% in the delta and alpha variants with the first dose of the vaccine.

The vaccine's efficacy is calculated [24] for hospitalization in delta or alpha variant infections. The author's analysis includes three categories of vaccination Pfizer, Astrazeneca, and any vaccine with respect to dose 1 and dose 2 against symptomatic disease, the hazard ratio for hospitalization, and vaccine effectiveness against hospitalization in case of alpha variant or delta variant. Pfizer's vaccine effectiveness against hospitalization is 83 percent upon the first dose and 95 percent after the two doses. AstraZeneca's is 76 percent upon the first dose and 86 percent after the two doses. Any vaccine's performance is 78 percent upon the first dose and 92 percent after the two doses. Pfizer's vaccine effectiveness against hospitalization is 94 percent upon the first dose and 96 percent after the two doses, AstraZeneca's is 71 percent upon the first dose and 92 percent after the two doses, and any vaccine's efficiency is 75 percent upon the first dose and 94 percent after the two doses. Authors found more protection against hospitalization with delta variant with a first or second dose of either vaccine. A recommendation system [25] was proposed to suggest patients for rapid diagnostic testing, quarantine period, and retesting in case of a negative report against SARS-CoV-2 with respect to symptomatic, asymptomatic, and patients with exposure to a variant of COVID-19. The recommendation includes as soon as early testing, quarantine till getting the test report, and retesting in case of negative RDT if the patient has a high chance of infection. The symptomatic patient should have testing as early as possible, quarantined until the testing report comes, and retested if they got a negative RDT report if the patient has a high possibility of SARS-CoV-2. Asymptomatic patients with symptoms of SARS-CoV-2 should have testing after 5 to 6 days. In case of a negative report, again have testing after 2 to 3 days. Unvaccinated patients with symptoms of SARS-CoV-2 should quarantine till getting the test report. In case of a positive report should isolate the negative report.

The cohort analysis of demographics of COVID-19 patients, risk of hospital admission, and vaccine effectiveness in Scotland using the EAVE-II platform [26] was presented. The author's used an extensive dataset, the national health care dataset of Scotland, which comprises 5.4 million people, around 99% population of Scotland, to analyze the demographics, risk factors, and vaccine effectiveness. The estimated risk factor contains the vaccine type and dose 1 or 2 against the Delta variant of concern (VOC) in various age groups. The vaccine efficacy analysis includes S gene-positive and S gene-negative cases to determine vaccination efficiency against those infected with the alpha variant and individuals infected with the delta variant in various age groups and sex. In their place, NHS Digital offered a system for monitoring and providing care to COVID-19 infected patients. The framework comprises remote monitoring of COVID-19 patients. A pulse oximeter was clipped to the patient's finger to observe oxygen saturation level thrice a day. Patient data is collected through various sources such as apps, web portals, and paper. Patients can directly submit their paper reading to the website if they are unfamiliar with using a digital solution to record their reading. Clinical staff at the local level assigned patients for further treatment and admitted them to the hospital if required. The framework suggests that patients infected with severe COVID-19 symptoms be admitted early to the hospital to avoid death.

The cohort analysis on the primary care data of the UK using the OpenSAFELY tool for mortality due to COVID-19 evaluated fatalities from other sources than COVID-19 [27]. Authors considered the associated factors to classify fatalities due to Coronavirus and mortalities due to non-coronavirus from 1st Feb 2020 to 10th Nov 2020 with respect to age greater than 18 and gender. Out of 17,456,515 persons, 17,063 died due to COVID-19 and 134,316 due to non-COVID-19. Most factors were similar for both cases, but older age (80 years), male, obesity, deprivation, and few comorbidities were more related to Coronavirus than mortality from non-COVID-19 (50-60 years). At the same time, smoking and alcohol, cancer, and liver disease had more involvement with mortality from non-COVID-19. All details of COVID-19 (B.1.1.7, B.1.617.1, and B.1.617.2), data source: Ministry of Health and Family Welfare, Government of India and COVID19India [28], analysis of active cases, recovered cases, testing, diseased, migrated cases or non-COVID death, vaccinated with 1 dose, fully vaccinated, vaccine doses allocation to the state, case positivity ratio of last seven days, fatality ratio, case growth over last week is done state wise/ union territory wise with respect to per lakh people, daily wise and weekly.

This previous supporting research helps analyze students' mental conditions and consider the symptoms to develop a model to predict the psychological distress of a particular student.

Proposed Methodology

This section discusses the proposed methodology implemented to identify students' psychological distress due to the recent emergence variant of COVID-19. Our approach includes two phases. In the first phase, we conducted the web-based survey, especially for university students in Odisha, considering the following characteristic such Name of the student, age, sex, branch, department, college, university, residence status (Apartment, duplex, hostel, farmhouse), vaccinated (dose 1 or dose 2). Time spent knowing COVID (1 hr, 1- 2 hrs, 2-3 hrs, > 3 hrs), mental illness history (Y, N), knowledge of COVID-19 (Mean, insufficient acquaintance, sufficient information), COVID Anxiety (Mean, Y, N), psychological discomfort (Mean, Y, N), dread of COVID (Mean, Y, N), etc.

The second phase generates a rule base to identify student psychological distress using an RSTconcept to save time, effort, and resources for patients and clinicians. A rough set concept [29] was introduced, a mathematical approach that helps make decisions more accurately and find hidden patterns in data.

It has the following essential attributes: communication system, organizational structure affects, indiscernibility, reduct, core, lower estimation, upper estimation, boundaries, external boundary area, approximate membership, and attribute dependence, which may be described as follows.

An information system is a pair (U, A), where U is a non-empty finite collection of objects (p1, p2,....p10) and A is a non-empty finite set of qualities (S1, S2,...S5) such that for any non-A. which can be defined as

$$p: U \text{x} A \rightarrow V \tag{1}$$

Where V is the collection of all input variables (Y/N).

Decision System- Based on this information, clinicians can identify the psychological distress.

$$\text{DS (Decision System): } T = (U, A \cup \{d\}) \tag{2}$$

d is a decision-making element, and d $\notin$A, whose constituents are conditionally variables.

Indiscernibility is a relationship among two or more elements in which all outcomes for a subset of examined characteristics are equivalent.

Assume $a \in A$, $v \in V$ and $t = (a,v)$ are entity pairs. A segment of t, indicated by [t], is a collection of all instances from U whose element a has the variable v.

Indiscernibility IND(B) is a binary association on U written for $x, y \in U$ as shown in:

$$(x,y) \in IND(B) \text{ if and only if } p(x,a) = p(y,a) \text{ for all } a \in B \quad (3)$$

Dispensable and Indispensable Attributes- a non-essential and redundant attribute that does not affect the decision after removal is called dispensable. The attribute is independent and involves the decision after removal is called indispensable.

Let $I = (U, A)$ denote a data system, $B \subseteq A$, and let $a \in B$. We conclude that an is avoidable in B if

$$IND(B) = IND(B - \{a\}) \quad (4)$$

if not, ‘a’ is indispensable in B.

Reduct- Any subset B' of B is called reduct if B' it is independent and

$$IND(B') = IND(B) \quad (5)$$

Core- Let B is a subset of A. The Core of B is the set of all indispensable attributes of B.

$$Core(B) = \cap Red(B) \quad (6)$$

Where Red(B) is the set of all reducts of B.

Choose a rough estimate - Let $T = (U, A)$ and let $B \subseteq A$ and $X \subseteq U$. We can estimate X by only the information included in B by building the B-lower and B-upper rough calculations of X, denoted $\underline{B}X$ and $\overline{B}X$, respectively, where

$$\text{Lower approximation: } \underline{B}X = \{x \mid [x]_B \subseteq X\} \quad (7)$$

$$\text{Upper approximation: } \overline{B}X = \{x \mid [x]_B \cap X \neq \Phi\} \quad (8)$$

Boundary region rough calculation

Boundary region of X- $BN_B(X) = \overline{B}X - \underline{B}X$ (9)

B-outside region of X- $U - \overline{B}X$ (10)

The lower approximation set of X's is a collection of all items of U that can be categorized as attributes of X. Upper approximation contains all data classified as fitting into the set X. Features may or may not belong to set X in the boundary region. Data certainly does Nt belong to set X in the outer region.

If a set's boundary area is non-empty, it's rough. The set is otherwise clean.

Rough Membership- We utilize rough membership to check the correctness of judgments whose function denotes the degree of crossover between set X and the equivalence class R(x) to which x belongs. This is how it is described:

$$\mu_X^R : U \rightarrow < 0,1 > \tag{11}$$

Where,

$$\mu_X^R(x) = \frac{|X \cap R(x)|}{|R(x)|} \tag{12}$$

And |X| deNtes the cardinality of X.

$$\underline{B}X = \{x \in U : \mu_X^R(x) = 1\}$$

$$\overline{B}X = \{x \in U : \mu_X^R(x) > 0\}$$

$$AN_B(X) = \{x \in U : 0 < \mu_X^R(x) < 1\}$$

The membership value of the lower approximation region's element will always be 1, the membership value of the upper approximation set element will be greater than 0, the membership value of the boundary region element will lie between 0 to 1, and the membership value of outside boundary region element will be 0.

Result Analysis

This section analyzes the implementation details and corresponding results of our implementations. Since our implementation includes two stages in the first phase, we analyze the web-based survey conducted from August 28 to October 18, 2021. The information on participation is presented in Table 1.

Table 1. Information of participants

Variable		Number (%)
Age, Years Mean (SD)		20 Years
Gender	Male	697 (63.4%)
	Female	403 (36.6%)
College/ Branch	Engineering	314 (28.5%)
	Science	233 (21.2%)
	Medical	464 (42.2%)
	Others	89 (8.1%)
Residence	Duplex	229 (20.8%)
	Apartment	510 (46.4%)
	Shared	260 (23.6%)
	Others	101 (9.2%)
Vaccination Status	Dose 1	1023 (93%)
	Dose 2	616 (56%)
	Nt Vaccinated	77 (7%)
Time Spent knowing about COVID-19	< 1Hr	264 (24%)
	1-2 Hr.	396 (36%)
	2-3 Hr.	297 (27%)
	> 3 Hr.	143 (13%)
Awareness about COVID-19	Adequate Knowledge	671 (61%)
	Average Knowledge	286 (26%)
	Inadequate Knowledge	143 (13%)
Fear of Infection	Y	869 (79%)
	N	231 (21%)
Anxiety	Y	693 (63%)
	N	407 (37%)
Tension/Worry	Y	935 (85%)
	N	165 (15%)
History of Mental illness	Y	121 (11%)
	N	979 (89%)

In the survey, 1100 students participated. Of the 1100 students, 697 (63.4%) were male, and 403 (36.6%) were female. Overall, 671 (61%) exhibited adequate knowledge and 286 (26%) average knowledge of COVID-19. 693 (63%) students were anxious, 869 (79%) from fear of infection, 935 (85%) from Tension or worry, 121 (11%) from a history of illness, and 561

(51%) were from psychological distress. Students are participated from engineering 314 (28.5%), science 233 (21.2%), medical 464 (42.2%) and others 89 (8.1%) respectively. Students were staying in duplex 229 (20.8%), apartment 510 (46.4%), shared 260 (23.6%) and others 101 (9.2%) respectively. 1023 (93%) students were vaccinated with dose 1, 616 (56%) with dose 2, and only 77 (7%) were Nt vaccinated. Students spent time learning about COVID 19, such as 264 (24%) with less than 1 hour, 396 (36%) between 1 and 2 hours, 297 (27%) between 2 to 3 hours, and 143 (13%) students with more than 3 hours.

College students who experienced coronavirus nervousness and spent more than three hours studying Coronavirus were more mentally affected. So, they were more cognitively upset. Students must demonstrate enough understanding of persons with a family history of depression. Less psychological distress was found in medical students and senior students. The online survey was conducted through various sources such as social media platforms and email, ensuring that information will be kept confidential.

To measure the knowledge about COVID-19 among students, we created a survey with 6 questions where 2 points were awarded for correct answers, 0.5 points were deducted for the wrong answer, and N issues were awarded for a blank response. Participants with scores 8 and above were rated "Adequate knowledge," whereas participants with scores>6 were rated "Average knowledge," and < 3 indicated "Inadequate knowledge" on COVID-19.

This scale was created to assess kids' fear of COVID-19 infection. Using a five-point scale, participants expressed their degree of agreement with statements. The lowest possible score of 1 denoted "N Fear." "Highest Fear" received the highest score, with three intermediate levels. By summing the scores for each item, the overall score was computed. The higher the score, the more fearful of COVID-19 you are.

The Panic Scale was used to assess pupils' anxiety about COVID-19. Using a six-point scale ranging from 0 (not at all) to 5 (occurring every day) over the last four weeks to score each item. Participants with a score of 10 or more were classified as having "severe COVID-19 anxiety," while those with less than 10 had "normal or non-COVID-19 anxiety."

This scale was used to determine if the students were in a Tension or worry state due to COVID-19. For this, the participants were asked 7 questions where the answers were accepted in the form of range (1-10). The results were calculated by finding the meaning of all the answers. The higher the results, the greater the Tension.

Increase the reliability of the research. The participants were asked about any history of suffering from any Mental illness so that their results of Anxiety and fear would be considered dispensable if found severe.

To identify the psychological distress in students due to COVID-19, proposing a rule using rough set theory. Considering anxiety, fear, knowledge about COVID-19, worry for pandemic due to the emergence of variants of COVID-19, and history of mental illness as symptoms to identify the psychological distress.

Subsequently, in the second phase, we applied the rough set concept to generate the rules to identify the psychological distress by using constraints in the future, which will help clinicians and patients. Considered symptoms are represented as conditional attributes in Table 2, as Information System.

Table 2. Information system of students decision table

	Attributes				
	COVID Anxiety	Fear	Knowledge of COVID	Tension	History of Mental Illness
S_1	H	Y	N	Y	Y
S_2	H	Y	N	Y	Y
S_3	VH	Y	N	Y	N
S_4	L	N	Y	N	N
S_5	VH	Y	Y	Y	Y
S_6	L	N	Y	N	N
S_7	VH	Y	N	Y	N
S_8	L	Y	N	N	N
S_9	L	Y	Y	N	N
S_{10}	VH	Y	N	Y	N

Table 3. Decision system of psychological distress

	Attributes					Decision
	COVID Anxiety	Fear	Knowledge of COVID	Tension	History of Mental Illness	Psychological Distress
S_1	H	Y	N	Y	Y	Y
S_2	H	Y	N	Y	Y	Y
S_3	VH	Y	N	Y	N	Y
S_4	L	N	Y	N	N	N
S_5	VH	Y	Y	Y	Y	Y
S_6	L	N	Y	N	N	N
S_7	VH	Y	N	Y	N	Y
S_8	L	Y	N	N	N	N
S_9	L	Y	Y	N	N	N
S_{10}	VH	Y	N	Y	N	Y

The decision table includes the decisional attribute and conditional features, with the help of dependent attributes corresponding to decisions.

Calculated indiscernibility relation of all subsets of given attributes to find dispensable and indispensable features. Indiscernibility of (COVID Anxiety, Fear, Knowledge of COVID, Tension, History of Mental Illness) is represented as A* here.

IND(A*) = {($S_{1,}$ $_{S2}$), (S_3, S_7, S_{10}), (S_4, S_6), S_5, S_8, $S_{9\}}$

An attribute is dispensable iff IND(A*) = {IND(A*)- (attribute)} otherwise attribute is indispensable. So, calculated dispensable and indispensable attribute as follows:

IND(A*) = {IND(A*)- (History of Mental Illness)}

IND(A*)- (History of Mental Illness) = {($S_{1,}$ $_{S2}$), (S_3, S_7, S_{10}), (S_4, S_6), S_5, S_8, $S_{9\}}$

Hence, History of Mental Element is dispensable attribute.
Similarly,

IND(A*) = {IND(A*) - (Tension)}

IND(A*) ≠ {IND(A*) - (Knowledge of COVID-19)

IND(A*) = {IND(A*) - (Fear)}

IND(A*) = {IND(A*) - (COVID Anxiety)}

Hence, Tension, Fear, and COVID Anxiety is also dispensable attributes, and Knowledge of COVID-19 is an indispensable attribute. So, Knowledge of COVID-19 can Nt be removed.

Now, calculate the dispensable attribute with the combination of another attribute.

IND(A*) = {IND(A*) - (Fear, Tension, History of Mental Illness)}

So, Fear, Tension, and History of Mental Illness are dispensable attributes.
Similarly,

IND(A*) = {IND(A*) - (Tension, History of Mental Illness)}

Thus, COVID Anxiety, Fear, Tension, History of Mental Illness, (Tension and History of Mental Illness) and (Fear, Tension, and History of Mental Illness) are dispensable in relation, and all other subsets are indispensable in relation.

This means classification defined by a set of 5 equivalence relations COVID Anxiety, Fear, Knowledge of COVID-19, Tension, History of Mental Illness is the same as the classification defined by relation (COVID Anxiety, Knowledge of COVID-19), (COVID Anxiety, Fear, Knowledge of COVID-19), (COVID Anxiety, Fear, Knowledge of COVID-19, Tension), (COVID Anxiety, Fear, Knowledge of COVID-19, History of Mental Illness), (Fear, Knowledge of COVID-19, Tension, History of Mental Illness), or (COVID Anxiety, Knowledge of COVID-19, Tension, History of Mental Illness).

Although we got more than one dispensable attribute and calculated a reduct to remove the dispensable attributes from the decision table, any subset B' of B is called a reduct if B' independent and IND (B') = IND(B).

Hence,

Reduct 1 = (COVID Anxiety, Fear, Knowledge of COVID-19, Tension)

Reduct 2= (COVID Anxiety, Fear, Knowledge of COVID-19, History of Mental Illness)

Reduct 3= (Fear, Knowledge of COVID-19, Tension, History of Mental Illness)

Reduct 4 = (COVID Anxiety, Knowledge of COVID-19, Tension, History of Mental Illness)

Reduct 5 = (COVID Anxiety, Fear, Knowledge of COVID-19)

Reduct 6 = (COVID Anxiety, Knowledge of COVID-19).

Now, Calculating the Core attribute, Core (A) = ∩Red(A), where A is the set of A* and Red(A) is the set of all reducts of A.

Core(A) = (COVID Anxiety, Fear, Knowledge of COVID-19, Tension) ∩ (COVID Anxiety, Fear, Knowledge of COVID-19, History of Mental Illness) ∩ (Fear, Knowledge of COVID-19, Tension, History of Mental Illness) ∩ (COVID Anxiety, Knowledge of COVID-19, Tension, History of Mental Illness) ∩ (COVID Anxiety, Fear, Knowledge of COVID-19) ∩ (COVID Anxiety, Knowledge of COVID-19) = (Knowledge of COVID-19).

Hence, Knowledge of COVID-19 is a Core attribute in the decision system which cannot be eliminated.

Remove the dispensable characteristics from the decision table after identifying the reduct and core attribute, and the new decision table is represented as Modified Decision Table.

Table 4. Modified decision system of psychological distress

	Attributes		Decision
	COVID Anxiety	Knowledge of COVID	Psychological Distress
S_1	H	N	Y
S_2	H	N	Y
S_3	VH	N	Y
S_4	L	Y	N
S_5	VH	Y	Y
S_6	L	Y	N
S_7	VH	N	Y
S_8	L	N	N
S_9	L	Y	N
S_{10}	VH	N	Y

Where H = High, L=Low, VH= Very High

Hence, rules can be generated from Table 4, such as follows:

if (COVID Anxiety= = "H" && Knowledge of COVID == "N")
then "Student is suffering from Psychological Distress";

else if (COVID Anxiety= = "VH" && Knowledge of COVID == "N")
then "Student is suffering from Psychological Distress";

else if (COVID Anxiety= = "VH" && Knowledge of COVID == "Y")
then "Student is suffering from Psychological Distress";

else
"Student is not suffering from Psychological Distress";

We roughly approximate the result as a student with psychological distress and students with non-psychological distress using the properties of set approximation such as B-lower approximation, B-upper approximation, boundary region of X, and outside the boundary region of X, where B⊆A, X

⊆U and T= (U, A), T represent decision table, U is set of a non-finite object (Students) and A is set of Attributes.

Lower approximation: $\underline{B}$ X= {x|[x]$_B$ ⊆X} = {S_1, S_2, ... S_{10}}

Upper approximation: $\overline{B}$ X= {x|[x]$_B$ ∩X ≠ Φ} = {S_1, S_2, ..., S_{10}}

Boundary region approximation:

B-Boundary region of X- $BN_B(X)$ = $\overline{B}$ X-$\underline{B}$ X = NULL

C-outside region of X- U-$\overline{B}$ X = NULL

There is no difference between this dataset's lower and upper approximation values. The lower rough calculation set of X's is a set of all elements of U. Which can be classified as elements of X. Here, Students that are identified with or without distress are {S_1, S_2, ..., S_{10}}, while in the case of upper approximation, all data which can be classified as belonging to the set X. Here, students possibly classified with or without stress are {S_1, S_2, ..., S_{10}}. Elements may be or may Nt belong to set X in the boundary region. None of the students is identified in the boundary region because N difference in decision possesses the same symptoms. In the outer region, data certainly does Nt belong to set X. In this dataset, N students belong to an outside region. Hence set is crisp.

We validate the accuracy of the decision using rough membership. The objective function denotes the percentage of approximate similarity between the set X and the quantification class R(x) toward that x corresponds. This is as follows.

Where,

$$\mu_x^R : U \to < 0,1 > \text{ and } \mu_X^R(x) = \frac{|X \cap R(x)|}{|R(x)|}$$

and |X| denotes the cardinality of X.

$$\underline{B}X = \{x \in U : \mu_X^R(x) = 1\}$$

$$\overline{B}X = \{x \in U : \mu_X^R(x) > 0\}$$

$$AN_B(X) = \{x \in U : 0 < \mu_X^R(x) < 1\}$$

The membership value of the lower approximation region's element is 1. In this dataset, Since the low to high approximation amounts are the same, the relationship of the higher approximation category is the same. Element is greater than 0. There is No value of membership value of boundary region element and membership value of outside boundary region element because None of the elements exists either in the boundary region or outside the boundary region.

Conclusion

We analyzed the web-based survey on university students in Odisha, conducted between August 28 and October 18, 2021, to find students' psychological distress due to the century pandemic COVID 19 and its variants. An online survey was conducted through various sources such as social media platforms and email to ensure that information would be kept confidential. COVID-19 awareness, nervousness, tension, panic, and psychiatric disorder in the past were used to screen the psychological distress. In the survey, 1100 students participated, 697 (63.4%) were male, and 403 (36.6%) were female. Overall, 671 (61%) exhibited adequate knowledge and 286 (26%) average knowledge of COVID-19. 693 (63%) students were anxious, 869 (79%) from fear of infection, 935 (85%) from Tension or worry, 121 (11%) from a history of illness, and 561 (51%) were from psychological distress. A scale was prepared to measure the symptom from various angles. Using RST, we then developed criteria for identifying mental health issues. We created a rule by applying RST to 10 students' data sets. Clinicians can use proposing rules to predict distress in the future. Our proposed rules aimed to get better healthcare effectiveness, minimize mistakes or unfavourable occurrences, and help participants of the care provider to become more effective

Future Work

In the future, apply a rough set concept to generate the rules on the full dataset and implement the proposed rules in a natural health care environment to validate the rules in real life and address the difficulties faced during implementation. Our proposed rules can be improved by considering the complete data set in this web-based survey.

Acknowledgments

This research work includes Kamakhya Narain Singh, Jibendu Kumar Mantri, Chinmaya Misra and Vijayalakshmi Kakulapati. Concept of authors and supervision by J K Mantri. Kamakhya Narain Singh and Jibendu Kumar Mantri designed and supervised the study. Kamakhya Narain Singh proposes the rough set theory. Chinmaya Misra carried out a Web-based survey. All authors analyzed the study. The scale was prepared to primary the symptom by Vijayalakshmi Kakulapati. Related study is done by Kamakhya Narain Singh and Jibendu Kumar Mantri. Kamakhya Narain Singh and Chinmaya Misra prepare the introduction. In conclusion, future work is written by Kamakhya Narain Singh and Vijayalakshmi Kakulapati. All authors make feature selection for predicting psychological distress. The work is completed with contributions from all authors.

References

[1] Saravanan, C., Mahmoud, I., Elshami, W., and Taha, M. H. (2020). Knowledge, anxiety, fear, and psychological distress about COVID-19 among university students in the United Arab Emirates. *Frontiers in Psychiatry*, 1057.

[2] World Health Organization. (2020). Mental health and psychosocial considerations during the COVID-19 outbreak, 18 March 2020 (N. WHO/2019-nCoV/Mental Health/2020.1). World Health Organization.

[3] KaNjia, A. (2020). *Impact of COVID-19 on Mental Health in India*.

[4] Ministry of Health and Prevention. Novel Coronavirus COVID-19. (2020). Available online at: https://www.doh.gov.ae/COVID-19 (accessed June 12, 2020).

[5] Odriozola-González, P., Planchuelo-Gómez, Á., Irurtia, M. J., and de Luis-García, R. (2020). Psychological effects of the COVID-19 outbreak and lockdown among students and workers of a Spanish university. *Psychiatry Research*, 290, 113108.

[6] Galal, Y. S., Labib, J. R., and Abouelhamd, W. A. (2014). Impact of an infection-control program on nurses' knowledge and attitude in pediatric intensive care units at Cairo University hospitals. *The Egyptian Public Health Association Journal*, 89(1), 22-28.

[7] Glasdam, S., and Stjernswärd, S. (2020). Information about the COVID-19 pandemic–A thematic analysis of different ways of perceiving true and untrue information. *Social Sciences & Humanities Open*, 2(1), 100090.

[8] Sun, N., Wei, L., Shi, S., Jiao, D., Song, R., Ma, L., Wang, H., Wang, C., Wang, Z., You, Y., Liu, S., and Wang, H. (2020). A qualitative study on the psychological experience of caregivers of COVID-19 patients. *American journal of infection control*, 48(6), 592-598.

[9] Ngwewondo, A., Nkengazong, L., Ambe, L. A., Ebogo, J. T., Mba, F. M., Goni, H. O., Nyunaï, N., Ngonde, M. C. and OyoN, J. L. E. (2020). Knowledge, attitudes, practices of/towards COVID 19 preventive measures and symptoms: A cross-sectional study during the exponential rise of the outbreak in Cameroon. *PLoS neglected tropical diseases*, 14(9), e0008700.

[10] Singh, K. N., Mantri, J. K., Kakulapati, V., Sharma, S., Patra, S. S., Misra, C., and Kumar, N. (2021). Analysis and Validation of Risk Prediction by Stochastic Gradient Boosting Along with Recursive Feature Elimination for COVID-19. In *Applications of Artificial Intelligence in COVID-19* (pp. 307-323). Springer, Singapore.

[11] El Safty, M. A., Zahrani, S. A., El-Bably, M. K., and El Sayed, M. (2021). Soft ζ-rough set and its applications in decision making of Coronavirus. *Computers, Materials, and Continua*, 267-285.

[12] Rashid, M. A., Hoque, M. T., and Sattar, A. (2014). Association rules mining-based clinical observations. arXiv preprint arXiv:1401.2571.

[13] Ilayaraja, M., and Meyyappan, T. (2013, February). Mining medical data to identify frequent diseases using the Apriori algorithm. In *2013 International Conference on Pattern Recognition, Informatics and Mobile Engineering* (pp. 194-199). IEEE.

[14] Stilou, S., Bamidis, P. D., Maglaveras, N., and Pappas, C. (2001). Mining association rules from clinical databases: an intelligent diagnostic process in healthcare. *Studies in health technology and informatics*, (2), 1399-1403.

[15] Harahap, M., Husein, A. M., Aisyah, S., Lubis, F. R., and Wijaya, B. A. (2018, April). Mining association rules based on the disease's population for a recommendation of medical needs. In *Journal of Physics: Conference Series* (Vol. 1007, N. 1, p. 012017). IOP Publishing.

[16] Bhapkar, H. R., Mahalle, P. N., Shinde, G. R., and Mahmud, M. (2021). Rough sets in COVID-19 to predict symptomatic cases. In *COVID-19: Prediction, Decision-Making, and its Impacts* (pp. 57-68). Springer, Singapore.

[17] Majumder, S., and Kar, S. (2021). Rough Set Theory-Based Multi-Class Decision-Making Framework for Cost-Effective Treatment of COVID-19 Suspected Patients.

[18] Vashist, R., and Garg, M. L. (2011). Rule generation based on reduct and core: A rough set approach. *International Journal of Computer Applications*, 29(9), 0975-8887.

[19] Ranjan, R. (2022). Omicron Impact in India: Analysis of the Ongoing COVID-19 Third Wave Based on Global Data.

[20] Twohig, K. A., Nyberg, T., Zaidi, A., Thelwall, S., Sinnathamby, M. A., Aliabadi, S., Seaman, S. R., Harris, R. J., Hope, R., Lopez-Bernal, J., Gallagher, E., Charlett, A., De Angelis, D., Presanis, A. M., Dabrera, G. (2022). Hospital admission and emergency care attendance risk for SARS-CoV-2 delta (B. 1.617. 2) compared with alpha (B. 1.1. 7) variants of concern: a cohort study. *The Lancet Infectious Diseases*, 22(1), 35-42.

[21] Singh, J., Rahman, S. A., Ehtesham, N. Z., Hira, S., and Hasnain, S. E. (2021). SARS-CoV-2 variants of concern are emerging in India. *Nature medicine*, 27(7), 1131-1133.

[22] Dhar, M. S., Marwal, R., Vs., R., Ponnusamy, K., Jolly, B., Bhoyar, R. C., ... and Cherian, S. S. (2021). Genomic characterization and epidemiology of an emerging SARS-CoV-2 variant in Delhi, India. *Science*, 374(6570), 995-999.

[23] Bernal, J. L., Andrews, N., Gower, C., Gallagher, E., Simmons, R., Thelwall, S., Stowe, J., Tessier, E., Groves, N., Dabrera, G., Myers, R., Campbell, C. N. J., Amirthalingam, G., Edmunds, M., Zambon, M., Brown, K. E., Hopkins, S., Chand, M. and Ramsay, M. (2021). Effectiveness of COVID-19 vaccines against the B. 1.617. 2 (Delta) variants. *New England Journal of Medicine*.

[24] Stowe, J., Andrews, N., Gower, C., Gallagher, E., Utsi, L., Simmons, R., Thelwall, Tessier, E., Groves, N., Dabrera, G., Myers, R., Campbell, C., Amirthalingam, G., Edmunds, M., Zambon, M., Brown, K., Hopkins, S., Chand, M., Ramsay, M. and Bernal, J. L. (2021). Effectiveness of COVID-19 vaccines against hospital admission with the Delta (B. 1.617. 2) variant. Public Health England.

[25] Drain, P. K. (2022). Rapid diagnostic Testing for SARS-CoV-2. *New England Journal of Medicine*.

[26] Sheikh, A., McMenamin, J., Taylor, B., and Robertson, C. (2021). SARS-CoV-2 Delta VOC in Scotland: demographics, risk of hospital admission, and vaccine effectiveness. *The Lancet*, 397(10293), 2461-2462.

[27] Bhaskaran, K., Bacon, S., Evans, S. J., Bates, C. J., Rentsch, C. T., MacKenna, B., Tomlinson, L., Walker, A. J., Schultze, A., Morton, C. E., Grint, D., Mehrkar, A., Eggo, R. M., Inglesby, P., Douglas, I. J., McDonald, H. I., Cockburn, J., Williamson, E. J., Evans, D., Curtis, H. J., Hulme, W. J., Parry, J., Hester, F., Harper, S., Spiegelhalter, D., Smeeth, L. and Goldacre, B. (2021). Factors associated with deaths due to COVID-19 versus other causes: population-based cohort analysis of UK primary care data and linked national death registrations within the OpenSAFELY platform. *The Lancet Regional Health-Europe*, 6, 100109.

[28] COVID19India: Available from: https://www.COVID19india.org/. Retrieved Jan 10, 2022. (2022). https://www.COVID19india.org/.

[29] Pawlak, Z. (1998). Rough set theory and its applications to data analysis. *Cybernetics & Systems*, 29(7), 661-688.

Chapter 5

Impact of Post-COVID Syndrome in Hospitalized Patients

Subhani Shaik[1,*], Vijayalakshmi Kakulapati[1] and Nagagopiraju Vullam[2]

[1]Sreenidhi Institute of Science and Technology,
Yamnampet, Ghatkesar, Hyderabad, Telangana, India
[2]Chalapathi Institute of Technology,
Guntur, Andhra Pradesh, India

Abstract

Major symptoms during coronavirus 2019 are dangerous, and the mass of patients recover a vital division of patients at the present more experience for long-term health care. In this context, spotlight on health-related measures after severe illness and hospitalization. This chapter is a theoretical study of health issues in initially obtainable patients with subtle symptoms of severe respiratory conditions and coronavirus infections. We mainly focus on moderate and severe COVID-19 in hospitalized patients. Almost 600 patients with respiratory syndrome and coronavirus infections were observed last year, with fatigue, anemia, and breathing problems. Among these symptoms, breathing is the most common symptom. These symptoms are projected on lengthy-term health issues post-COVID-19. This type of symptom is measured by uni or multi-logistic regression model techniques. We observed more than 600 patients over one year after COVID-19. So many issues like breathing issues, anosmia, and long-time symptoms in hospitalized patients were experiential one-year post-infection. The evaluation will be

*Corresponding Author's Email: subhanicse@gmail.com.

In: Data Science Applications of Post-COVID-19 Psychological Disorders
Editor: Vijayalakshmi Kakulapati
ISBN: 979-8-88697-165-1

continued for post-COVID-19 conditional patients. It will become a critical mission to describe and lessen the socioeconomic and long-term medical effects of COVID-19.

Keywords: Post COVID-19, a univariable and multivariable logistic regression model, hospitalized patients

Introduction

Coronavirus is one of the viruses that can root disease in your sinuses, nose, and upper throat. Most of the cases are not dangerous. If anyone gets Coronavirus with mild symptoms, it damages the respiratory system [1]. Different coronaviruses are hazardous because particular treatment for viruses is not yet available to prevent multi-organ failure [2]. So a variety of viruses causes dangerous illnesses in mammals and birds. The virus causes respiratory syncytial difficulties and, in rare circumstances, mortality [3].

Most people infected with COVID-19 infection get better within 10 days of illness. People who continue to experience mild symptoms post-recovery are called Post-COVID Syndrome or Long COVID. These people may experience post-COVID conditions and also develop long-term complications that affect the organs

Post-COVID complications are a wide range of novel, continuing health situations. People can gain knowledge more than twenty-eight days after being infected with Coronavirus

Post-acute COVID syndrome is after four weeks from the acute symptoms characterized by the determination of clinical signs. These include

- Long COVID unrelenting post-COVID syndrome.
- Multi-organ issues of COVID.
- Hospitalization of COVID-19 purpose.

Classified post-acute COVID based on symptoms of infection affected as follows

- COVID symptoms with Subacute.
- Post-COVID symptoms are after those twelve weeks. There is no alternative diagnosis for attributable [4].

These works describe the occurrence, system-based manifestation, proper clinical investigation, dealing, and significance of inter proficient team move toward the administration of monitoring patients with post-acute COVID syndrome.

The Coronavirus is not new to humans. It was discovered in the 1960s, and the virus was designed like crown spikes. The Latin word Crown name as Corona and such viruses is a massive cluster of viruses that infect bats, pigs, mammals, etc. Scientists identified those types of viruses transfer from one to another quickly. Scientists have practically recognized that there are two probable reasons for the Coronavirus [5]:

- The Coronavirus is eating wild animals: the infection of most common cause come across for eating bats and snakes [6].
- *Animal pathogens*: The architecture and behavior of every animal are different from one another. Some detailed micro-organism resides in their body — if eating them affects the inappropriateness in the being and the possibility of customary suffering diseases.
- *Transmission*: Transmission of Coronavirus occurs by touching your nose, eyes, or mouth before making contact with a surface.
- Symptoms are classically mild to moderate when most people get infected with coronaviruses at one point in their lives.
- The first phase of Coronavirus usually affects the respiratory system in humans, so the various symptoms usually experiential in human beings are:- A common emotion of being unwell, Respiratory system problems, running of the nose, Throat problems, Cough, chills, fever, and kidney issues.
- Proper procedure of corona prevention is not availed but suitable safety measures taken from experts [7]:
- *Lab tests*: CT scan is the best appropriate measure for Coronavirus.
- *Self-safety*: At the time of the beginning, there was no vaccine for Coronavirus. After that, most health care companies develop the vaccine for adults only by preventive measures like washing hands with soap and warm water. To maintain distance from each other (social distance).
- *Food management*: After curing Coronavirus, take healthy and robust food to develop immunity power in your body to fight the virus.
- *Drugs*: Drug management is entirely set by the doctors. If not, you get side effects, which cause death after Corona is free from our body.

- *Convalescent plasma treatments*: The plasma treatment can save the patient's life for some time, it is not helpful for long-time prevention, but at the beginning of Corona, most doctors follow the plasma treatment.

Causes of Post-COVID Syndrome

Currently, researchers cannot define the causes related to the long-term effects of Coronavirus. As per a recent report, possible long COVID causes identified in recovery from COVID-19 patients may include:

- Reduced or lack of response from the immune system
- Reinjection of the virus
- Multisystem inflammatory syndrome (MIS)
- Prolonged hospitalization due to severity
- Post-traumatic stress

Objectives

- Post-acute COVID-19 syndrome is the explanation for long-term symptoms in patients.
- Post-acute COVID-19 syndrome is a system-based manifestation.
- Symptoms of post-acute COVID-19 with a summary of methods are recognizing signs and conversing about the administration.
- Design inters professional squad for post-acute COVID-19 syndrome.

Motivation

Post-coronavirus disease syndrome includes crucial virus symptoms for novel infection of diseases within a month after preliminary scientific and biological cure. Post-discharge follow-ups are the essential qualities in COVID patients. It is very dangerous to people towards death [8]. After three weeks, only 10% of patients recovered from COVID, and new symptoms were developed in patients. The mechanism of this post-disease syndrome is unclear. A standard method was developed to handle care completely for this situation.

This chapter should be arranged. Section 1 outlines the introduction. Section 2 discusses the Background. Section 3 gives relative work. Section 4 provides a Design procedure. Section 5 addresses the findings, material, and methods of COVID. The related topic is discussed in Section 6. Section 7 outlines the study and future directions for the study

Background

COVID-19 survivors are relatively far above the long-term symptoms that have been observed. These symptoms return after post-COVID, so take minor precautions in our daily life automatically to overcome this issue [9]. If you do not follow up on these things, joining the hospital for mild, moderate, and severe is necessary.

Some observations are conducted predominantly on hospitalized patients for acute COVID. After hospitalization, check the symptoms regularly for up to three months [10]. According to the report, 20-80 percent of those impacted have issues after six months. 23 percent of patients were readmitted after six months [11], and 90% of patients were set back within two months after post-COVID [12]. This research gives essential information regarding categories of patients that may be affected in children, young and old [13]. Due to this reason, require more advanced health care services to control the situation. Most countries have to set up dedicated clinics for treatment [14], groups of people handle similar symptoms, and follow the network to monitor patients' health conditions. Enhance the facilities for controlling the situation of post-COVID to get better results [15].

Some other people live in quality life. After post-COVID, they follow strict rules regarding post-COVID, which also affects our socioeconomic life. So many issues raise after post-COVID, and it cannot handle our real-life works—so many symptoms available for detecting COVID, all these rules designed by WHO. Based on WHO guidelines, most counties take the pre-and post-COVID situation. From our research, different treatment procedures are followed by doctors for COVID patients [16]. It includes other post-COVID like acute, post-acute, and long-term treatments [17].

In a specific time frame, COVID recovery people require more assistance for not getting Corona in the future to rest and eat healthy food. Anybody can't expect a situation after recovery from the COVID. It can be hard to differentiate symptoms caused by post-COVID states from symptoms that happen for other reasons. Patients get many side effects after curing COVID-

19 for many reasons based on the immunity power of patients, weather conditions, area of living, and interaction of different people.

Systematic study of post-COVID conditions gives proof-based information on COVID patients. It is also possible to categorize in different ways. These processes support handling the COVID situation at any cost and a comprehensive understanding of patient care. Our knowledge is beyond the case of post-COVID and to let somebody know research priorities. Based on this knowledge, improve infrastructure for COVID treatment and develop integrated multi-specialty services to the patients. COVID acute symptoms have been observed after three to four weeks of recovery, so take precautions regarding these symptoms to overcome post-COVID issues [18, 19]. SARS-Cov-2 is not a replication of post-COVID symptoms after three weeks [20]. The SARS-CoV-2 disease is affected after four weeks. It is a long-term disease based on research studies. It is further divided into two kinds of infections.

1. Subacute symptomatic COVID-19: symptoms present in the body for four to twelve weeks.
2. Post-COVID-19 syndrome: symptoms present in the body for three to twelve weeks.

Related Works

In a specific time frame, COVID recovery people require more assistance for not getting Corona in the future to rest and eat healthy food. Anybody can't expect a situation after COVID of the people. Due to other reasons, symptoms are not easy to separate from each other. Patients get many side effects after curing COVID-19 for many reasons based on the immunity power of patients, weather conditions, area of living, and interaction of different people [21, 22]. Post-COVID Syndrome is different from secret codes and symptoms that expand during constant infection that continue for a long time [23]. Post-intensive care conditions can also include various health special effects after a critical illness. Extreme weakness and post-stress disorder are as a result of such situations.

Asymptomatic patients mean COVID-19 patients get a tough time for good health. In the first phase, 20%–30% of patients were hospitalized with severe COVID19. 50% of patients are hospitalized in the second phase, and below 10% are hospitalized in the third phase. All the patients in different stages suffer different health issues [24]. Phase to phase patient rate of COVID hospitalized is different. Multiple mechanisms are used to predict the various illness of hospitalized patients. In a few severe cases, patients are given the death penalty for various side effects of the post-COVID [25].

The average multiple phases are at a higher risk of developing long-term cardiovascular complications. Who are the patients who suffer different diseases before COVID; they get more side effects after post-COVID. Patients with diabetes, hypertension, obesity, dyslipidemia, and kidney disease would complicate their recovery after the risk phase. Among these issues, Chest pain has been reported in ~20% of COVID-19. Palpitations have been reported in ~10% of COVID-19. Chest pain and palpitations have been reported in 5% and 9%, respectively. Stress cardiomyopathy is 4-5 times more general during the COVID-19 pandemic compared to before pandemic periods [26].

In a specific time frame, COVID recovery people require more assistance for not getting Corona in the future to rest and eat healthy food. Anybody can't expect a situation after COVID of the people. It can be hard to differentiate symptoms caused by post-COVID states from symptoms that happen for other reasons. Patients get many side effects after curing COVID-19 for many reasons based on the immunity power of patients, weather conditions, area of living, and interaction of different people. Some patients with post-COVID conditions do not have positive but suffer from other reasons for health problems that require consideration. Improve anti-bodies in our body to fight with Corona effectively.

Effects of COVID-19 hospitalization are more in the first phase, after which it may be reduced due to less danger. Long-term diseases affected people can't tolerate COVID symptoms. Some of the symptoms are similar to regular patients suffering from respiratory systems. Post-intensive care conditions can also include a range of health effects after a critical illness. Due to such conditions, severe weakness and post-traumatic stress disorder [27].

Post-COVID Conditions

Weeks after infection with COVID-19, changes in body behavior like abnormal, and after recovery from COVID, few people get side effects in their health conditions. In a specific time frame, COVID recovery people require more assistance for not getting Corona in the future to rest and eat healthy food. Anybody can't expect a situation after COVID of the people. It can be hard to differentiate symptoms caused by post-COVID states from symptoms that happen for other reasons. Patients get many side effects after curing

COVID-19 for many reasons based on the immunity power of patients, weather conditions, area of living, and interaction of different people. Some patients with post-COVID conditions do not have positive but suffer from other reasons for health problems that require consideration.

Multi-Organ Effects of COVID-19

After affecting the COVID, in our body, so many changes occur. They can affect multiple organs and then cause the failure of different systems in our body. Sometimes it may cause the death penalty. These types of conditions only occur after the post-COVID of the patients. The multi-initiative system can show the way to more prolonged symptoms due to unsettled complications from the diseases. This type of system is currently unavailable globally, but investigations worldwide. WHO support such kind of activities to save a life from different viruses? Few health issues are solved using this system to keep multiple organs. We can't expect how much time is taken to implement such strategies in our health care.

Effects of COVID-19 Hospitalization

Effects of COVID-19 hospitalization are more in the first phase, after which it may be reduced due to less danger. Long-term diseases affected people can't tolerate COVID symptoms. Some symptoms are similar to regular patients suffering from the respiratory system. Post-intensive care conditions can also include a range of health effects after a critical illness due to infections, severe weakness, and post-traumatic stress disorder.

It can be hard to differentiate symptoms caused by post-COVID states from symptoms that happen for other reasons. Patients get many side effects after curing COVID-19 for many reasons based on the immunity power of patients, weather conditions, area of living, and interaction of different people. Some patients with post-COVID conditions do not have positive but suffer from other reasons for health problems that require consideration.

Novel Symptoms

Novel symptoms can occur after post-COVID; these symptoms are present in the inpatient health care system for various causes. Based on the previous health of the patients, they may be dependent. Person to person is different for these new symptoms for their health profile. After hospitalization, these novel symptoms impact the health of the COVID patient. WHO supports such types of activities to save a life from different viruses? Few health issues are solved using this system to save multiple organs. We can't expect how much time is taken to implement such systems in our health care. Post-COVID, the most generally reported symptoms include the following symptoms are [28]:

- Respiratory effort problem
- weariness
- Cognitive impairment
- Dry Cough
- Chest ache
- Headache
- Abdominal soreness
- Diarrhea
- Difficulties in sleeping
- Fever
- Abnormal feeling
- tenderness
- skin complaint
- the frame of mind changes

Design Procedure

Baseline information of patients collected for analysis of post-COVID can construct, such as oxygen saturation, demographics, and clinical signs. On employment, routine lab tests such as blood count, random blood sugar, C-reactive protein, and CT scan were advised. The initial positive test for COVID-19 was RT-PCR performed after the result. Whom guidelines for clinical development were defined for at least three days on average body temperature and check the respiratory symptoms, oxygen saturation stage > 93% and no need for hospital care for any clinician assessment. RT-PCR test was conducted after fourteen days due to limited facilities. At the beginning of the COVID situation, there were no proper facilities for quick action against the pandemic. This research supports post-COVID-19 syndrome as well-thought-out [29].

Materials and Methods

Who required immediate hospital and such patients were admitted for care smoothly? Based on the physician's advice, particular investigations were performed on the rules of the WHO guidelines. From the advice of physicians, all patients are treated with standard care. In general, Patients' conditions were followed up every day and recorded. After the patient's condition is normal, perform the RT-PCR test again for COVID conditions in the patient body. After discharge of the patient, follow up one month through telephone and give suggestions regarding the patient's condition. Most patients recover successfully, and only below 1% suffer after post-COVID. Identified such types of patients and immediately admitted to the hospital again, and treatment started immediately with previous conditions of patients.

COVID-19 patient study is crucial for the next step of enhanced treatment for COVID patients. >18 age patients follow up the standard guidelines of WHO and <18 also issue few guidelines regarding COVID. In some cases, like <12, children have not properly affected COVID symptoms. Check the hospitalized patients' history regularly and gain more information regarding their condition. The general formula for determining the post-COVID Studies is Z^2pq/a^2, Where $z = 1.93$; $p = 50\%$, in India Post-COVID symptoms happening is not recognized.

After discharge from the hospital, the COVID patient's symptoms compare with a corresponding organized cluster from the standard population. Now easily understand the problems after COVID recovery. That means a follow-up of 180 days. Almost 98% of the patients discharged from hospitals, only 1-2% died. From these statistics, patients with respiratory problems ($P < 0.002$), diabetes ($P < 0.002$), and cardiovascular disease ($P < 0.001$) significantly raised in patients with COVID. 96% of the patients were happy after readmitting to the hospital. Also, from phase to phase, Effect COVID with an age difference in people. Age 60 years person affects more in phase I and phase II, all ages except children. The significant difference for respiratory disease is 12.5% for age less than 60 years, and for age ≥ 60 is 4% -5%.

Statistical Analysis

The following table represents 450 patients data, who give at least 93% in the binary time examination using a p-value of <0.05andnotice a 50% occurrence of post-COVID syndrome. Variables are obtainable unconditional as n (%), in general, disseminated incessantly are obtainable as mean, and continuous skewed variables are accessible like median. Numerical consequence was set @ p <0.05. In statistical analysis, two clusters with post-COVID developed symptoms compared with variables and without developed post-COVID symptoms. Chi-square test was standard for measuring categorical variables were compared using continuous and discrete variables were sample Student's t-test. Cross tab analysis used comparative danger with a 96% self-assurance time calculated. Developing the post-COVID symptoms with the conditional forward method to assess the impact of different variables, monitor the likelihood, and develop a logistic regression model. In this process, so many independent variables like health condition, age, sex, present characteristics of COVID, the duration of enhancement and adaptation to the next level of sternness, and positivity steady for the virus symptoms.

Table 1. Post-COVID-19 symptoms Spectrum

Trait	Total patients (450)	Symptomatic Patients
increased respiratory effort	33	0.73
Fatigue	43	0.95
"Brain fog," or cognitive impairment	2	0.04
Cough	37	0.82
Chest pain	5	0.01
Headache	26	0.57
Abdominal pain	2	0.04
Diarrhea	4	0.08
Insomnia and other sleep difficulties	23	0.51
Fever	43	0.95
Lightheadedness	2	0.04
Impaired daily function and mobility	3	0.06
Pain	38	0.84
Rash	21	0.46
Mood changes	12	0.26

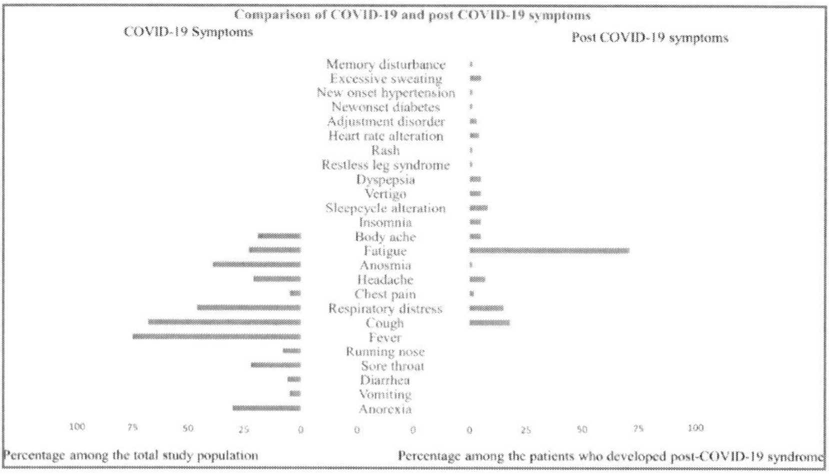

Figure 1. Comparison of COVID-19 and post-COVID-19 symptoms [36].

Post-COVID-19 Prediction of syndrome based on uni and multi models gives different results. We calculated and adjusted the odd regression on uni and multi models. If you check the table below, find the zero hospitalization patients after post-COVID-19.

Post-COVID-19 syndrome was 29% among 450 patients, and most of the patients exaggerated the symptoms after seven days of primitive recovery from COVID. The symptoms were diverse from Post-COVID to primary COVID symptoms. Post-virus weariness was the best part of the general symptom, followed by persistent symptoms like dry cough, sleep disorders, and headache. The post-COVID conditions were different in India to Europe countries. The crucial feature is the age and previous health history of the patient. In this research, 70% of patients were <40 years old and 10% were >60 years old. Most patients have symptoms like fever, cough, tiredness, and respiratory problems.

In the post-COVID-19 condition, there is no harmony regarding the determination enhancement of symptoms, and the state is not defined correctly regarding post-COVID. WHO standard guidelines for post-COVID patients are two weeks and 12 weeks for observation, respectively. Post-COVID-19 symptoms patients were hospitalized. Approximately 10% of patients showed. In this situation, the patient must take a long time to rest better to meet the WHO guidelines for recovery from COVID. The study did not consider patients developing novel symptoms of mild COVID-19 because there was no need to take the drug. This study also did not have a significant proportion of mild sternness patients. Such types of patients did not require hospitalization. Whatever it may be, this research considers a sample of Post-COVID patients. The number of COVID cases is different from symptoms and hospitalization based on the patient's condition. Some patients admitted to the ICU may construct symptoms like post-traumatic stress disorder, anxiety, depression, and decision-making dysfunction due to post-ICU symptoms. After post-COVID, patient readmitted to intensive care is most dangerous to patient health, and 90% of the patients get the death penalty. So observe and join intensive care initially, then automatically avoid critical situations.

From the advice of physicians, all patients are treated with standard care. In general, Patients' conditions were followed up every day and recorded. After the patient's condition is normal, perform the RT-PCR test again for COVID conditions in the patient body. After discharge of the patient, follow up one month through telephone and give suggestions regarding the patient's condition. Most patients recover successfully, and only below 1% suffer after post-COVID. Identified such type of patients and immediately admitted to hospital again and treatment started immediately with previous conditions of patients [30].

Different studies generate various post-COVID-19 symptoms in different ways to affect humans. Mild cases also develop different symptoms after Post-COVID-19. The majority of COVID symptoms, such as fever, cough, bodily discomfort, and respiratory issues, are indications of the disease. However, specific symptoms may be added to COVID patients based on past health conditions. The primary symptom in the first phase is respiratory system problems, second phase throat problems, and third phase without any symptoms affecting COVID. Viral infection plays a significant role in the immunity system and may cause weakness [31].

In previous studies, danger factors connected to the post-COVID-19 situation were not predictable. Due to lack of recognition, doctors do not adequately control a significant connection between post-COVID-19 states and COVID after scientists' RT-PCR test was developed and recognized the symptoms correctly. Most symptoms like fever, cough, body pain and respiratory problems indicate COVID, but post-COVID, some other symptoms are added to the COVID patients based on previous health conditions. Person-to-person symptoms vary post-COVID, so observation is mandatory for COVID patients after recovery from COVID. Most of cases, a similar type of problem arises after COVID. Less than 5% of cases differ from each other. This study brings weakness, cough, fever, chest pain, headache, etc. [32].

Predicts of the Post-COVID-19 Symptoms

Post-COVID-19 Prediction of syndrome based on uni and multi models gives different results. We calculated and adjusted the odd regression on uni and multi models. If you check the table below, find the zero hospitalization patients after post-COVID-19. Every time, compare post-COVID symptoms with ordinary people for accurate predictions to find better results and enhance the treatment of post-COVID. So observation is mandatory for COVID patients after recovery from COVID. Most of cases, a similar type of problem arises after COVID.

Table 2. Post-COVID predictions of syndrome based on uni and multi-variety models

Symptoms during Acute Phase		Post-COVID Syndrome		Uni-variate Regression		Multi-variate Regression	
		No (n = 395)	Yes (n = 55)	OR (95% CI)	P Value	aOR (95% CI)	P Value
	Male	178	25	0.49	0.02	0.59	0.04
	Female	187	19	0.50	0.01	0.61	0.03
	Cough	105	28	1.37	0.17	0.94	0.82
	Fever	154	31	0.78	0.26	-	-
	Median Age	103	98	0.99	0.43	-	-
	Preconditions	95	91	0.88	0.62	-	-
	Hospitalization	12	0	-	-	-	-
	Sore throat	65	43	1.27	0.27	-	-
	Headache	156	121	1.44	0.40	0.84	0.53
	Diarrhoea	21	17	2.19	0.10	1.50	0.27
	Anosmia	123	109	-	-	-	-
	Asia	87	63	-	-	-	-
IgG Level	IgG<= 1	29	23	1.92	0.054	2.05	0.051
	IgG<= 2 -3	77	55	1.78	0.021	1.90	0.015
	IgG<= 4	123	39	-	-	-	-

Discussion

In the post-COVID last six months, vast numbers of COVID-19 patients with inexorable symptoms are not easy to handle, particularly after recovery from COVID. These conditions are handled carefully with the most profound observations and compared with ordinary people. These observations are not only for strict COVID patients but also for mild and moderate. Current preliminary information also observed and understood long-term COVID symptoms in children, men, and women with age. Women's risk is double for long-term COVID symptoms after age 60. Below 60 is a low risk for any gender. Most studies give similar risks for males and females [33]. Different immune arrangements retort during and after COVID-19. It is possible that these gender differences. Immunity power is low; Long term COVID symptoms increase in persons.

In the Cohort study, we observe that most people do not recover quickly from long-term COVID infection. Most of the people who suffered symptoms of fatigue are found in our study. 25% of people suffered from some degree of dyspnea. These two symptoms and many problems raised in the long term COVID, based on immunity power and course of medicines also impact patients. These results are most important for further studies of the post-COVID syndrome. It needs a broad range of healthcare services to support its requirements.

In post-COVID, multi-organ infection is detected with 201 low-risk symptoms issues in our body, this research found in the UK. 18% of people admitted to hospitals with different issues in post-COVID. The harm to the kidneys (12%), lungs (33%), heart (32%), and liver (10%) was expected [34]. These percentages find in our research with potential estimated results. Most of the patients discharge from hospitals too quickly. This type of research in all countries worldwide, based on virus variants, affects populations with different criteria like age, male, female, and children [35]. Although we found that readmission occurs commonly for COVID-19 patients admitted to the hospital, we did not examine the most common reasons for readmission because it differs from patient to patient.

Conclusion

Major symptoms during coronavirus 2019 are dangerous, and the mass of patients recover entirely an essential division of patients at the present more experience for long-term health care. In this context, spotlight on health-related measures after severe illness and hospitalization. This chapter's theoretical study of health issues in patients is initially obtainable with minute symptoms of acute respiratory condition coronavirus infections. We mainly focus on moderate and severe COVID-19 in hospitalized patients. Almost 600 patients with respiratory syndrome coronavirus infections were observed last one year. In that observation, fatigue, anosmia, and breathing problems. Among these symptoms, breathing is the most common symptom. These symptoms are projected on lengthy-term health issues post-COVID-19. This type of symptom is measured by uni or multi-logistic regression model techniques. We observed more than 600 patients over one year after COVID-19. So many issues like breathing issues, anosmia, and exhaustion as long-term symptoms even in hospitalized patients were experiential at one-year post-infection. The evaluation will be continued for patients with the post-COVID-19 condition and will become a critical mission to describe and lessen the socioeconomic and long-term effects of COVID-19.

Future Enhancement

More ordinary people get multi-organ risks than people who take precautions from the world health organization for this issue to take immediate action and research regarding improving medical infrastructure facilities and develop the vaccine. Every time observe the symptoms of patients and follow up the medical treatment. Post-COVID-Syndrome is more dangerous than primary COVID infection due to this multi-organ damage. Rehabilitative therapies should begin early to enable a quick return to work.

References

[1] Ke, R., Sanche, S., Romero-Severson, E., & Hengartner N. (2020). Fast spread of COVID-19 in Europe and the us suggests the necessity of early, strong and comprehensive interventions. *medRxiv*, 2020.

[2] Chopra, V., Flanders, S. A., O'Malley, M., Malani, A. N., Prescott, H. C. (2020) Sixty-day outcomes among patients hospitalized with COVID-19. *Ann Intern Med*, 2020.

[3] Salzberger, B., Buder, F., Lampl, B., Ehrenstein, B., Hitzenbichler, F., Holzmann, T. (2020). SARS-CoV-2/COVID-19-epidemiology and prevention. *Nephrologe*, 2020, 1–7.

[4] Nalbandian, A., Sehgal, K., Gupta, A., Madhavan, M. V., McGroder, C., Stevens, J. S., Cook, J. R., Nordvig, A. S., Shalev, D., Sehrawat, T. S., Ahluwalia N, Bikdeli B, Dietz D., Der-Nigoghossian, C., Liyanage-Don, N., Rosner, G. F., Bernstein, E. J., Mohan, S., Beckley, A. A., Seres, D. S., Choueiri, T. K., Uriel, N., Ausiello, J. C., Accili, D., Freedberg, D. E., Baldwin, M., Schwartz, A., Brodie, D., Garcia, C. K., Elkind, M. S. V., Connors, J. M., Bilezikian, J. P., Landry, D. W., Wan, E. Y. Post-acute COVID-19 syndrome. *Nat Med.*, 2021 Apr, 27(4), 601-615.

[5] Gildings school global public health, (2020). "*Researchers map how coronavirus infection travels through cells of nasal cavity and respiratory tract*, June 2,

[6] Dhama, K., Patel, S. K., Sharun, K., Pathak, M., Tiwari, R., Yatoo, M. I., Malik, Y. S., Sah, R., Rabaan, A. A., Panwar, P. K., Singh, K. P., Michalak, I., Chaicumpa, W., Martinez-Pulgarin, D. F., Bonilla-Aldana, D. K., & Rodriguez-Morales, A. J. (2020). SARS-CoV-2 jumping the species barrier: Zoonotic lessons from SARS, MERS and recent advances to combat this pandemic virus. *Travel medicine and infectious disease*, *37*, 101830. https://doi.org/10.1016/j.tmaid.2020.101830.

[7] https://www.who.int/csr/resources/publications/whocdscsreph200212.pdf.

[8] arfi, A., Bernabei, R., Landi, F. for the Gemelli Against COVID-19 Post-Acute Care Study Group. Persistent Symptoms in Patients after Acute COVID-19. *JAMA*., Published online July 09, 2020. pmid:32644129.

[9] COVID Symptom Study. How long does COVID-19 last? Kings College London, 2020. https://COVID19.joinzoe.com/post/COVID-long-term?fbclid=IwAR1RxIcm mdL-EFjh_aI-.

[10] Huang, C., Huang, L., Wang, Y., Li, X., Ren, L., Gu, X., et al. 6-month consequences of COVID-19 in patients discharged from hospital: a cohort study. *Lancet*., 2021, 397, 220–232. pmid:33428867.

[11] Donnelly, J. P., Wang, X. Q., Iwashyna, T. J., Prescott, H. C. Readmission and Death After Initial Hospital Discharge Among Patients With COVID-19 in a Large Multihospital System. *JAMA*., 2021, 325, 304. pmid:33315057.

[12] Chopra, V., Flanders, S. A., O'Malley, M., Malani, A. N., Prescott, H. C. Sixty-Day Outcomes Among Patients Hospitalized With COVID-19. *Ann Intern Med*., 2020, M20-5661. pmid:33175566.

[13] Davis, H. E., Assaf, G. S., McCorkell, L., Wei, H., Low, R. J., Re 'em, Y., et al. Characterizing Long COVID in an International Cohort: 7 Months of Symptoms and Their Impact. *medRxiv*. 2020; 2020.12.24.20248802.

[14]. National Health Service (NHS) England. Long COVID patients to get help at more than 60 clinics.

[15] Norton, A., Olliaro, P., Sigfrid, L., Carson, G., Paparella, G., Hastie, C., et al. Long COVID: tackling a multifaceted condition requires a multidisciplinary approach. *The Lancet Infectious Diseases*., 2021, pmid, 33548193.

[16] Barker-Davies, R. M., O'Sullivan, O., Senaratne, K. P. P., Baker, P., Cranley, M., Dharm-Datta, S., et al. The Stanford hall consensus statement for post-COVID-19 rehabilitation. *Br J Sports Med*., 2020, 54(16), 949–59. https://doi.org/10.1136/bj sports-2020-102596.

[17] Liebl, M. E., Gutenbrunner, C., Glaesener, J. J., Schwarzkopf, S., Best, N., Lichti, G., et al. Frühe Rehabilitation bei COVID-19 – Best Practice Empfehlungen für die frühe Rehabilitation von Patient/innen mit COVID-19 [Early rehabilitation in COVID-19 - Best practice recommendations for the early rehabilitation of patients with COVID-19]. *Phys Rehab Kur Med*., 2020, 30(03),129–34. https://doi.org/ 10.1055/a-1162-4919.

[18] Datta, S. D., Talwar, A. & Lee, J. T. A proposed framework and timeline of the spectrum of disease due to SARS-CoV-2 infection: illness beyond acute infection and public health implications. *J. Am. Med. Assoc.*, 324, 2251–2252 (2020).

[19] Greenhalgh, T., Knight, M., A'Court, C., Buxton, M. & Husain, L. Management of post-acute COVID-19 in primary care. *Brit. Med. J.*, 370, m3026 (2020).

[20] Van Kampen, J. J. A. et al. Duration and key determinants of infectious virus shedding in hospitalized patients with coronavirus disease-2019 (COVID-19). *Nat. Commun.*, 12, 267 (2021).

[21] Shah, W., Hillman, T., Playford, E. D. & Hishmeh, L. (2021). Managing the long term effects of COVID-19: summary of NICE, SIGN, and RCGP rapid guideline. *Brit. Med. J.*, 372, n136.

[22] Characterisation WHOWGotC. Management of C-i. (2020). A minimal common outcome measure set for COVID-19 clinical research. *Lancet Infect Dis*, 2020, 20(8), e192-e7.

[23] Neuhauser, H., Kuhnert, R., & Born, S. (2017). 12-Month prevalence of hypertension in Germany. Robert Koch-Institut, Epidemiologie und Gesundheitsberichterstattung, [Robert Koch Institute, Epidemiology and Health Reporting] 2017.

[24] Xie, M., Liu, X., Cao, X., Guo, M., & Li, X. (2020). Trends in prevalence and incidence of chronic respiratory diseases from 1990 to 2017. *Respir Res*, 2020, 21(1), 49.

[25] Management of Post-COVID Cardiovascular Sequelae, Directorate General of Health Sciences Ministry of Health and Family Welfare Government of India, Sep 2021.

[26] National Comprehensive Guidelines of Management of post-COVID Sequelae, Ministry of Health and Family Welfare Government of India, Oct 2021.

[27] Mattioli, F., Marchioni, A., Andreani, A., Cappiello, G., Fermi, M., & Presutti, L. (2021). Post-intubation tracheal stenosis in COVID-19 patients. *European archives of oto-rhino-laryngology: official journal of the European Federation of Oto-Rhino-Laryngological Societies (EUFOS): affiliated with the German Society for Oto-Rhino-Laryngology - Head and Neck Surgery*, 278(3), 847–848. https://doi.org/10.1007/s00405-020-06394-w.

[28] Clinical Spectrum of SARS-CoV-2 Infection, October 19, 2021, http://www.COVID19treatmentguidelines.nih.gov.

[29] Mahmud, Reaz, et al. "Post-COVID-19 syndrome among symptomatic COVID-19 patients: A prospective cohort study in a tertiary care center of Bangladesh." *PloS one* vol. 16, 4 e0249644. 8 Apr. 2021, doi:10.1371/journal.pone.0249644.

[30] Mahmud, R., Rahman, M. M., Rassel, M. A., Monayem, F. B., Sayeed, S. K. J. B., Islam, M. S., et al. (2021). Post-COVID-19 syndrome among symptomatic COVID-19 patients: A prospective cohort study in a tertiary care center of Bangladesh. *PLoS ONE*, 16(4), e0249644. https://doi.org/10.1371/journal.pone.0249644.

[31] Post-COVID Conditions: Information for Healthcare Providers, CDC, COVID-19, July 9, 2021.

[32] Ayoubkhani, D., Khunti, K., Nafilyan, V., Maddox, T., Humberstone, B., Diamond, I., Banerjee, A. Post-COVID syndrome in individuals admitted to hospital with COVID-19: retrospective cohort study. *BMJ.*, 2021 Mar 31, 372, n693. DOI: 10.1136/BMJ.n693. PMID: 33789877; PMCID: PMC8010267.

[33] British Society for Immunology. *Long-Term Immunological Health Consequences of COVID-19.* Available online at: https://www.immunology.org/sites/default/files/BSI_Briefing_Note_August_2020_FINAL.pdf (accessed August 13, 2020).

[34] Dennis, A., Wamil, M., Kapur, S., et al. Multi-organ impairment in low-risk individuals with long COVID. *medRxiv [Preprint]* 2020. https://www.medrxiv.org/content/10.1101/2020.10.14.20212555v1doi:10.1101/2020.10.14.20212555.
[35] McCarthy, C. P., Murphy, S., Jones-O'Connor, M., et al. Early clinical and sociodemographic experience with patients hospitalized with COVID-19 at a large American healthcare system. *E Clinical Medicine*, 2020, 26, 100504. doi:10.1016/j.eclinm.2020.100504. pmid:32838244.
[36] Reaz Mahmud, Md. Mujibur Rahman, Mohammad Aftab Rassel, et al., "Post-COVID-19 syndrome among symptomatic COVID-19 patients: A prospective cohort study in a tertiary care center of Bangladesh", *PLoS one*, 8, April-2021.

Biographical Sketch

Dr. Subhani Shaik

Affiliation:
Sreenidhi Institute of Science and Technology (Autonomous), Hyderabad

Education:
1998-2002 Graduated with the CSE Faculty of Andhra University
2009-2011 Post Graduatein CSE from JNT, Hyderabad
2013-2019 CSE Doctorates from Acharya Nagarjuna University, Guntur.

Business Address:
Department of Information Technology, Block-2, Yamnampet, Ghatkesar, Hyderabad-501301.

Research and Professional Experience:
Associate Professor position at Sreenidhi Institute of Science and Technology since 2017.

Professional Appointments:
Coordinator of the NAAC. Reviewer of the several Journals on international.

Honors:
Academic excellence Professional recognition in SSRN- Elsevier (2020).

Publications from the Last Year:

Sujan Reddy, Renu Sri, and Subhani Shaik, "Sentimental Analysis using Logistic Regression," *International Journal of Engineering Research and Applications (IJERA)*, Vol. 11, Series-2, July-2021.

Mamatha, Srinivasa Datta and Subhani Shaik, "Fake Profile Identification using Machine Learning Algorithms," *International Journal of Engineering Research and Applications (IJERA)*, Vol.11, Series-2, July-2021.

Vijaya Kumar Reddy, Subhani Shaik, B. Srinivasa Rao, "Machine learning-based outlier detection for medical data" *Indonesian Journal of Electrical Engineering and Computer Science*, Vol. 24, No. 1, October 2021.

Swapna, D. and Subhani Shaik, "IOT Based Face mask identification and temperature detection" *Design Engineering*, Issue 7, Nov-2021.

Vijay Kumar Reddy and Subhani Shaik, "The General Design of the Automation for Multiple Fields using Reinforcement Learning Algorithm," *Paper accepted in Indonesian Journal of Electrical Engineering and Computer Science*, Dec-2021.

Chapter 6

Computational Intelligence Models for Stress

P. Selvi Rajendran* **and K. R. Kartheeswari**
Department of Computer Science and Engineering,
Hindustan Institute of Technology and Science, Tamil Nadu, India

Abstract

Stress is characterized as unpreventable tension and distress. This is a psychological term for a form of psychological tension and strain. Pressure also has adverse consequences. Good thinking can focus on empowering us to work much harder. Distress can be bad for health. Stress response will lower our consciousness. COVID-19 is a coronavirus-caused severe deadly disease that has become highly infectious in 2020. COVID-19 harmed the general populace's psychological well-being significantly. COVID-19 has triggered a worldwide shutdown. Disorder, anxiousness, and pressure ailments were observed. It caused numerous issues in almost every aspect of life. Consequently, people experience greater unpredictability and unsafe working conditions, which cause stress.

Keywords: stress, COVID-19, psychological, pressure, characteristics, consequences, patients

*Corresponding Author's Email: p.selvirajendran@gmail.com.

In: Data Science Applications of Post-COVID-19 Psychological Disorders
Editor: Vijayalakshmi Kakulapati
ISBN: 979-8-88697-165-1

Introduction

In the Chinese city of Wuhan, the World Health Organization SARA-Cov-2 stated that the virus causes Coronavirus Disease 2019 is extremely Spreadable (COVID-19). This global health crisis had psychological repercussions for the whole population. A range of stressors associated with COVID-19 was frustration, a lack of information, fear of contagion, and the quarantine's length. The educational community has also been significantly impacted, and several explicit circumstances must be considered. A person's stress level increases when their surroundings outweigh the resources available to deal with the threat. The imprisonment scenario and COVID-19 marked a significant change in landscape. In this way, there was a change in the university structure. Other considerations unique to the system of education were exposed to students, including changes in terms of teaching methodologies, changes in the examination environment (This was carried out via the internet), issues with technology encountered to reduce physical activity and sleeping hours while utilizing virtual platforms, and so on. As a result, attributing high-stress ratings only to confinement is now impossible scores like this may already exist in society. These findings highlight the need to examine current stress levels and other relevant variables and compare them to previous conditions to the extent that research design allows for such comparisons. Artificial intelligence has also been used to examine several characteristics that define the epidemic and fight against COVID-19. Although predictive models have been promoted as useful tools for meeting psychological needs, their application in disciplines such as economics, medicine, and transportation are more widespread.

Various artificial intelligence tools and techniques to reduce stress in a working environment are outlined in detail in this chapter. There is also a discussion of the causes of stress and its reasons.

What Does Stress Mean?

Stress affects everyone from time to time. Stress is a normal response to both positive and harmful situations. It affects our bodies, emotions, attitudes, and behaviours. Stress can have either positive and harmful effects or a mix of both. For example, stress can either boost student motivation and concentration or cripple their capacity to do anything.

Stress is caused by an occurrence or idea that makes us angry, upset, or worried.

Stress occurs when our bodies react to a challenge or demand. Stress can be good in small quantities, such as when it helps us avoid danger or meet a deadline. On the other hand, stress can be damaging if it lasts for an extended period.

It has significantly impacted our lives in dealing with the pandemic of COVID-19.

Sometimes children and adults face challenging situations that cause strong emotions and are stressful.

Implementing public health measures such as social separation is essential for preventing the spread of COVID-19. Still, it can also create feelings of loneliness, tension, and worry. If we learn to manage stress healthily, we will become more resilient and the people around us. COVID-19 has most likely influenced how we work, whether from home or at the workplace. Burnout is caused by various factors, including professional stress, fear about this new disease, and other strong emotions. We must recognize the signs of stress during this pandemic, take actions to increase our resilience and manage job stress, and know where to get help if needed.

Definition of Stress

A typical physiological response to a potentially harmful scenario is stress. When suddenly stressed, our brain releases chemicals and hormones like adrenaline and cortisol into our systems.

As a result, our hearts beat quicker, providing blood to muscles and vital organs. We feel energized and more aware of our surroundings, allowing us to concentrate on our current requirements. Below is a list of the various types of stress and how many people survive them.

Hormones of Stress

The hypothalamus, located at the base of the brain, reacts when we are in danger. During this period, many hormones are stimulated in our adrenal glands, which transfer nerve and hormone impulses to them. The body uses these hormones to prepare us for danger and increase our chances of survival.

One of these hormones is named adrenaline. Another name for it is epinephrine, also known as the fight-or-flight hormone.

Different Types of Stress

There are various sorts of stress [1, 2, 3, 4, 5], such as:

1. Acute stress
2. Episodic acute stress
3. Chronic stress

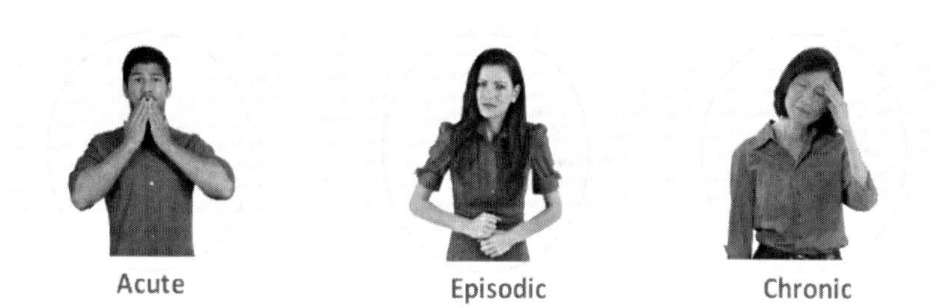

Figure 1. Types of stress.

Acute Stress

Acute stress is something that everyone experiences [1, 2, 3] at some point in their lives. Anxiety is the body's response to a novel and changing environment, such as the kind we might experience after narrowly avoiding an accident. Acute stress can occasionally be caused by doing something we enjoy. We get a frightening yet thrilling sense when we ride a roller coaster or ski down a steep mountain slope.

We are mostly not hurt by acute stress attacks. We are mostly not hurt by acute stress attacks. Sometimes they might even be good for our health. Stress clarifies how our bodies and minds respond to future stressful events in the most effective way possible. Once the dangerous stress is passed, our bodies should return to usual. A different story is told in the case of severe acute stress. This type of stress, such as that experienced when challenged with a situation that threatens life, can develop into post-traumatic stress disorder (PTSD) or other mental health issues. A different story is told in the event of extreme acute stress. Stress can develop into post-traumatic stress disorder or other mental health issues when faced with a life-threatening circumstance.

Episodic Acute Stress

We are said to be enduring episodic acute stress when we experience acute stress regularly. This may arise if we are frequently nervous and concerned about occurrences that we believe may occur. Our lives may appear to be in disarray, and we may appear to be bouncing from crisis to crisis. Specific vocations, such as enforcement or fire fighting, can expose you to high-stress circumstances daily. Acute stress that occurs regularly can have a severe influence on both physical and mental health.

Chronic Stress

Stress that remains high for a prolonged period is chronic. Long-term stress like this might be dangerous to our bodies. It might be helpful for: Anxiety, cardiovascular disease, depression, high blood pressure, and a weakened immune system are all signs of an immune system falling. Headaches, gastrointestinal difficulties, and sleep problems are classic symptoms of chronic stress. Understanding the many types of stress and how to recognize them can be good.

Workplace Stress

Work can be highly stressful for a variety of reasons [6, 7, 8]. This type of stress might be short-term or long-term. Workplace stress can take the following forms:

- It is the feeling that we have little or no control over what happens to us
- being compelled to perform something, we don't want to do
- quarrelling with a co-worker
- being overworked or expected to do too much

Stress appears unavoidable if we are stuck in a work we despise or continuously answering to others' expectations with little checking. Quitting or battling for a better work-life balance is sometimes the best option. This is how we can tell whether we're about to burn out at work.

Of course, specific vocations are inherently riskier than others. Some professions, such as emergency first responders, require us to risk our lives. Then there are jobs where we hold someone else's life in our hands, such as those in the medical industry, like doctors or nurses. Maintaining our mental health requires finding balance and controlling our stress.

Stress Management

There are various variables to consider when discussing stress management approaches.

Recognize the Source of Stress

It can be different for each individual. When the person understands what stress looks like for him, they can better prepare to reach for our stress management toolbox.

Identify the Sources of Our Stress

The root cause of stress must be identified. Work, family, change, or tens of thousands of additional potential triggers are all possibilities.

Develop the Ability to Recognize and Respond to Stress Signals

Everyone will react to stress differently, so being aware of our stress is critical. The identification for those is low tolerance, headaches, stomach problems, or combinations of the aforementioned are examples of stress symptoms.

Recognize the Stress Management Work Techniques

We need to analyze our go-to stress-relieving technique. These are frequently learned habits that aren't necessarily the best choices. Some people, for example, self-medicate with alcohol or overeat to cope with stress.

Use Stress-Reduction Practices That Are Both Healthy and Effective

It's critical to be conscious of any existing harmful coping mechanisms so that we can replace them with a better option. If overeating is our coping mechanism, they could attempt medication or call a friend to chat about our issues. According to the American Psychological Association, the most efficient strategy to achieve positive change is to modify one behavior at a time.

Make Self-Care a Priority

The well-being of others should be prioritized when we set aside time for ourselves. This may appear self-centred at first, but it's similar to the airplane analogy: we must first put on our oxygen masks before assisting others. The most fundamental parts of health, such as getting adequate sleep, eating healthy, resting, and exercising, are frequently overlooked.

Seek Assistance
If the person is feeling overwhelmed, they should reach out to a friend or family member who can assist them. Speaking with a healthcare professional can also assist us in developing suitable coping mechanisms.

Techniques and Strategies for Stress Management

These are divided into three categories [9, 10]:

- Action-Oriented Approaches: These are approaches that are utilized to take action to modify a stressful circumstance.
- Emotion-focused Tactics: Changes the way we perceive a stressful situation.
- Acceptance-based Approaches are utilized to deal with stressful events beyond our control.

Action-Oriented Approaches

Action-oriented techniques allow for changing a stressful situation.

Be Self-Confident
Being self-confident necessitates effective and clear communication. When we're aggressive, we can ask for what we want or need and communicate what's bothering us. The idea is to do so reasonably and firmly while remaining compassionate toward others around you. Once we've discovered what we need to say, we can stand up for ourselves and aggressively try to improve the unpleasant situation.

Reduce the Amount of Noise
Turning off the technology, screen time, and constant stimulus can help us slow down. Set aside sometime each day for quiet. Then we can predict that our urgent tasks become essential and crisis-like. That to-do list will be there when we are ready to return to it. Remember that rechanging is an excellent way to cope with stress.

Keep Track of Our Time

When we allow our days to consume us, we become overwhelmed. Prioritizing and organizing our tasks can make our lives less stressful and more joyful.

Establishing Limits

On a personal level, boundaries are the rules we set for ourselves. They define the behaviours we need or need not tolerate how much time and space we require from others, and our priorities.

Get Our Heads Out of Our Asses

It's sometimes better not to try to deal with racing thoughts at all. Occasionally we all require some time to relax. We need to divert our attention away from ourselves. Watch a movie, talk on the phone or text with a friend, go for a walk, or do something else that we know will keep us occupied.

Emotion–Oriented Approaches

Emotional techniques are employed to alter our perceptions of stressful events.

Visualizations and Affirmations

Positive images and affirmations have now been scientifically proven to increase positive emotion. When our thinking is pleasurable, our brain interprets it as a reality. So, by replacing those negative ideas with positive affirmations, we may challenge and change how we view and experience the world.

Cognitive Restructuring

This approach was combined for decoding the negative feelings and addressing the often inaccurate assumptions that underlie them. The cognitive restriction is a crucial component of cognitive behavioural therapy (CBT).

The ABC Method

A - Adversity or a stressful situation is represented by the letters ABC. B – our views, or how we react to the situation. Then there's C - consequences, which are the results of our beliefs leading to our actions and the event's outcome. A favourable outcome will come about as a result of a high degree of optimism on our part.

Acceptance-Oriented Methodologies

In stressful situations over which we have little control, acceptance-oriented approaches can help.

Exercise and Diet

We've heard it before: what we consume shapes our personalities. Attempt to eat a healthy, well-balanced diet. Simple dietary changes, such as cutting, and less on alcohol, coffee, and sweets, have been demonstrated to help people feel less anxious. Exercising is another practical approach to de-stress. It has also been demonstrated to be equally helpful as antidepressants in treating mild depression.

Physical and Mental Relaxation through Meditation

You can relieve stress in many ways, including deep breathing, guided visualizations, yoga, and guided body scans. These activities aid in physical relaxation. Below are a few examples for us to consider.

Develop Resiliency

Whether we can bounce back from stressful or unfavourable circumstances is called resiliency. To put it another way, People who possess resilience can recognize that a circumstance has occurred, learn from it, and move on.

Discuss It

Don't keep everything to yourself. Discuss our concerns or the issues that upset us with someone close to us. Sharing our worries can help us reduce them while also allowing us to laugh at potentially embarrassing situations.

When we voice our worries out loud, they sound much less frightening. We can write down our thoughts even if we aren't interested in sharing them. Alternatively, you might work with a freelancer. There are numerous services available, including some that are free, and we can simply Google what is accessible in our city to see what is available.

Get Some Rest

Sleeping is essential to reloading energy and coping with stressful situations. While a good amount of sleep necessary varies from person to person, 8 hours of uninterrupted sleep is generally recommended.

Stress Management in the Workplace

Workplace stress is one of the leading causes of job loss and a drop in employee productivity; workplace stress levels are rising worldwide, and businesses must find a way to help their employees healthily cope with stress if they want to succeed [11, 12, 13, 14]. This is connected to better performance, higher retention rates, and creativity. Flexible working hours and psychiatric counselling are examples of employee-friendly practices that might help with stress management. This section demonstrates how artificial intelligence (AI) can aid in the reduction of workplace stress.

Many people have experienced workplace stress, whether it's as a result of long hours, impossible deadlines, demanding co-workers, or unappreciative managers.

The world health Organization defines occupational or work-related psychosocial stress as "the reaction people may have when presented with work demands and pressures that are not matched to their knowledge and abilities and that challenge their ability to manage."

On the other hand, occupational stress has complications outside of the job, affecting our relationships, home lives, and overall productivity. Figure 2 from the WSH Institute (2018) displays the various causes of workplace stress and the organizations' and individuals' roles in coping with these threats.

According to a report from Oracle and Workplace Intelligence, employees worldwide are battling mental health concerns and wanting support. The analysis also looked at how artificial intelligence and technology could be utilized as solutions. The research surveyed 12,000 workers, HR managers, and C-level executives between the ages of 22 and 74 from across the globe during July and August 2020. The findings reflect a workforce struggling with unprecedented levels of stress and worries and would gladly turn to artificial intelligence (AI) and technology to help improve their mental health.

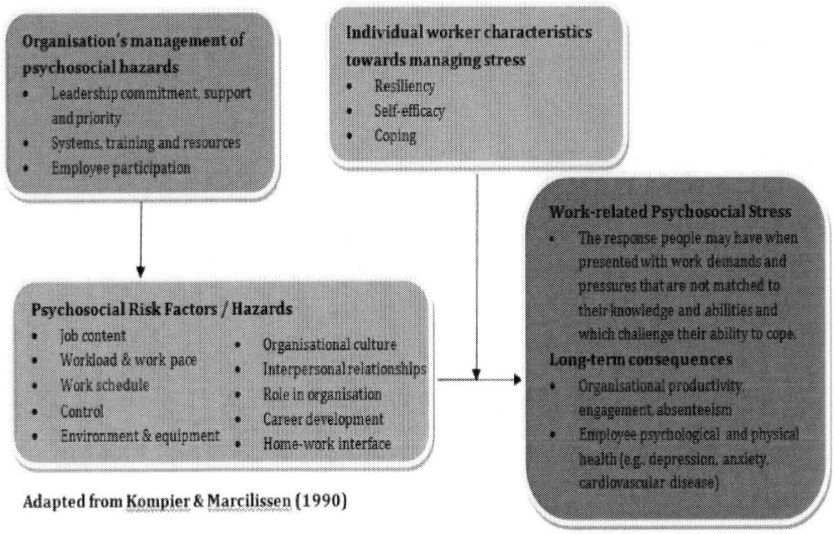

Figure 2. Stress factors.

Seventy percent of respondents claimed 2020 was the most stressful year of their professional careers, with 40 percent struggling to satisfy day-to-day job expectations like meeting performance requirements, conducting mundane and repetitive chores, and dealing with unmanageable workloads. Over three-quarters (78%) felt the COVID-19 epidemic had harmed their mental health by increasing stress (38%) and causing burnout (25%) and sadness (25%) as well as disrupting a good work-life balance (14%), and eroding a healthy work-life balance (35 percent).

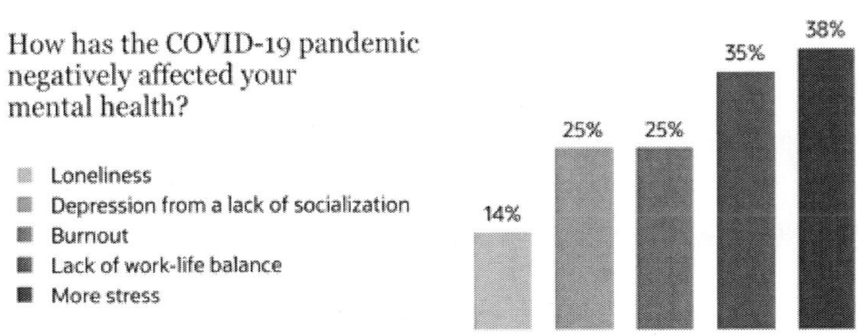

Figure 3. Impact report of COVID-19.

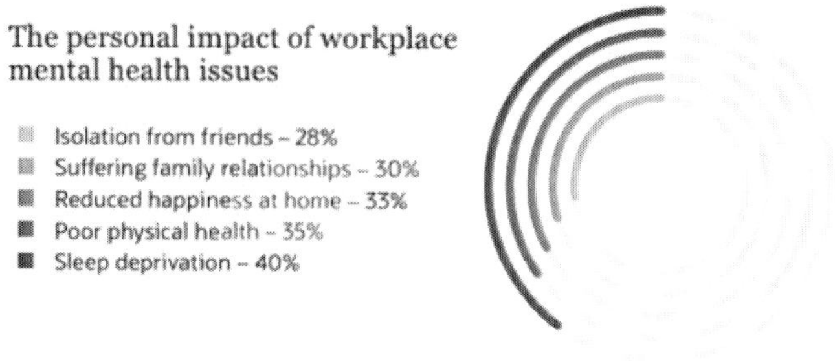

Figure 4. Survey report of workplace impact on individuals.

More than eighty percent of those polled say that work-related mental health issues harm their personal lives, including sleep deprivation (40%), reduced home happiness (33%), strained family relationships (30%), poor physical health (30%), and social isolation (30%). These effects extend beyond the workplace as well (28%).

While mental health services have been on the rise for years, the pandemic has brought these challenges to a head. Companies must offer and enhance benefits and support services as quickly as feasible to sustain their workforce's well-being, productivity, and performance. One method to swiftly and efficiently implement much-needed solutions is through technology. 82 percent of respondents believe AI is superior to people at giving help, according to the report. Chatbots, wellness and meditation apps and fitness tracking are examples.

Employment, Earnings, and Technical Innovation: A Relationship

Economists have warned about the risk of 'technological unemployment' since the Industrial Revolution, in which jobs are lost due to technical advancement. Since the 1980s, much research by labour economists has found that the emergence of skill-biased technology development, favouring predominantly highly skilled people, has led to a widening wage gap in recent years. There have been forecasts that new information technologies, such as artificial intelligence (AI), could steal many workers' jobs, resulting in even wider wage disparities. Employment, unemployment, and salaries are a few consequences of technological progress. It impacts many issues, including work activities, office atmosphere, job satisfaction, stress, and health. Because new information technologies can be applied to a diverse variety of tasks, there are bound to be positive and negative implications in numerous directions. Due to the spread of new information technology, job satisfaction, and stress levels have increased.

The Japan Science and Technology Agency's Research Institute of Science and Technology for Society (RISTEX) project explores the impact of new information technologies on work practices and well-being. They performed an original survey of approximately 10,000 workers. One interesting finding is that, as seen in Figure 1, new information technologies, such as AI, are adopted for job satisfaction evaluation. Work-related stress, on the other hand, has a propensity to rise.

Artificial Intelligence in the Environment

Artificial intelligence's versatility, which allows it to be sculpted into any shape or size, is another essential trait. The best example is AI in the Internet of Things.

AI may now be employed at our workplace to understand our lifestyle patterns better and make intelligent judgments using the same approach based on the knowledge obtained [15, 16, 17, 18]. Employees can benefit from the workplace's artificial intelligence (AI), such as emotion detection sensors, which can help them reduce stress and be more innovative, resulting in better performance.

The state of our immediate environment dramatically impacts how we manage our mental health. Employees can concentrate better on their work while maintaining a calm mindset by using lights that alter their brightness according to the time of day or night. In addition to introducing environmentally-friendly measures, combining them with AI improves the workplace and boosts productivity like never before.

Artificial Intelligence Role in Stress Management

Today, Chatbots are messaging platforms companies use for customer service, client follow-up, and even automated telemedicine platforms for doctors. This reduces unneeded workload and relieves workers of a considerable strain [19].

By automating tedious tasks like filling out reports, responding to emails, and providing customer support, workers could use their brains and skill set for creative jobs, emotional intelligence, decision-making, and social relationships, which AI cannot automate. Conversational bots for customer service, for example, can converse with consumers autonomously and accurately answer more than 80% of their questions. Customer service agents will have less work to do due to this.

Automated Technologies for Mental Health

Mental health care will have to rely on ever-evolving technology to progress. Natural language processing (NLP) is now being used by various applications to create Chatbots that can speak with humans and deliver customized responses. This is beneficial while performing Cognitive Behavioural therapy (CBT) [20, 21].

Employees may talk with these Chatbots on a low-intensity day and feel revived by receiving some affection.

In the event of increased workload, companies might leverage these technologies to assist employees in providing stress-relieving services. We can better understand our employees' feelings and start thinking positively by interacting with affection Chatbots.

Automation

Reducing staff responsibilities can significantly influence stress levels and free up time for jobs that AI cannot automate. According to Forbes, 72 percent of working professionals attribute low-stress levels to productivity-enhancing tools and technology, and 64 percent believe automation technology helps reduce workload and workplace stress. Employees are enthusiastic about AI-powered automation since it will allow them to work more efficiently and minimize stress. According to a Verint study, there is a clear link between workplace technology and employee stress levels, indicating that AI automation technology may just be the first step toward ensuring employee pleasure.

Employees Can Benefit From AI

AI has a crucial influence in reducing workplace stress, as seen by the examples and use cases mentioned above. Burnout among employees is a problem that many people face daily. Employees are more likely to work in a healthy environment if there are measures to help them overcome burnout.

Companies must understand the importance of employee mental health and provide resources to help them overcome it. Statistics show that 72 percent of employees are happy when working in a low-stress environment, highlighting the importance of a healthy workplace.

Human Error Risks are Reduced

The colour in someone's face fades as soon as they realize they've missed a chore. Marketing mistakes, such as forgetting to post on social media, or accounting errors that are preventable by using automation, are just a few examples. Workers can use automation to schedule their work, set reminders, and automatically check for errors.

As a result, the risks of human error are reduced, lowering employee stress.

Stress Sensors and Emotion Recognition

With various unique technologies designed to monitor and improve employee health and wellness, well-being technology also upends the workplace.

A wearable gadget powered by artificial intelligence can, for example, track employee behaviour and emotions using deep learning methods, speech and image recognition, and natural language processing [22, 23, 24]. Employees with difficulty performing their job duties or who are afflicted with mental illnesses such as depression or anxiety can be identified in this way.

Boston-based Cognition has developed a way to identify anxious customer service representatives using a platform that records and analyses customer service conversations.

These are the solutions used in machine learning techniques and speech recognition to track employees' stress levels by recognizing tone and pace of speech.

Artificial Intelligence (AI) Chatbots

Woe bot, for example, interprets a user's input and generates customized responses using natural language processing and sentiment analysis. It measures the user's ideas and mood by asking straightforward questions and helps them re-evaluate their cognitive patterns. This Chatbot employs cognitive behavioural therapy (CBT) techniques to provide individualized responses to assist people with mental health issues to change their emotions and behaviours by making helpful recommendations [25, 26, 27, 28, 29].

The Mood kit program includes four tools: a thought checker that regulates one's terrible ideas and mood and encourages the user to think positive thoughts, and a Mood kit notepad where the user may keep track of their thoughts and mood throughout the day.

Getting it might be difficult for those who require professional care for mental health difficulties. A person must go through several steps before making an appointment with a professional on call. Employees can employ therapeutic AI Chatbots to assess their mental health in a confidential and secure environment. AI Chatbots use NLP and sentiment analysis to assess cognitive and behavioural data and provide users with customized responses. These Chatbots interact with people to help them think more positively, determine when they require assistance, and provide a safe environment where they may express themselves. These Chatbots assist users in altering their mentality and outlook by urging them to think positively and feel good about themselves. Sanvellois, another mental health Chatbot, takes it a step further by incorporating mindfulness elements like meditation and yoga.

The AI-Based application Bio base uses Bio beam, a wearable gadget that collects information about the user's sleep habits, activity level, mood, and heart rate variability. The software analyses this data to provide a complete picture of the user's health. Then there are automated suggestions for reducing stress and improving one's mental health.

Rendering Repeated Work Moot

Automating repetitive procedures that may be template, such as filling out reports, planning meetings, and sending emails, can save our staff time and effort. This reduces stress, gives them more time to focus on more important tasks, and allows them to manage their time better.

Ability to Work More Independently

Reporting to a supervisor and being reminded of your goals might be stressful. When employees are extensively monitored or micromanaged, they are more likely to focus on meeting the deadline than the task. It also limits the potential of personnel to think creatively and grow. Workflow management allows employees and employers to function more freely by explicitly outlining responsibilities and increasing interaction by giving notifications as and when needed.

Improved Workflow Management

Merging our operations can help provide a unified perspective of the workflow process and make it more efficient for personnel across departments. A content strategy that is systematic and organized can help employees work more efficiently and successfully. This allows administrators to keep their eyes on employees without engaging them regularly, and it encourages employees to work in a more collaborative setting. Finally, by removing complexity and saving time, using automation to structure workflows can help to reduce stress.

Potential Power of Integrated Digital Tools

Digital data from connected wearable devices and Smartphone apps can be used to investigate the complex and dynamic biological stress response in its natural state (Figure 5). By 2020, it is estimated that 50 billion people will own linked cell phones, each owning over six connected devices. Many physiological proxies of the autonomic nervous system stress response, such as resting heart rate, heart rate variability, body temperature, electro dermal activity, and relative blood pressure, can be collected longitudinally using smart watches and rings. 11-13 Cortisol14 and inflammatory cytokines15, as well as eye-tracking glasses and wireless EEG caps, are getting closer to measuring Addison's disease [30, 31, 32].

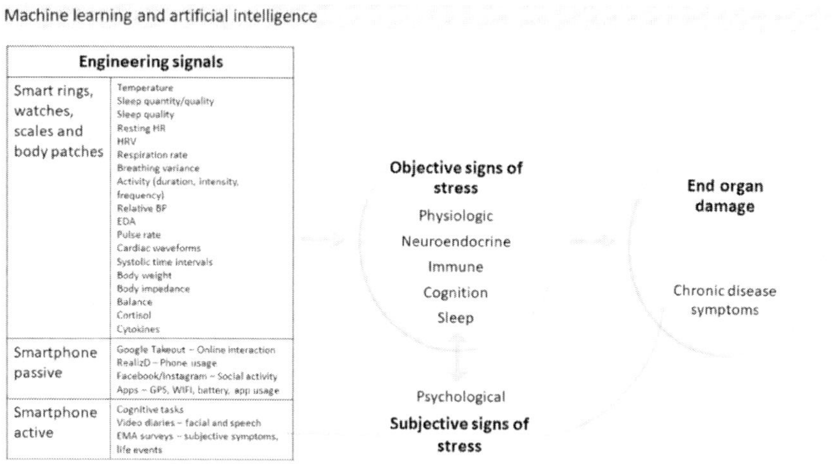

Figure 5. Engineering signals ranging from wearable devices through stress indications to end-organ damage.

A growing body of evidence suggests that connected digital gadgets may be capable of detecting stress indications utilizing a range of digital biomarkers. A GPS sensor, for example, may detect shifts in movement patterns, activity, and the amount of time spent in various locations. At the same time, Smartphone applications can gather passive data such as changes in device or app use, the number of calls or messages received, and so on. These digital markers have been linked to subjective stress and mood changes in university populations [12, 13, 17], various psychiatric populations [18-20], and Parkinson's disease [21]. Smartphone audio recordings' rate of speech, pitch shifts, and pauses have been linked to objective stress measures acquired by smart watches during stressful real-time situations [22, 33, 34]. These aspects have been linked to objective stress measures acquired by smart watches during stressful real-time situations [23]. Furthermore, video-captured cell phones include facial expression detection capabilities, which detect changes in subjectively reported mood states [24, 35, 36, 37, 38]. However, there has been little proof that stress social comparisons [39], different online interactions and views ("likes"), and other proxies of social support are associated with health outcomes, and certain kinds of online activity may cause damage.

Interaction with people with solid connections, on the other hand, has been linked to a boost in self-reported happiness [25, 40, 41, 42, 43, 44].

The use of these digital objective stress metrics in conduction with Smartphone apps that collect subjective stress experiences regularly could provide a mechanism to establish whether or not feeling anxious and the body's biological acute and long-term stress response agree.

This potential also opens the door to new concerns about new models of stress and disease, such as the role of a fleeting feeling of control or uncertainty [26] during stress exposure and how this experience corresponds to objective stress and negative consequences.

New statistical approaches are necessary to put this knowledge into a helpful form for both individuals and healthcare predictors. In high-dimensional data [30, 45, 46, 47, 48], modern machine learning and AI algorithms are practical tools for evaluating and learning from complicated relationships (unknown, unknown, as defined in the Cynefin framework [27]). As a result, the goal is to go to more complex interactions, where cause and effect may be described using AI's "expert" help. Machine learning and AI experts are finding it challenging to develop approaches capable of generating interpretable individual-level sickness trajectories due to the massive amounts of data provided by wearable devices and smartphone applications. While supervised approaches such as recurrent neural networks can predict future disease based on previous occurrences, their interpretability is limited, leaving uncertain molecular pathways of disease progression and discoveries pertinent to population-level interpretation. Methodological limitations are being addressed by recent developments in machine learning and artificial intelligence (AI) for more complex data structures, such as high-frequency longitudinal individual-level data with a lot of variation between individuals as well as the generation of individual predictions for impending disease [31, 32, 49] and making individual predictions for impending disease [50, 51, 52]. Using machine learning and artificial intelligence, new insights into disease trajectories could lead to revisions to the current categorical nosology, which could lead to new endotypes defined as disease subtypes that reflect the underlying pathophysiology rather than observable characteristics, which were first used in the context of asthma [53, 54, 55, 56, 57, 58, 59].

Challenges

Although the promise of employing digital devices to promote health and well-being is widely recognized, there are several cautions regarding their use. [60, 61] Although the characteristics of digital tool users and non-users are primarily unknown, online surveys show that people more likely to utilize wearable devices for health monitoring are younger and from higher socioeconomic backgrounds [62, 63, 64].

From a practical and ethical standpoint, this raises concerns about equal access and addressing vulnerable people who will gain the most from new tools [65, 66, 67, 68, 69, 70]. Big data, which involves a significant volume, variety, velocity, and variability of data across various venues, as well as extra feasibility and ethical challenges, revolves around the information created by integrated Smartphone apps and wearable gadgets. Because of the volume of data generated by integrated digital instruments, data privacy, security, and sophisticated ETL pipelines must be carefully considered.

Connected digital technology can restore human agency but is not without risk. The likelihood of unpleasant or dangerous reactions to the recurrence of symptoms, primarily objective symptoms, or experts monitoring symptoms is mostly unknown [71, 72, 73, 74, 75]. In addition, connected digital devices designed to detect, track, and reduce stress may inadvertently cause stress by disrupting daily life, sleep, and real-world social interactions and relationships, as well as by increasing daily hassles related to connectively, battery life, and device malfunction. Parallel to pilot testing these technologies, these potential hazards should be investigated.

Finally, stress is a natural and essential part of the human experience. Defining the line between adaptive and harmful stress via connected digital devices would necessitate careful thought and consideration to avoid another way of de-stressing persons from everything conflictual or disruptive that may be required for resilience. This possible devaluation of stress will be especially crucial to examine in the context of digital devices aimed at young or vulnerable people.

Wearable gadgets, Smartphone apps, machine learning, and artificial intelligence (AI) are advancing digital technologies, providing a unique opportunity to expedite stress research and use this technology for evidence-based care. In a realistic situation, these alternative methods may find previously unknown patterns of stress response complexity. In the short term, the ability to identify digital biomarkers of impending chronic conditions could benefit the scientific and medical communities in understanding the stress-related origins of disease through individual trajectories and developing and testing interventions based on this information [76, 77, 78, 79]. In the long run, these innovative approaches may bridge the gap between symptom change and healthcare visits by enabling and empowering individuals to monitor their stress outside the hospital setting and by providing healthcare workers with continuous information to identify early warning signs. The ramifications for the return of agency and tailored treatment are numerous, indicating an exciting moment with numerous possibilities.

References

[1] Prince Kumara, Shruti Garga, Ashwani Gargb, "Assessment of Anxiety, Depression, and Stress using Machine learning models, *Procedia computer science*," 2019.

[2] Cohen S, Janicki-Deverts D, Miller GE. "Psychological stress and disease." *JAMA* 2007; 298:1685–1687.

[3] Halfon N, Larson K, Lu M, Tullis E, Russ S. "Lifecourse health development: past, present and future. Matern." *Child Health J.* 2014;18:344–365.

[4] Sapolsky RM. Stress and the brain: "Individual variability and the inverted-U. *Nat. Neurosci.*" 2015; 18:1344–1346.

[5] Selye, H. Stress Without Distress. (J. B. Lippincott Co, Philadelphia, PA, 1974).

[6] Joels M, Baram TZ. "The neuro-symphony of stress." *Nat. Rev. Neurosci*. 2009; 10:459–466.

[7] McEwen BS. Stress, adaptation, and disease. "Allostasis and allostatic load." *Ann. N. Y. Acad. Sci.,* 1998;840:33–44.

[8] Juster RP, McEwen BS, Lupien SJ. "Allostatic load biomarkers of chronic stress and impact on health and cognition," *Neurosci. Biobehav. Rev*. 2010; 35:2–16.

[9] McIntyre, Christa K, Teiko Miyashita, Barry Setlow, Kristopher D Marjon, Oswald Steward, John F Guzowski, and James L McGaugh "Memory-influencing intra-basolateral amygdala drug infusions modulate expression of Arc protein in the hippocampus," *Proc. Natl Acad. Sci. USA.*

[10] Shannon M, King TL, Kennedy HP. Allostasis: "a theoretical framework for understanding and evaluating perinatal health outcomes." *J. Obstet. Gynecol. Neonatal Nurs*, 2007;36:125–134.

[11] Topol EJ, Steinhubl SR, Torkamani A. "Digital medical tools and sensors." *JAMA*. 2015; 313:353–354.

[12] Muaremi A, Arnrich B, Troster G. "Towards measuring stress with smartphones and wearable devices during workday and sleep," *Bio nanoscience*. 2013; 3:172–183.

[13] Sano, A. & Picard, R. W. "Stress recognition using wearable sensors and mobile phone," In *2013 Affective Computing and Intelligent Interaction—Humaine Association Conference*. 671–676 (IEEE, 2013).

[14] Sano, Akane, Sara Taylor, Andrew W McHill, Andrew JK Phillips, Laura K Barger, Elizabeth Klerman, and Rosalind Picard. "Identifying objective physiological markers and modifiable behaviors for self-reported stress and mental health status using wearable sensors and mobile Phones," observational study. *J. Med. Internet Res*. 2018;20: e210.

[15] Parlak O, Marais KS, Curto A, Salleo VF. A.," Molecularly selective nanoporous membrane-based wearable organic electrochemical device for noninvasive cortisol sensing. " *Sci. Adv.* 2018;4: eear2904.

[16] Hladek, Melissa D., Sarah L. Szanton, Young-Eun Cho, Chen Lai, Caroline Sacko, Laken Roberts, and Jessica Gill. "Using sweat to measure cytokines in older adults compared to younger adults: a pilot study." *J. Immunol. Methods*, 2018;454: 1–5.

[17] G. tec. Human-Centered Research with Eye-Tracking and Brain-Computer Interface Technologies, http://blog.gtec.at/human-centered-research-eye-tracking-and-bci/ (2017).

[18] DaSilva, Alex W, Jeremy F Huckins, Rui Wang, Weichen Wang, Dylan D Wagner, and Andrew T Campbell. "Correlates of stress in the college environment uncovered by the application of penalized generalized estimating equations to mobile sensing data." *JMIR Mhealth Uhealth*, 2019;7: e12084.

[19] Faherty, Laura J, Liisa Hantsoo, Dina Appleby, Mary D Sammel, Ian M Bennett, and Douglas J Wiebe. "Movement patterns in women at risk for perinatal depression: use of a mood-monitoring mobile application in pregnancy," *J. Am. Med Inform. Assoc.* 2017; 24:746–753.

[20] Ben-Zeev D, Scherer EA, Wang R, Xie H, Campbell AT, "Next-generation psychiatric assessment: using smartphone sensors to monitor behavior and mental health," *Psychiatr. Rehabil. J.* 2015; 38:218–226.

[21] Fraccaro, P., Beukenhorst, A., Sperrin, M., Harper, S., Palmier-Claus, J., Lewis, S., Van der Veer, S. N. and Peek, N. "Digital biomarkers from geolocation data in bipolar disorder and schizophrenia: a systematic review," *J. Am. Med. Inform.* Assoc. (2019) Nov 1; 26(11): 1412-1420. DOI: 10.1093/jamia/ocz043.

[22] Schwab, P. & Walter, K. Phone MD: "learning to diagnose Parkinson's disease from smartphone data," *arXiv*:1810.01485 (2018).

[23] Slavich GM, Taylor S, Picard RW, "*Stress measurement using speech: recent advancements, validation issues, and ethical and privacy considerations Stress,*" 2019;22:408–413.

[24] Lu, Hong, Denise Frauendorfer, Mashfiqui Rabbi, Marianne Schmid Mast, Gokul T. Chittaranjan, Andrew T. Campbell, Daniel Gatica-Perez, and Tanzeem Choudhury. Stress Sense: Detecting stress in unconstrained acoustic environments using smartphones. In *Proceedings of the 2012ACM Conference on Ubiquitous Computing*. 351–360 (ACM, 2012).

[25] Verduyn, Philippe, David Seungjae Lee, Jiyoung Park, Holly Shablack, Ariana Orvell, Joseph Bayer, Oscar Ybarra, John Jonides, and Ethan Kross. Passive Facebook usage undermines affective well-being: Experimental and longitudinal evidence. *J. Exp. Psychol. Gen.* 2015; 144:480–488.

[26] Burke, M. & Kraut, R., "The relationship between Facebook use and well-being depends on communication type and tie strength," *J. Comput. Mediat. Commun.* 21, 265–281 (2016).

[27] Peters A, McEwen BS, Friston K.," Uncertainty and stress: why it causes diseases and how it is mastered by the brain," *Prog. Neurobiol.* 2017; 156:164–188.

[28] Cappon G, Acciaroli G, Vettoretti M, Facchinetti A, Sparacino G. Wearable continuous glucose monitoring sensors: a revolution in diabetes treatment. *Electronics*. 2017; 6:65.

[29] Catarina Godinho, Josefa Domingos, Guilherme Cunha, Ana T Santos, Ricardo M Fernandes, Daisy Abreu, Nilza Gonçalves, Helen Matthews, Tom Isaacs, Joy Duffen, Ahmed Al-Jawad, Frank Larsen, Artur Serrano, Peter Weber, Andrea Thoms, Stefan Sollinger, Holm Graessner, Walter Maetzler, Joaquim J Ferreira. A systematic review of the characteristics and validity of monitoring technologies to assess Parkinson's disease. *J. Neuroeng. Rehabil.* 2016; 13:24.

[30] Snowden DJ, Boone ME. A leader's framework for decision making. *Harv. Bus. Rev.* 2007; 85:68.

[31] Obermeyer Z, Emanuel EJ. Predicting the future—big data, machine learning, and clinical medicine. *N. Engl. J. Med.* 2016; 375:1216–1219.

[32] Harini Suresh, Nathan Hunt, Alistair Johnson, Leo Anthony Celi, Peter Szolovits, Marzyeh GhassemiClinical intervention prediction and understanding using deep networks. *arXiv*:1705.08498 (2017).

[33] Systematic review of smartphone-based passive sensing for health and well-being. *J Biomed Inform.* 2018.

[34] Review New dimensions and new tools to realize the potential of RDoC: digital phenotyping via smartphones and connected devices. *Transl Psychiatry*. 2017.

[35] Digital medical tools and sensors. *JAMA*. 2015.

[36] Review A systematic review of the characteristics and validity of monitoring technologies to assess Parkinson's disease. *J Neuroeng Rehabil*. 2016.

[37] Ray PP, Dash D, De D. A systematic review of wearable systems for cancer detection: current state and challenges. *J. Med. Syst.* 2017; 41:180.

[38] Surwit, Richard S., Miranda A.L. van Tilburg, Nancy Zucker, Cynthia C. McCaskill, Priti Parekh, Mark N. Feinglos, Christopher L. Edwards, Paula Williams, and James D. Lane. Stress management improves long-term glycemic control in type 2 diabetes. Diabetes *Care*. 2002; 25:30–34.

[39] Bazrafkan, S., Nedelcu, T., Filipczuk, P & Corcoran, P., "Deep learning for facial expression recognition: A step closer to a smartphone that knows your moods," In *2017 IEEE International Conference on Consumer Electronics (ICCE)*. 217–220 (IEEE, Las Vegas, Nevada, 2017).

[40] A leader's framework for decision making. A leader's framework for decision making. *Harv Bus Rev*. 2007.

[41] Predicting the Future - Big Data, Machine Learning, and Clinical Medicine. *N Engl J Med*. 2016.

[42] A targeted real-time early warning score (TREW Score) for septic shock. *Sci Transl Med*. 2015.

[43] Galatzer-Levy IR, Ma S, Statnikov A, Yehuda R, Shalev AY., "Utilization of machine learning for prediction of post-traumatic stress: a re-examination of cortisol in the prediction and pathways to non-remitting PTSD." *Transl. Psychiatry*, 2017;7(3):e0.

[44] Review Asthma endotypes: a new approach to classification of disease entities within the asthma syndrome. *J Allergy Clin Immunol*. 2011.

[45] Using sweat to measure cytokines in older adults compared to younger adults: A pilot study. *J Immunol Methods*. 2018.

[46] Identifying Objective Physiological Markers and Modifiable Behaviors for Self-Reported Stress and Mental Health Status Using Wearable Sensors and Mobile Phones: Observational Study. *J Med Internet Res.* 2018.

[47] Correlates of Stress in the College Environment Uncovered by the Application of Penalized Generalized Estimating Equations to Mobile Sensing Data. *JMIR Mhealth Uhealth.* 2019.

[48] Movement patterns in women at risk for perinatal depression: use of a mood-monitoring mobile application in pregnancy. *J Am Med Inform Assoc*. 2017.

[49] Ghassemi M, Wu M, Hughes MC, Szolovits P, Doshi-Velez F. Predicting intervention onset in the ICU with switching state-space models. *AMIA Jt. Summits Translat. Sci. Proc*. 2017; 2017:82–91.

[50] Lötvall, Jan, Cezmi A Akdis, Leonard B Bacharier, Leif Bjermer, Thomas B Casale, Adnan Custovic, Robert F Lemanske Jr, Andrew J Wardlaw, Sally E Wenzel, and Paul A Greenberger. "Asthma endotypes: a new approach to classification of disease entities within the asthma syndrome," *J. Allergy Clin. Immunol*. 2011; 127:355–360.

[51] Henry KE, Hager DN, Pronovost PJ, Saria S., "A targeted real-time early warning score (TREW Score) for septic shock." *Sci. Transl. Med*. 2015; 7:299ra122.

[52] Schulam, P. & Saria, S.," A framework for individualizing predictions of disease trajectories by exploiting multi-resolution structure." *Adv. Neural Inf. Process.*, Syst. 748–756 (2015).

[53] Lim B. & van der Schaar, M. Disease-Atlas: "Navigating Disease Trajectories using Deep Learning." *arXiv preprint arXiv*:1803.10254.

[54] Memory-influencing intra-basolateral amygdala drug infusions modulate expression of Arc protein in the hippocampus. *Roc Natl Acad Sci USA*. 2005.

[55] Review Allostasis: a theoretical framework for understanding and evaluating perinatal health outcomes. *J Obstet Gynecol Neonatal Nurs*. 2007.

[56] Digital medical tools and sensors. *JAMA*. 2015.

[57] Towards Measuring Stress with Smartphones and Wearable Devices During Workday and Sleep. *Bionanoscience*. 2013.

[58] Identifying Objective Physiological Markers and Modifiable Behaviours for Self-Reported Stress and Mental Health Status Using Wearable Sensors and Mobile Phones: Observational Study. *J Med Internet Res.* 2018.

[59] Molecularly selective nanoporous membrane-based wearable organic electrochemical device for noninvasive cortisol sensing. *Sci Adv.* 2018.

[60] Hunter, B., Henley, J., Fenwick, J., Sidebotham, M. & Pallant, J. Work, *Health and Emotional Lives of Midwives in the United Kingdom: The UK WHELM study* (Cardiff University, Wales, 2017).

[61] Cornet VP, Holden RJ. Systematic review of smartphone-based passive sensing for health and well-being. *J. Biomed. Inform.* 2018; 77:120–132.

[62] Torous J, Onnela JP, Keshavan M. New dimensions and new tools to realize the potential of RDoC: digital phenotyping via smartphones and connected devices. *Transl. Psychiatry*. 2017;7.

[63] Review Stress, adaptation, and disease. Allostasis and allostatic load. *Ann N Y Acad Sci*. 1998.
[64] Review Allostatic load biomarkers of chronic stress and impact on health and cognition. *Neurosci Biobehav Rev*. 2010.
[65] Nielsen, C. Tech-styles: are consumers really interested in wearing tech on their sleeves, http://www.nielsen.com/us/en/newswire/2014/tech-styles-are-consumers-really-interested-in-wearing-tech-on-their-sleeves.html.2014 (2014).
[66] Digital Phenotyping: An Epistemic and Methodological Analysis Stress-related consequences of the coronavirus disease 2019 pandemic on symptoms of Crohn's disease, *European Journal of Gastroente*.
[67] The growing field of digital psychiatry: current evidence and the future of apps, social media, chatbots, and virtual reality, *World Psychiatry*. 2021.
[68] Artificial intelligence in prediction of mental health disorders induced by the COVID-19 pandemic among health care workers, *Croatian Medical Journal*. 2020 Jun; 61(3)279.
[69] Review Stress and the brain: individual variability and the inverted-U. *Nat Neurosci*. 2015.
[70] Review The neuro-symphony of stress. *Nat Rev Neurosci*. 2009.
[71] e-Addictology: An Overview of New Technologies for Assessing and Intervening in Addictive Behaviours. *Front Psychiatry*. 2018.
[72] The Age of Artificial Intelligence: Use of Digital Technology in Clinical Nutrition. *Curr Surg Rep*. 2021.
[73] Data-driven modeling and prediction of blood glucose dynamics: Machine learning applications in type 1 diabetes, *Artif Intell Med*. 2019.
[74] What Are We Measuring When We Evaluate Digital Interventions for Improving Lifestyle? A Scoping Meta-Review, *Frontiers in Public Health*. 2022.
[75] An Alternative to the Light Touch Digital Health Remote Study: The Stress and Recovery in Frontline COVID-19 Health Care Workers Study, *JMIR Formative Research*. 2021.
[76] Topol, E. *The Topol Review*. Preparing the Healthcare Workforce to Deliver the Digital Future. 1–48 (Health, Education, England, Leeds, 2019).
[77] Articles from NPJ Digital Medicine are provided here courtesy of Nature Publishing Group.
[78] Identifying Objective Physiological Markers and Modifiable Behaviors for Self-Reported Stress and Mental Health Status Using Wearable Sensors and Mobile Phones: Observational Study. *J Med Internet Res*. 2018.
[79] Using reality mining to improve public health and medicine. *Stud Health Technol Inform*. 2009.

Chapter 7

Multimodality Analysis of Psychological Disorders

S. Chandra Sekarn[1,*] and M. Senbagavalli[2,†]
[1]P. S. V. College of Engineering and Technology, Krishnagiri, Tamilnadu, India
[2]Alliance College of Engg. and Design, Alliance University, Bangalore, India

Abstract

In persons and communities all around the world, the COVID-19 outbreak has caused and will cause enormous personal problems connected to psychological disorders consequences such as melancholy, sleeplessness, appetite, nervousness, and stress disorder. We relate pandemic difficult variables, detrimental mental health effects, and appropriate treatment options through a thorough evaluation of the expanding empirical data on the COVID-19 outbreak and research on earlier corona virus outbreaks. This chapter describes how societal risks and outbreak stressors would wreak havoc on psychological disorders. The globe has undoubtedly failed to protect COVID-19-induced physiological treatments, while confidentiality issues regarding the mental health aspect have been ignored or ignored.

COVID-19-related emotional anguish affects upwards of 83 percent of the participants, resulting in irritability, insomnia, and family strife. The public healthcare answer and psychological health service revisions consume almost all focused on preventing contagion, reconfiguring access to analysis and treatment, ensuring continuity of attention for

*Corresponding Author's Email: chandrudpi@gmail.com.
†Corresponding Author's Email: senba1983@gmail.com.

In: Data Science Applications of Post-COVID-19 Psychological Disorders
Editor: Vijayalakshmi Kakulapati
ISBN: 979-8-88697-165-1

mental well-being practitioners, and paid care to the current instances of psychological unkind health and societies at great danger of psychological disorders issues. Specialists, patients and clinicians should collaborate to build long-duration variations of supply methods for emotional health treatment that are explicitly geared to decrease differences in health-care conditions.

In order to better satisfy today's patients and prevent any future problems from occurring, those who urgently require adequate treatment with multimodality analysis of psychological disorders and management, as well as those who frequently lack adequate support systems. The approach will assist people in managing the outbreak and improving psychological disorders in order to combat privacy issues related with COVID-19 and upcoming epidemics. This chapter's outline comprises the following: an introduction to intelligent psychological disorders care systems, a review of the role of recent technologies (AI, ML, DL, and IoT) in smartly handling psychological health care systems, contains multimodality analysis of Psychological disorders, the Importance of multimodality analysis and tools, Conclusion and References.

Introduction

Artificial Intelligence is a system of program a workstation, automaton, or some other object to reflect like a human being in a smart way. AI works to resolve tribulations and it is the learning of how the person brains think, learn, and makes decisions. Lastly, this study produces smart software systems. The aim of Artificial Intelligence is to advance computer operations that are associated to person perceptive, such as interpretation, knowledge, and solving problems.

Mental health practitioners will be able to more objectively identify psychological sickness than is at present finished in the DSM-5, recognize these illnesses at a former or prodromal stage when interventions may be more effective, and personalize treatments based on an individual's unique characteristics as AI techniques are refined and improved. However, prudence is requisite to keep away from overinterpreting preliminary data, and more work is required to bridge the gap between AI research and mental health clinical care. We've talked about how artificial intelligence can be used to track psychological problems. The evaluation includes a total of 28 original research studies on Artificial Intelligence and psychological healthiness.

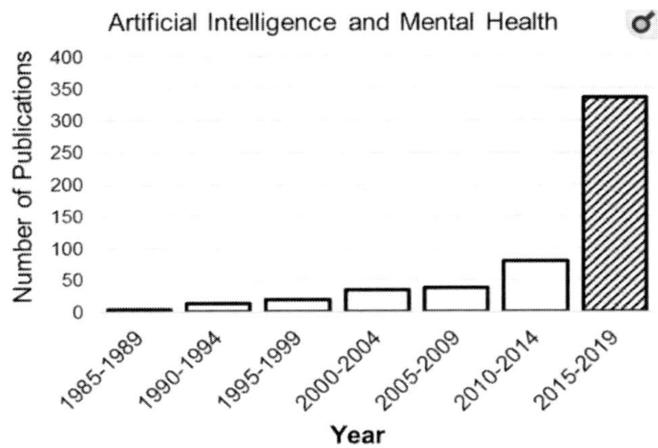

Source: https://www.ncbi.nlm.nih.gov/pmc/articles/PMC7274446/.

Figure 1. Frequency of publications by year in PubMed using search terms artificial intelligence and mental health.

Psychological Disorders

There are a variety of psychiatric disorders that affect the COVID-19 population, including the following mental illnesses.

Neurodevelopmental Disorders

Neurodevelopmental disorders are those that are identified throughout childhood, adolescence, or adulthood. This form of empirical complaints occurs before the age of eighteen and is marked by impairments in both cognitive functioning and adaptive behaviour. The use of Command tests is widely used to link limitations in intellectual ability.

Bipolar and Affiliated Disorders

Before the age of eighteen only this form of empirical complaint occurs and is marked by impairments in both cognitive performance and flexible behaviour. The use of Command tests is widely used to link limitations in intellectual ability.

Anxiety Disorders

Worry disorders are characterised by excessive and persistent fear, solicitude, anxiety, and associated behavioural problems in patients. 5 Fear is an emotional reaction to a threat, whether that threat is genuine or imagined. Anxiety is the fear of something bad happening that hasn't happened yet.

Stress-Related Disorders

Trauma and stressor-related disorder that is caused by being exposed to a traumatic or stressful experience. These were previously included with anxiety disorders, but they are now recognized a separate illness category.

Dissociative Disorders

Dissociative disorders are a type of neurological condition in which certain parts of cognition, such as identity and memory, are dissociated or interrupted. As a result of separation, this issue comprises a brief loss of memory. This memory loss, which can persist for a short time or multiple times, is frequently caused by some form of brain trauma.

Physical Symptom Disorders

Physical symptom complaints are characterized by a fixation with physical problems, making it difficult to treat normally. This concern with symptoms causes emotional torment and makes it difficult to function during the day. It's crucial to emphasise that physical effects do not imply that people are lying about their pain, exhaustion, or other problems.

Eating Disorders

Consuming disorder is defined by compulsive weight-loss and eating practises that have a severe impact on natural and psychological health. Battening and consuming disorders that used to be identified during childhood and adolescence are now being diagnosed in adults.

Sleep Disorders

Narcolepsy is a syndrome in which people experience an irrepressible need to sleep. Sleep disorders involve a disturbance in sleeping habits that causes agony and has an impact on day-to-day performance. People who are awake may experience an unexpected reduction of muscle tone.

Disruptive Disorders

Impulse-control illnesses are characterised by an inability to regulate one's feelings and behaviours, sometimes to one's disadvantage or that of others. Conduct that violates others' rights, such as destroying property or physical aggressiveness, as well as conduct that is inconsistent with social morality, authority numbers, and laws, describe these behavioral and emotional regulatory issues.

Review on Multimodality Analysis of Psychological Disorders

There has been a poor level of replication of findings in the research of personality and psychophysiology [1]. This is due in large part to the incompatibility of the methodologies utilised in different programmes. The study of personality as it relates to physiological processes is based on a solid foundation of previous research and theory, and it continues to pose a unique challenge to those who want to perform meticulous theory-driven research on complicated processes.

It is believed that treatment should be based on an understanding of the mechanisms that generate or perpetuate obesity [2]. This hypothesis suggests that behavioral interventions are unlikely to improve, and instead points to direct changes in the biological systems that regulate body weight. Binge eating and other obesity-related maladaptive behaviors can be reduced with cognitive-behavioral therapy. It has the potential to improve diet and physical activity, resulting in considerable health advantages, even if weight loss is not achieved.

MultiSense, a real-time computing framework for context-based nonverbal behavior analysis, was introduced [3]. It provides adaptable and effective synchronization methodologies for context-based non-verbal behavior assessment. When interpreting nonverbal behaviors, MultiSense is designed to use interaction signals from both workstation and the participants and combine this circumstantial knowledge.

The goal of this study is to use Decision Rule Set Formation to better detect and diagnose the existence of three important and common psychological disorders: Major Depressive Disorder, Bi-Polar Affective Disorder, and Schizophrenia (RST) [4]. To confirm this prediction, it is compared to the results of machine learning models that predict the psychiatric condition based on the patient's fMRI image and PET pictures collected from the EHR [5, 6].

This work is significant and novel in two ways: 1) It exposes YinYang into biomedical science for the awareness of such neurobehavioral abnormalities and nurtures a new benchmark prototype for clinical, therapeutic, and pharmacological research and applications; and 2) it provides a mathematical formalism for the categorization of emotional regulation in individuals and/or a group of patient populations with biomedical engineering application areas and potential nanotechnology implementations [7]. This study examines the features of three different types of mental diseases and applies them to large-scale datasets [8]. These findings aid in the identification of social network users who may be suffering from mental illnesses.

Proposes a model that uses multicriteria approach and a specialized system to facilitate the progression of early on detection of a variety of psychiatric disorders based on qualitative and proportional examination of events and criteria [9]. The first increased actuality system for the therapy of cockroach phobia is shown [10, 11]. The AR Toolkit software was used to create our system. It has only been experienced on only one patient, and the outcomes have been excellent. The patient was unable to move toward an actual cockroach at the start of the publicity session, but after using our improved reality technology, she was able to approach an actual cockroach, engage with it, and destroy it on her own.

On irregularities of self-related processing in patients from many dimensions of the Self, classical scientific psychology paradigms are used, and speech signal processing and Machine Learning approaches are used for depressed speech [12]. We hope that by using this strategy, we will be able to better capture the psychological characteristics of depressed individuals and make significant progress in increasing diagnosis accuracy. Participants' self-reports for sentiment and questionnaire about psychological character as well as electrocardiography (ECG) (physiological signal) were collected and analyzed non-invasively [13, 14]. This work describes a system that automatically scans online crisis hotline talks to (1) extract fine-grained distress indicators that correspond to DSM IV codes and (2) perform triage categorization depending on the intensity of distress [15, 16].

In a universal context, a multimodal psychological computational technology was presented [17]. The proposed work develops a naturalistic mental disorder collection of databases which include long-term ubiquitous interpretable psychological execution model based on previous information and multimodal information fusion. The proposed mental disorder database which achieves long-term complex mental health status, intricate emotion detection, efficiently reduces systematic and accuracy-related challenges under recognition and prophecy.

Focuses on developing a multimodal deep learning structure for automatically extracting salient features from recorded speech samples in order to detect mental diseases such as depression, bipolar disorder, and schizophrenia [18]. To extract embeddings from both audio and text segments, we use a range of pre-trained models.

The suggested methodology intends to supplement traditional subjective self-report predictors of mental health illnesses with objective metrics, aligning with recent literature on artificial intelligence-based predictive modelling [19]. This method can be used by anyone who has been exposed to high amounts of stress during the COVID-19 epidemic, and it may help mental health professionals establish diagnoses more quickly and accurately.

Present the main phases of MHMS and suggest a categorization taxonomy to aid the review of related research [20]. This paper reviews recent research on mental health monitoring systems (MHMS) that employ sensor data and machine learning techniques. We concentrated on studies on mental diseases and ailments such as depression, anxiety, bipolar disorder, stress, and so on.

Artificial intelligence (AI)-based solutions for psychiatric research and diagnostics are rapidly being created, but there is no systematic overview of their uses [21]. As a result, this paper looks at three important brain observation methods used to research psychiatric disorders MRI, EEG, and kinesics diagnoses as well as related AI technologies and methods.

As AI techniques are refined and improved, mental health practitioners will be able to more objectively define mental illnesses than DSM-5 [22].

Artificial intelligence (AI) methods were developed to assist psychiatrist and psychologists in producing judgments based on the health data for example medical proceedings, behavioral data, social media data, etc. [23]. Deep learning is a relatively new AI technology, has demonstrated improved routine in a variety of real-world outcomes, ranging from computer vision to healthcare.

Learning human activities patterns, identifying psychosomatic symptoms and hazard factors, creating illness succession predictions, and customizing and humanizing therapies are all possible with machine learning technologies [24, 25]. Regardless of the possible reimbursement of using machine learning in mental health, this is an innovative turf of study, and creating victorious ML-enabled apps that can be used in practice is riddled with a host of complex, interrelated challenges.

About Psychological Disorders

The functioning of various learnedness within one medium is referred to as multimodality. Figure 2 depicts the multimodal model's architecture for predicting psychiatric disorders in COVID-affected mortal creatures. Multimodal emulsion is a method of merging several colored data modalities for analysis purposes. In this chapter, the early emulsion system will be used to extract the features of alluni-modal data prior combining them into a supervector form representation. The positive feelings vectors was focused alongside the neutral sentiments vector and the negative feelings vector due to the multimodality. After feelings normalisation, the system also receives the early emulsion vector, which is used as the input for a classifier. The vaticinator will be obtained via a fully focused subcaste, in which the input learns the semantic idea for the early emulsion method.

The presented multimodal approach caters to various crucial rudiments, such as landing the semantic and resolving the nebulosity from psychological disease, as well as exercising good and negative sensations for profiling and better understanding of emotion and gets of COVID afflicted folks. This chapter focuses on using COVID instances to exercise various forms of psychological disorders. Positive feelings, neutral feelings, and negative feelings will be among the data modalities used. Positive feelings data analysis will be based on stationary descriptor or, in particular, negative feelings analysis with negative psychological disorder problems, whereas neutral feelings data analysis will be based on stationary descriptor or, in particular, negative feelings analysis with negative psychological disorder problems.

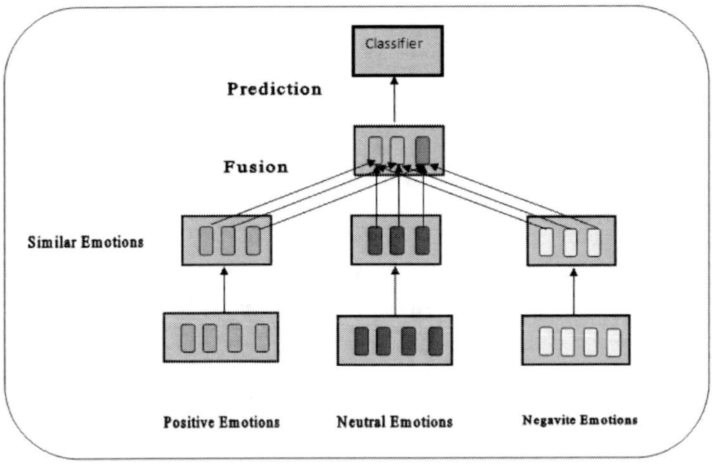

Figure 2. Design of multimodal model to predict psychological disorder.

Machine Learning Model Training

By means of the introduction of information system and communication, the amount of information is generated on a daily basis, and it is rapidly increasing. In the year 2017, 2.5 quintillion bytes of information are generated in each day, and this rate will only increase as new detectors and bias are developed. Because machine computing power has increased in latest years, it can be possible to employ that processing capacity to dissect massive amounts of data in order to correct informative information. Machine Learning can be defined as a collection of computer systems algorithm that automatically uncover intriguing formats and connections from massive amounts of information.

Types of Models

Supervised Learning, unsupervised Learning, semi-supervised Learning, transfer Learning, and reinforcement Learning are the five main types of machine learning algorithms.

Supervised Learning

The algorithms in supervised learning are given a collection of instruction exemplifications. Each case consists of a pair of I/O (Input/Output) values. The input is typically signified as an collection that numerically characterizes the cases. The point vector is the name given to this array. The issue is the value we're trying to predict, such as an order or an actual number. The scandal is commonly referred to as the class when it comes to bracket issues.

Unsupervised Learning

The Unsupervised learning is that the affair variable y is unknown at the outset of training; thus, the aim is to discover the various sorts of ordering that could be naturally build up from parallelism in the input information.

Semi-Supervised Learning

There is a lot of sampled and training information but only a small percentage of samples have the relevant variable (marker), semi-supervised learning is used. Semi-supervised methods use both labelled and unlabeled cases to train models. Because it's frequently complex to tag information with their matching ground verity type, semi-supervised learning is useful for internal country finding (class).

Transfer Learning

The transfer learning, information from same or distinct fields with labelled data is utilised to learning a new in different sector where there is no or a lot of sampled training data. For example, the skills learned when learning to fete nags from photographs may be applied to trying to fete cows. A more exact example is a model that learnt to recognize distinct pictures orders based on veritably simple circumstances such as pussycats, tykes, buses, and so on, and is also used to learn how to tell if an image has a particular complaint or not.

Reinforcement Learning

An agent learns through sample testing relationships with its terrain in reinforcement learning. The agent's job is to maximize prices and decide on a stylish course of action based on the present situation. We wish to evaluate how well a machine learning model will perform in real-life circumstances, such as when making prognostications on unseen data, once it has been trained.

Research Challenges in Multimodality Analysis of Psychological Disorders

Although there have been significant advancements in the autonomous monitoring of internal health, there are still difficulties to overcome before fully effective and automated systems can be implemented. These difficulties present a number of exploration opportunities for improving parts of structure autonomous internal state monitoring systems at various stages. Following that, we give a list of some of the MHMS exploration problems and opportunities.

Data Labeling

Data labelling, or linking a set of detector data with the matching genuine internal state during that time span, is one of the most difficult aspects of constructing internal monitoring systems. This is termed as ground verity of data, and it is required for machine learning models to be trained. The quality of the ground verity data will determine the models' final performance. Carrying this data is difficult and time-consuming; for example, in cases of bipolar disorder, a professional examination is required to determine the current status, which necessitates a visit to the sanitarium. Transfer learning is one system that could be utilized when there isn't enough labelled data. One possible strategy to alleviate internal health issues is to adopt semi-supervised Learning styles, which we believe have a good chance of being useful for internal health monitoring.

Inter-User Friction

Because each person is different, drug addicts' physiological and behavioural tendencies will differ. While this is valuable for a few tasks that require stoner authentication/identification, such as behavioral biometrics, it presents a challenge for internal monitoring systems because one size does not fit all. As a result, stoner-independent models tend to underperform stoner-dependent models.

Intra-User Friction

It indicates to the variability of a stoner's physiological and behavioral characteristics, particularly across time. This could be attributed to changes in diurnal habits such as starting a new work, relocating to a different megacity, enrolling in a new conditioning programme, and so on. Natural changes such as metabolism, vocal change throughout puberty, ails, and in women, intra-user friction has been observed to alter with the menstrual periods phase in various studies on detecting stress in voice and domicile-rate. Actors' short-term behavioral changes can also be seen. Based on GPS, cell halls, and WiFi data is an example, some authors noticed various position change patterns on weekdays and weekends. Indeed, because to intra-user friction, a stoner-dependent model that is currently doing well may begin to deteriorate over time. Time adaptive models are quite desirable in this type of situation.

Detector Data Emulsion

As the model seen, there are a variety of information sources from which physiological disorders and behavioral data can be gathered in order to draw conclusions. Software or tackle can be used as data sources. Each information source has its own template, measurement units, and rates, and other characteristics, necessitating the use of multiple preprocessing methods. The input data for predictive models must be in a specific format. Aggregation (also known as early emulsion) is typically used to do this, which entails creating point vectors including aggregated data from all viewing modalities. The models are also trained and prognosticated using these aggregated point vectors. One of the issues with this method is that the dimension of point vectors can rapidly expand, slowing down the training phase. This may not be a problem when models are trained on the garçon side, but if models are trained locally in a wearable device, it can take a long time and consume a lot of battery (smartphone).

Integration with Other Systems

Although the difficulties we've outlined thus far have focused primarily through the machine learning components, these systems are expected to perform with a variety of other processes and within a greater ecosystem.

Stoner databases, executive tools and system interfaces for caregivers and croakers, as well as health care involvement and support systems (whether web-based, smartphone-based, or others) are all included. Communication mechanisms between different modules and systems must be relinquished and developed if stable and scalable outcomes are to be achieved.

Clinical Confirmation

One goal of EMAs is to provide just-in-time actions based on the acquired detector data, therefore clinical confirmation that the information indicates form it's supposed to measure and that it's clinically significant is critical. The clinical validity of the data may be harmed by noise in the environment, poor data collecting, and low adherence. A clinical expert, acting as the gold standard, can label the detector information may be as regular or irregular in order to determine the clinical validity. Even so, there is a continuum in the realm of internal health, and the threshold for abnormality varies depending on context and individuality. As a result, clinical professionals are unable to identify all detector data. Rather than finding unequivocal countries, as Grünerbl et al., argue, volition is to detect changes from a baseline.

The most popular strategy in medical research is the substantiation-based approach, in which information is developed based on the most up-to-date clinically useful substantiation gleaned by methodical investigation. Methodical evaluations on the use of machine Learning in neuroscientific and psychiatric and research underline the need for a proposition-driven machine learning method, which is based on getting information and thesis, in order to generate useful results and a longer understanding. To put it another way, this is the model for obtaining high-quality ground verity information. Similarly, Anila Umar et al., novel's explanation method has the potential to facilitate additional scientific knowledge by providing insight into, as well as reasons for, the classifiers' predictions.

Conclusion

In this chapter, the lot of survey research works on physiological disorders and it is focus on user sensors to collect behavioral information with machine learning to analyze the huge information from the sample disorders collected from COVID affected areas.

The proposed system model identified the key characteristics of the classification taxonomy and it is believed that a lot of research gives overall structure of this their model.

But in this chapter which identified the important cycles of physiological disorders using machine learning the information are collected analyses, and evaluation. The physiological disorders like positive emotions, negative emotions and neutral emotions. The different levels of emotions collected and analyzed give correct indication to the medical representation or doctors. Up to the knowledge by the surveyed literature, the application of multimodal physiological disorder model using with machine learning methods which leads a great prospect in the advancement of provided that mental health care information technology tools for treatment.

References

[1] Geen, R. G., "Psycho physiological Approaches to Personality," *Handbook of Personality Psychology*, 1997, Pages 387-414.

[2] Wilson, G. T., "Behavioral treatment of obesity: thirty years and counting," *Advances in Behaviour Research and Therapy*, Volume 16, Issue 1, 1994, Pages 31-75.

[3] Stratou, G., Louis-Philippe Morency, "MultiSense - Context-Aware Nonverbal Behavior Analysis Framework : A Psychological Distress Use Case," *IEEE Xplore, IEEE Transactions on Affective Computing*, Volume : 8, Issue : 2, April-June 1 2017.

[4] Umar, A., Usman Qamar, "Detection and Diagnosis of Psychological Disorders Through Decision Rule Set Formation," *IEEE 17th International Conference on Software Engineering Research, Management and Applications (SERA)*, 2019.

[5] Aryal, Y., Angelika Maag, Nirosha Gunasekera, "Application of Machine learning algorithms in diagnosis and detection of psychological disorders," *IEEE*, 2021.

[6] Nunes, L. C., Plácido Rogério Pinheiro, Tarcísio Cavalcante Pequeno, "An expert system applied to the diagnosis of psychological disorders," *IEEE*, 2009.

[7] Zhang, W. R., Anand K. Pandurangi, Karl E. Peace, "Yinyang dynamic neurobiological modeling and diagnostic analysis of major depressive and bipolar disorders," *IEEE Transactions on Biomedical Engineering,* Volume : 54, Issue : 10, Oct. 2007.

[8] Lavhare, J. N., M. A Kulkarni, Mental Disorders Detection using Social Networking Sites," *IEEE*, 2021.

[9] Nunes, L. C. Plácido Rogério Pinheiro, Mirian Calíope Dantas Pinheiro, Marum Simão Filho, Rafael Espíndola Comin Nunes, "Automatic Detection and Diagnosis of Neurologic Diseases," *IEEE Access*, 2019, Volume : 7.

[10] Juan, M. C., C. Botella, M. Alcaniz, R. Banos, C. Carrion, M. Melero, J. A. Lozano, "An augmented reality system for treating psychological disorders: application to phobia to cockroaches," *IEEE,* 2005.

[11] Panagiotakopoulos, T. C., Dimitrios Panagiotis Lyras, Miltos Livaditis, Kyriakos N. Sgarbas, George C. Anastassopoulos, Dimit, "A Contextual Data Mining Approach Toward Assisting the Treatment of Anxiety Disorders," *IEEE*, 2010, Volume : 14 Issue : 3.

[12] Lu, X., Aibao Zhou, Hongwu Yang, "A novel method design for diagnosis of psychological symptoms of depression using speech analysis," *IEEE*, 2018.

[13] Hsieh, D. L., Tzu-Chien Hsiao, "Heart rate variability of internet gaming disorder addicts in emotional states," *IEEE Xplore*, 2016.

[14] Daluwatte, C., Judith H. Miles, Shawn E. Christ, David Q. Beversdorf, Andrew Lofgreen, Nathan Berliner, Gang Ya, "Age-dependent pupillary light reflex parameters in children," *2012 Annual International Conference of the IEEE Engineering in Medicine and Biology Society*, 2012.

[15] Chen, W., Bin Han, "Psychological intervention treatment in psychiatric rehabilitation," *Proceedings 2011 International Conference of Human Health and Biomedical Engineering*, 2011.

[16] Pacula, M., Talya Meltzer, Michael Crystal, Amit Srivastava, Brian Marx, "Automatic detection of psychological distress indicators and severity assessment in crisis hotline conversations," *2014 IEEE International Conference on Acoustics, Speech and Signal Processing (ICASSP)*, 2014.

[17] Sun, X., Yezhen Song, Meng Wang, "Toward Sensing Emotions With Deep Visual Analysis: A Long-Term Psychological Modeling Approach," *IEEE MultiMedia*, Volume : 27, Issue : 4, Oct.-Dec. 1 2020.

[18] Naderi, H., Behrouz Haji Soleimani, Stan Matwin, "Multimodal Deep Learning for Mental Disorders Prediction from Audio Speech Samples," 2020, *cornell university*.

[19] Ćosić, K., Sinisas Popović, Marko Šarlija, Ivan Kesedžić, and Tanja Jovanovic, "Artificial intelligence in prediction of mental health disorders induced by the COVID-19 pandemic among health care workers," *PMS US National Library of medicine national institutes of health* 2020.

[20] Garcia-Ceja, E., Michael Riegler, Tine Nordgreen, Petter Jakobsen, Ketil J. Oedegaard, Jim Tørresen, "Mental health monitoring with multimodal sensing and machine learning: A survey," *Pervasive and Mobile Computing*, 2018.

[21] Liu, G. D., Yu-Chen Li, Wei Zhang, Le Zhang, "*A Brief Review of Artificial Intelligence Applications and Algorithms for Psychiatric Disorders*," Elsevier-Engineering, 2020.

[22] Graham, S., Colin Depp, Ellen E. Lee, Camille Nebeker, Xin Tu, Ho-Cheol Kim and Dilip V. Jeste, "Artificial Intelligence for Mental Health and Mental Illnesses: an Overview," *Psychiatry In The Digital Age*, 2019.

[23] Su, C., Zhenxing Xu, Jyotishman Pathak & Fei Wang, "Deep learning in mental health outcome research: à scoping review," *Journal of Neurology*, 2020

[24] theime, A., Danielle belgrave, gavin Doherty, "Machine Learning in Mental Health: A Systematic Review of the HCI Literature to Support the Development of Effective and Implementable ML Systems," *ACM DL digital library*, 2020.

[25] Graham, S., Colin Depp, Ellen E. Lee, Camille Nebeker, Xin Tu, Ho-Cheol Kim, and Dilip V. Jeste, "Artificial Intelligence for Mental Health and Mental Illnesses: An Overview," *PMC US national library of medicine National institutes of health*, 2019.

Chapter 8

Mathematical Modeling and Analysis of Psychological Disorders

A. Paramasivam*, P. Vidhushini and N. Arunprakash
Rajalakshmi Engineering College, Chennai, Tamil Nadu, India

Abstract

In general, a psychological disorder is a syndrome with significant rapid variability in control of emotions, cognitive control, and behaviors that reflect dysfunction in the biological, psychological, or development process underlying the function of cognitive behavior. Psychological disorders are occurring more prominently in post-COVID-19 patients. This work aims to investigate a detailed literature review on psychological disorders and mathematical models of the system to predict and forecast the psychological and mental illnesses and the spread of COVID-19 during the pandemic. A systematic statistical analysis was more appreciable to determine the significant level to suggest an appropriate medical direction to overcome the psychological disorders. The mathematical models, such as the system dynamics model used to predict the growth rate and causes of the various disorders such as depression, bipolar disorder, eating disorders, personality disorders, stress disorders, psychotic disorders, etc., propose the medical precautions and treatment methods for the dynamic combination of psychological disorder patients effectively with a systematic approach. Further, the extended work on machine learning approaches enhances its accuracy. It matches the scenario in real-time to predict the effects of disorders in post-COVID-19 patients. A set of massive data from the open-source will substantiate the model's effectiveness in predicting

*Corresponding Author's Email: paramasivam.a@gmail.com.

In: Data Science Applications of Post-COVID-19 Psychological Disorders
Editor: Vijayalakshmi Kakulapati
ISBN: 979-8-88697-165-1

disorders of various levels and simulate the data using the system dynamics model using VenSim to foresee its future growth rate to design and develop the methodology to minimize the psychological disorders. The planned contents are: stating the various psychological disorders, mapping the psychological disorders of post-COVID patients with the standard, and work performed in the multimodal analysis of psychological analysis in the literature to date with the mapped psychological disorders. A questionnaire survey from doctors on psychological disorders was quantified and analyzed using statistical methods. Various mathematical models, such as Markov chain, Monte Carlo simulation, SIR model, and simulation models of multimodal analysis of psychological disorders, substantiate the model using the system dynamics using the VenSim package to predict the effects. Using open-source data, the researchers proved the accuracy of the computational modelling and stochastic mathematical modelling results in building the models to predict the disorders and viable proposed solutions for patients' healthy well-being by minimizing the effect of the disorder at the earliest.

Keywords: psychological disorder, post COVID-19, data analysis, system dynamics, VenSim, multimodal analysis, statistical methods, machine learning

Introduction

Psychological disorders are depression, anxiety, stressful feelings, abnormal thinking, mental distress, actions, and feelings. Furthermore, depression, psychosis, sleep, anxiety, and other psychological illnesses can all be linked, affecting people in different ways with differential severity. The dysfunctional pattern with emotion determines psychological disorder, thought, or behavior which results in adequate discomfort and is observed as aberrant in the culture of the individual. Abnormal thoughts, feelings, and behavior significantly result in the indication of psychological disorder. A mental illness is a behavioral pattern that causes mental stress or impairs personal feelings and functions. This can also be called a psychiatric problem.

The behavioral state that impairs perception, emotion, and behavior is called mental illnesses such as autism, schizophrenia, and depression. The approach of formal clinical changing from a limited perspective to a holistic perspective shifted from a partial perspective to a holistic perspective with the change of focus from curing illness to improving health conditions. Over the past six decades, mental illness has been caused due to limited mental disorder (schizophrenia and depression), which is treated and diagnosed with stated standard medical procedure collected from National statistical data. In 1980 and 1990, the national care centers failed to support the needs of the mentally ill patients due to the increasing trend of admitted patients, which resulted in releasing many patients with mental illnesses. Few community health service centers addressed the patients' needs but could not meet the entire patient. The National Institute of Mental Health's objective is to diagnose and cure patients with mental illness. This incident changed the standard operating procedure for mental illness patients, extending with duration, disability, and threshold period.

Psychiatric illnesses result from unchecked emotional, behavioral, or cognitive dysfunctions. The Individual suffers from such disorder due to the life losses and life stress factors in the living culture of society. Concerning the development in technology and culture change, the factors that lead to mental illness/disorder are increasingly added at an exponential rate. The factors are (i) history of family and genes, (ii) experiences in life -stress, abuse in childhood or later, (iii) imbalance of chemicals in the brain, (iv) injury in the brain, (v) during pregnancy – toxic chemicals or virus exposure (vi) medical conditions such as cancer, (vii) fewer friends (viii) lonely or isolated living feeling, etc. It's not limited to this added due to the family's change of culture and relationship culture. Flaws in character and a lazy attitude do not lead to mental illness. However, the primary cause of most probable mental illness is still fuzzy and unable to predict. In general, it's the combination of factors related to the environment of the culture or family (death, abnormal lifestyle and family relationships, anxiety, loneliness, change of work, expectation of social, lack of self-esteem), biological factors such as (circuits of the nerve cells – abnormal function, damage of the brain due to trauma, heredity of family, stress, abuse, infections leading to brain damage, pediatric autoimmune neuropsychiatric disorder (PANDAS), poor nutrition, loss of oxygen to the brain, and psychological factors (physical/emotional/sexual abuse, poor ability).

Classification of Psychological Disorder

The classification of psychological disorders is shown in Table 1 in detail. Liang et al. (2020) and Alharb et al. (2022) predicted the post-COVID effect on the mental health of the younger generation in China and Saudi Arabia.

Logistic regression of collected samples reveals that 40.4% of youth are prone to psychological disorders, and 14.4% are affected by PTSD. It is specified that COVID-19 shows remarkable evidence of psychological disorder. Qu et al. (2014) stated that one of the significant disorders that vitally impact psychological and depression problems is post-traumatic stress disorder (PTSD).

Table 1. Classification of psychological disorders

Psychological Disorder Classification

1.Neurological Development Disorder

- ✓ Intellectual Disability
- ✓ Global Development Delay
- ✓ Communication Disorder
- ✓ Autism Spectrum Disorder
- ✓ Attention Deficit Hyper activity Disorder (ADHD)

2. Sleep Disorder

- ✓ Narcolepsy
- ✓ Insomnia disorder
- ✓ Hypersomnolence
- ✓ Parasomnias
- ✓ Breating related sleep disorder
- ✓ Restless leg syndrome

3.Bipolar Related Disorder

- ✓ Mania
- ✓ Depressive Episode

4. Anxiety Disorder

- ✓ General Anxiety Disorder (GAD)
- ✓ Agoraphobia
- ✓ Social Anxiety Disorder (SAD)
- ✓ Specific Phobia
- ✓ Separation Anxiety Disorder
- ✓ Panic

5. Eating Disorder

- ✓ Anorexia nervosa
- ✓ Bulimia nervosa
- ✓ Rumination disorder
- ✓ Pica
- ✓ Binge eating disorder

6. Stress related Disorder

- ✓ Acute Stress Disorder
- ✓ Adjustment disorder
- ✓ Post-Traumatic Stress Disorder (PTSD)
- ✓ Reactive Attachment Disorder

7. Disruptive Disorder

- ✓ Kleptomania
- ✓ Pyromania
- ✓ Intermittent explosive disorder
- ✓ Conduct disorder
- ✓ Oppositional defiant disorder

8. Substance related Disorders

Alcohol, Cannabis, Inhalant-Use, Stimulant use, Tobacco Use Disorders

9. Somatic Symptom Disorders

- ✓ Acute Stress Disorder
- ✓ Illness Anxiety Disorder
- ✓ Conversion Disorder
- ✓ Factitious Disorder

10. Dissociative Disorder

- ✓ Dissociative Amnesia
- ✓ Dissociative Identity Disorder
- ✓ Depersonalization disorder

11.Obsessive Compulsive Disorders

Alcohol, Cannabis, Inhalant-Use, Stimulant use, Tobacco Use Disorders

12.Neuro Cognitive Disorders

Delirium

13. Schizophrenia Disorders

14. Depressive Disorder

Claudia et al. (2021) investigated psychological disorder/distress during COVID 19. Furthermore, the psychological disorder patients affected by COVID-19 are strongly affected by mental illness compared with other COVID patients. It is suggested that COVID-19 patients be monitored for mental disorders such as stress, sleep disorders, etc., during the COVID post period.

Sanaz et al. (2021) investigated and evaluated post-COVID-19 mental and physical health problems. Also, psychological problems like anxiety, depression, PTSD, and fatigue affected the post-COVID 19 patients.

Anand et al. (2021) investigated the factors that affected the psychological distress of the Indian population during the pandemic of COVID 19. The snowball method was used to study the Indian population of 1543 people, using elements such as socio-demographic, community, health-related risk factors, intrapersonal factors, and psychological components. A machine learning algorithm was used to model and analyze the data to determine the most critical factors.

Matsumoto et al. (2022) investigated the post-COVID effect on the human mental health of Swedish and Japanese populations. In this study, anxiety, depression, and post-traumatic stress are measured by looking at the answers to questions about demographic factors.

Xiong et al. (2020) investigated the post-COVID impact on patients in countries such as Denmark, Turkey, Spain, Italy, China, Iron, Turkey, Nepal, and the U.S. conducted a systematic review to determine the physical and mental health of post-COVID patients. It is similar to the previous study where the patients were affected by anxiety, depression, PTSD, psychological disorders, and stress, which affect human physical and mental health.

Delfina Janiri et al. (2020) proposed that the patients who suffered from COVID-19 were affected by psychological distress, depression, and stress from the detailed study using the questionaries review conducted with a sample size of 61 aged above 60.

Rogers et al. (2020) stated that insomnia, anxiety, memory loss, depression, fatigue, stress, and irritation are the significant post-COVID illness psychological impacts that patients suffer irrespective of age and gender from the detailed metadata. The patients are affected by this for three consecutive months, which differs based on age and gender.

Murch et al. (2021) investigated the supply and decisions during the first COVID-19 wave pandemic through an exploratory modelling approach using the UK health care system under uncertain conditions. Further developed the discrete simulation model to determine the optimal decision and supply and decision using a multi-server queuing network.

Maarten et al. (2022) used the computation and mathematical modelling approach to understand the complex behavior of psychological disorders by integrating the inter and intra-individual factors. This agent-based modelling is carried out to determine the factors affecting the psychological disorder.

Cassidy et al. (2019) developed a system-dynamic and agent-based approach to simulate health behavior at the macro and micro levels to identify the problems.

Darryl et al. (2009) developed a generalized framework to determine the effect of bipolar disorder and the optimal sequence of biological treatment to reduce the effect.

Subit et al. (2021) developed the mathematical model to determine and predict the psychological stress effect due to the dynamic behavior of COVID-19 patients. The proposed model shows the mode of propagation of patients before being affected during COVID and post-COVID in India. The effects of the empirical analysis, numerical simulation, significant psychological factors, and theoretical results are analyzed.

The initial literature review is pertinent during the post-COVID period when patients are affected by mental disorders caused by various psychological factors. The proposed mathematical model in India's geographical region determined an effective method to predict the effects of post-COVID and remedial standard operating procedures.

COVID-19 Impact on Mental Health

Impact of COVID-19 pandemic created the consequences such as loneliness, stress, immobility, monotony, social distance, closure of schools and university, mental stress due to online mode of work culture, depression due to not meeting the relationships, laziness due to not playing in outdoor, sleepless nights, suicidal thinking, the poor habit of day activities, etc., not limited to this, extends much more. The world population in the context of genders and age categories got affected by various psychological changes in behavior due to the pandemic environment. Further, the patients with COVID-19 suffered more from the psychological disorder during and post COVID (lasted for three to six months. Some affected long-lasted with the psychological disorders).

Several researchers predicted and forecasted psychological disorders during the COVID and post COVID-19 using various empirical and statistical studies. Some investigations focused on studying human wealth before and after COVID pandemic lockdowns, resulting in a massive fall in economic growth due to loss of jobs, layoff, and partial payroll, which affects psychological disorders such as distress and depression, low self-esteem, and anxiety. Researchers stated that women's mental health prediction results due to pandemics. Women are affected with more anxiety, depression, and stress due to childcare, parent care, and house financial management than men.

In the current COVID-19 scenario, people's health is affected by self-medication, which leads to overdoses and harmful side effects that cause severe and long-term health problems. People with chronic diseases are highly likely to be affected by severe physical and mental illnesses, including psychological disorders. Further, the people screened for COVID-19 and diagnosis confirmed with a positive test are affected with mood disorders, anxiety, distress, vulnerable behavior, mental disorder, etc.

COVID-19 causes anxiety in patients, non-patients, caregivers, and healthcare professionals because of its infectious potential, the uncertainty of symptoms and prognosis, and government restrictions, all of which lead to social, occupational, psychological, and familial dysfunction, economic, and other domains. Rumors, a deluge of information in the media and on the internet, changes in everyday life and routine, economic instability, discrimination, stigma, a sense of isolation, and guilt add to thc anxiety. Patients and their families must deal with the final three factors. Anxiety is characterized by concern, brooding, the dread of being infected or infecting others, and uneasiness, jitteriness, tremors and palpitations, chest discomfort, and breathing difficulties.

People who are depressed may experience dull mood, weariness, pessimistic, vague sleeping order, and hunger, with feelings of weakness, guilt, and desperateness, steady loss in work output. Elderly adults are highly vulnerable, and they need special care and attention.

Anyone unhappy or exhibits the symptoms listed above should get help from a health professional in the field of mental health, known as a psychologist or psychiatrist. Therapy's first and most crucial step is being conscious, admitting, and understanding that one has psychological issues. Talking to a psychologist professional, living a routine and sound lifestyle, eating good food, avoiding tobacco, and engaging in innovative and creative activities such as singing, painting, writing, music, and dance helps them cope with anxiety. Restriction or blocking access to electronic media is appropriate if one is vulnerable and distressed. The data must be obtained from reliable sources.

Most COVID-19 individuals are asymptomatic, with minor issues that improve over time. Panic should be avoided at all costs. The current situation should be viewed positively, considering that the odds of contracting an infection are extremely low. Simple precautions such as wearing masks, social distancing, and hand washing are sufficient to avoid infection. Be cautious but not alarmed. From the above study, factors such as loneliness, mental stress, distress, anxiety, childcare, depression, and low self-esteem are the source of psychological disorders.

Mathematical Modeling Techniques to Determine the Post-COVID-19 Effect and Its Spread

The new coronavirus illness (COVID-19) is a widespread infectious pandemic disease. Several times, including this year's pandemic, the world has been hit by coronaviruses, including SARS-CoV, SARS-CoV-2, and MERS-CoV. All coronavirus patients have the same symptoms: respiratory problems, fever, dry cough, and so on; however, COVID-19 is more contagious than its predecessors. This disease has afflicted almost every country, and its severity is growing by the day. The disease spreads from country to country primarily due to travel by air, as many people move between the countries.

The countries are severely affected by corona illness. Many persons have been confirmed as COVID-19 positive, and many more are in quarantine, asymptomatic stage. Because asymptomatic and exposed people are affected easily, more people are getting infected daily.

However, because of many cases infected by COVID and inadequate medical capability in most countries, the diagnostic test for confirmation of COVID-19 infection in the exposed, asymptomatic, and quarantined classes is poor. This fact also helps to increase the number of afflicted people. COVID-19 is so dangerous that approximately 42 lakh people have been infected with it since 11 May 2020, with 287,131 dying. Because the disease spreads through interaction and there is currently no effective treatment, reducing social distance and interaction is the only strategy to prevent disease spread. The Chinese government implemented a lockdown program to maintain social distance and can control the disease's spread.

In densely populated nations such as India, Bangladesh, and others, many individuals commute from one location to another for work, and more people migrate from infected countries to these countries. As a result, these countries face a high risk of spreading the disease. The Indian government implemented a lockdown strategy for twenty-one days in the first phase, beginning on March 25, 2020, and lasting until May 17, 2020, to control and stop population movement.

COVID-19 is a highly infectious pandemic disease that is spreading throughout the world. No appropriate specific vaccination, medication, or antiviral therapy can protect or cure this virus. As a result, the current significant challenge worldwide is defending human society against infection. In this case, several preventive measures can protect humans from infection, including maintaining social distance, wearing masks, frequent handwashing with soap and water, etc.

Maintaining social distance is an essential part of the COVID-19 prevention strategy. Maintaining a safe space among people, not members of their household, is social distance. This social distance should be at least six feet in length. Due to their awareness, a section of society maintains distance in social gatherings to avoid infection during the pandemic. It is included to investigate the impact of this significant element (social distance) on illness dynamics.

This work's primary objective is to explore the various mathematical modeling approaches feasible to determine and predict the COVID-19 pre- and post-COVID-19 psychological disorder. Model parameters are evaluated, assessed the adequate reproduction number, and made some predictions regarding the disease's prevalence using daily reported cases from India. The model has been developed. The basic properties, as well as the primary reproduction number, are mentioned. The steady-state analysis of the infection-free equilibrium point is investigated. The following steps are completed: fitting the model, estimation of parameters, validation of the model, and prediction. The primary and adequate reproduction numbers are computed from the actual growth rates.

Many models for the propagation of COVID-19 in India have been presented. Exponential/Poisson-type regression models and compartmental epidemiology models are the two types of models that can be found. The susceptible-infected-removed (SIR) model is one of the compartmental models. A series of differential equations about the number of vulnerable persons, infected people (cases), and people who have been removed (either recovered or dead) at any given moment guide these models. The susceptible-exposed-infected-removed (SEIR) model expands the SIR model that includes an additional compartment of actually exposed people to offer an early thorough review.

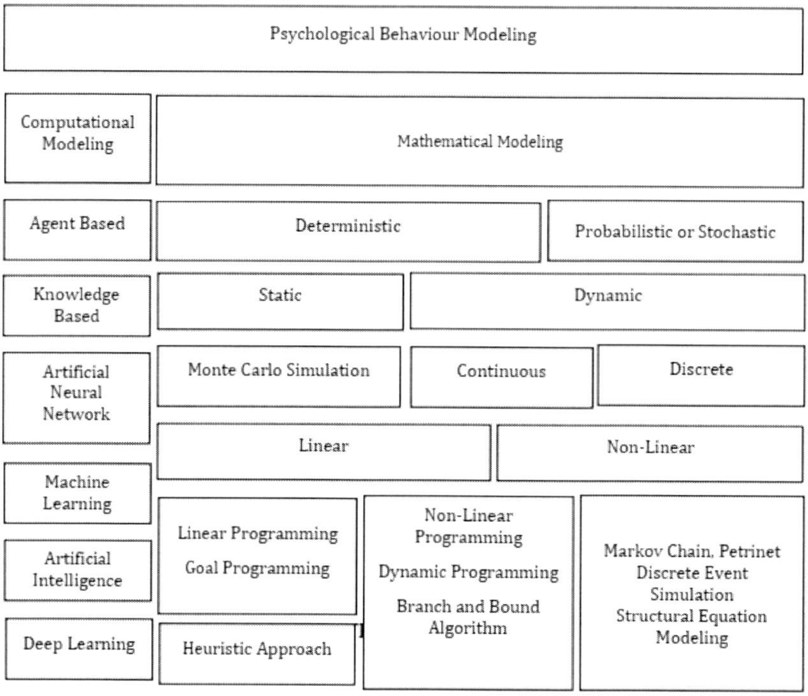

Figure 1. Psychological behavior modeling techniques.

These models' data vary, from simple case counts to age sex demographics, age-specific contact networks, and mobility data. Some, but not all, models are transparent, expressing their assumptions publicly, sharing their code, and updating their predictions regularly. Given how quickly the ground reality changes, such continual recalibration and updating is essential. Psychological behavior is modelled using the list of models given in Figure 1.

Related Works

Mansell Warren and Huddy Vyv (2020) stated that human psychological behavior is a closed-loop model. There is significant interaction, and effects exist between them. Hence closed-loop modeling systems are predicted more accurately than the open-loop system models. Computation modeling techniques are closed-loop systems used to model the complex interaction factors in the system with mathematical and statistical techniques. Further, the model is optimized and validated with the whole system.

Shamil et al. (2020) developed the model to simulate COVID-19 spread in countries using the agent-based modelling technique. Validated the model with the real-time data of the USA, ford county, and KS scenarios and predicted the COVID-19 spread for every hour by tracing the smart mobile of patients.

Thenral and Arunkumar (2020) investigated the literature review on the role of artificial intelligence in potential mental health. Further, developed the thematic framework and its analysis and mapping with concepts from 253 research articles.

Hueniken et al. (2021) developed the machine learning model to determine the identified collection of factors concerning the mental illness symptoms. Further, to predict and monitor the dynamic changes during the pandemic of COVID 2019 based on Canadian population and geographical factors. In addition, this principal component analysis of the data reveals that significant factors such as anxiety and depression impact psychological disorders during the post COVID-19 pandemics.

Zu et al. (2022) developed the continuous-time Markov chain model to determine the spread trend of COVID-19 and to forecast the dynamic distribution of the epidemic with the immunity threshold. The Markov model is more effective than the susceptible-infectious-recovery model in predicting and forecasting given geographic locations.

Patric Glynn et al. (2014) stated the importance of mathematical modelling of psychological disorders to predict the significant factors which cause mental illness and forecast the psychological disorder concerning various pandemic diseases and situations.

Structural equation modeling is a collection of methods for describing assumptions about observable data’s means, variances, and covariances using fewer structural factors given by an underlying conceptual or theoretical model. Gallagher et al. (2020) investigated the significant mental illness factors due to COVID-19 in the specific geographic location of American adults with a sample size of 565. To the study, anxiety and depression are the functional weakening factors of psychological and mental illness using the structural equation modelling shown in Figure 2.

Yao et al. (2020) emphasized that stress, sadness, anxiety, and mental stress are the most aggravating variables for the COVID-19 patients. Richard and eric's (2022) students' knowledge of COVID-19 and attitudes toward the pandemic disease were used to determine the determinants of COVID-19 preventative measures. An online survey of university UG and PG students were used to obtain the study's data. Structural equation modeling explored the association between students' knowledge, attitude, and COVID-19 prevention actions.

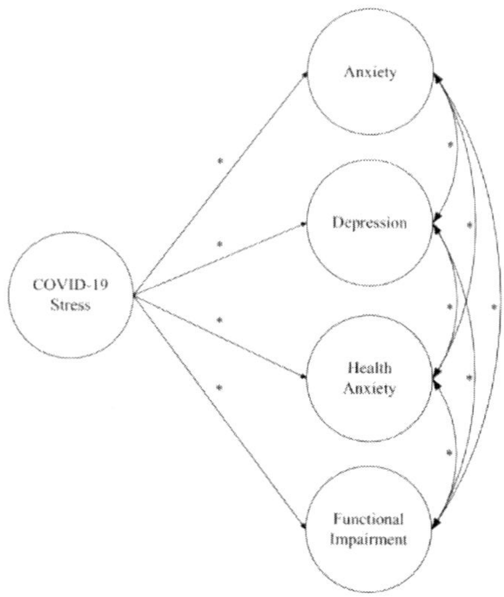

Latent effects of COVID-19 associated stress on outcomes in SEM analysis

Outcome	b	*se*	*p*	*B*	95% CI *B*	R^2
Anxiety (OASIS)	0.190	0.011	< 0.001	0.683	0.627: 0.739	0.467
Depression (ODSIS)	0.202	0.012	< 0.001	0.631	0.576: 0.687	0.398
Health anxiety (HAI-SF)	0.452	0.033	< 0.001	0.550	0.490: 0.610	0.302
Functional impairment (WSAS)	0.634	0.041	< 0.001	0.601	0.546: 0.655	0.361

b represents unstandardized beta coefficient and *B* represents completely standardized beta coefficient

Note: *OASIS* Overall Anxiety Severity and Impairment Scale, *ODSIS* Overall Depression Severity and Impairment Scale, *HAI-sf* Health Anxiety Inventory Short Form, *WSAS* Work, and social modification Scale.

Figure 2. Structural equation model (Gallagher et al. (2020).

Kermack and McKendrick established the epidemic model in 1927. SIR (Susceptible, Infectious, and Recover/Removed) epidemic model is another name for this epidemic model. Avian influenza, Cholera, SARS, Ebola,

Plague, Yellow fever, Meningitis, MERS, influenza, Zika, Rift Valley Fever, and Lassa fever have all been effectively treated with this approach. The SIR model is beneficial for forecasting the end and peak of epidemic diseases and other outbreak-related behavior.

Ramjeet (2020), using the SIR model, the spread of the COVID-2019 was estimated as an outbreak in India and its conclusion. Using Euler's technique, the spread of the COVID-2019 outbreak using the Euler method is a solution method with ordinary differential equations. Three ordinary differential equations are combined in the SIR model. The data from the COVID-2019 outbreak in India on May 8, 2020, is used for the investigation. The introductory level of experimental need identified 135710 sensitive cases, 54340 infectious cases, and 1830 reward/removed cases. The SIR model was applied to examine data from various infectious diseases.

Mohamadou et al. (2020) investigated a complete review of the methodology utilized in these studies and a collection of available datasets in open-source concerning COVID-19 to the scientific community. COVID-19 was investigated and reviewed in 61 academic publications, papers, fact sheets, and websites. The most common mathematical models used were the Susceptible-Exposed-Infected-Removed (SEIR) and Susceptible-infected-recovered (SIR) models, with Convolutional Neural Network (CNN) on X-ray and CT images being the most common AI implementation. Aggregated case reports, medical pictures, management techniques, healthcare personnel, demography, and migration during the outbreak are among the datasets accessible. Mathematical modeling and artificial intelligence have been shown to be effective instruments in the fight against the pandemic.

Saad et al. (2020) proposed intelligent health care services, a mechanism for predicting and preventing the spread of COVID-19. Cloud computing, artificial intelligence, fog computing, machine learning, cognitive computing, deep learning, and edge computing are all advanced intelligent computing. This research proposes a way of forecasting COVID-19 using SIR and machine learning for innovative health care and the well-being of KSA citizens. For mathematical modeling to determine the behavioral effects of the pandemic, knowing the number of susceptible, infected, and recovered patients each day is crucial. It describes the situation for the next 700 days. COVID-19 will expand throughout the population or die off in the long run, according to the proposed system. Scenarios: "no actions," "lockdown," and "new treatments," mathematical modeling, and simulation results are offered here as a means of forecasting the outbreak's course and possible end. The impact of interventions such as lockdown and new medications is compared to the "no action" scenario. The shutdown case changes the area equality rule of the infected curves and delays the peak point by decreasing infection. On the other hand, new treatments significantly impact the curve of infection by reducing the infected people rate over the period. The most significant number of instances is expected to occur between 15 and 30 November 2020, according to COVID-19 projection data.

System Dynamics is a strategy and policy formulation method that uses computers. The primary purpose is to help people make better decisions when facing difficult situations and dynamic systems. Modeling and analyzing dynamic systems can be done using the methods and tools. The model's outputs can share significant findings and help everyone understand how the system operates.

It uses simulation modeling based on feedback systems theory to augment systems thinking approaches. It can be applied to social, managerial, economic, and ecological systems to tackle dynamic challenges. It applies to social, managerial, economic, environmental, and physiological systems. System Dynamics's objective is to encourage people to make improved judgments when faced with complex, dynamic systems. The discipline offers philosophy-based methods for modeling and analyzing dynamic systems. This field includes methodologies and techniques to investigate present decision-making and improve decision-makers learning.

A variety of assumptions underpin System Dynamics modeling.

- It is possible to provoke a structural description of dynamic-oriented complexity articulated as a system dynamics model with a process of indirect/direct link with domain experts using the following methods: i) Interviews, ii) Group model building workshops, and iii) Documentation analysis
- Simulation models are factorized to recreate current and historical behavior; these are known as reference modes of behavior. By running a simulation ahead of time, they can predict.

The proximity of the behavior model to the data in the first scenario provides some confidence in the second. Modelling gives insight into where it may act in the system and the effects of such interventions, which are likewise modelled as a check. Intervention can change existing feedback patterns by removing specific feedback channels or adding new paths.

- Interventions in policy that have an exogenous effect on system behavior.

An endogenous theory of behavioral dynamics has this quality. The models produced by System Dynamics must account for all the dynamic complexity we experience in a system to be helpful.

When external causes dominate dynamic complexity, for example, if oil price thoroughly influences traffic volume, System Dynamics modeling provides more vision into interventions to affect traffic size. When possible, System Dynamics modelers strive for endogenous explanations of the complexity of dynamic nature.

Jeanne et al. (2021) investigated the uncertainties with testing and optimizing strategies for detecting and diagnosing infected people. Researchers used a system's dynamics epidemiology model, as shown in Figure 3, with other interconnected system models in public health, such as hospitals, intensive care units, masks, contact tracing, social distancing, and newly developed testing and diagnostics model. 54 simulations with two scenarios of 10% and 30% asymptomatic people, altering crucial inputs for testing and social distancing, using an orthogonal array Latin Hypercube experimental design. Systems dynamics modeling can deliver speedy and quantitative decision-making results when combined with experimental computer design and statistical analysis. Our findings imply that identifying asymptomatic people in the public and widespread testing, contact tracing, and quarantine can aid in pandemic containment.

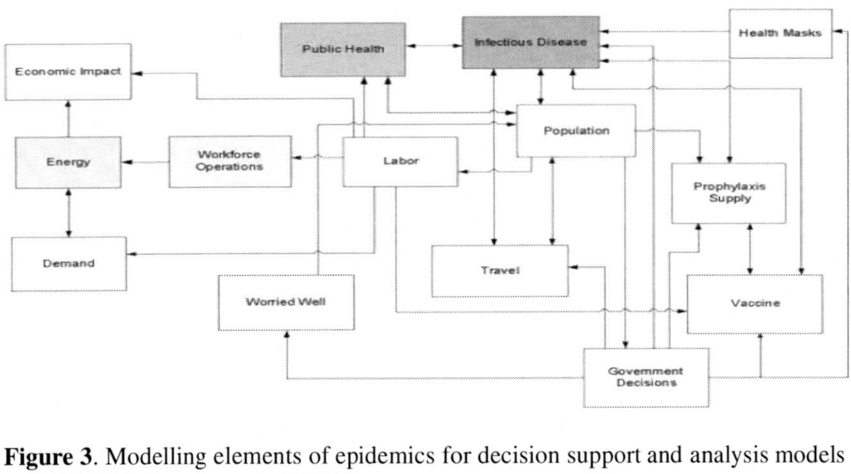

Figure 3. Modelling elements of epidemics for decision support and analysis models – COVID-19 (Jeanne et al. (2021).

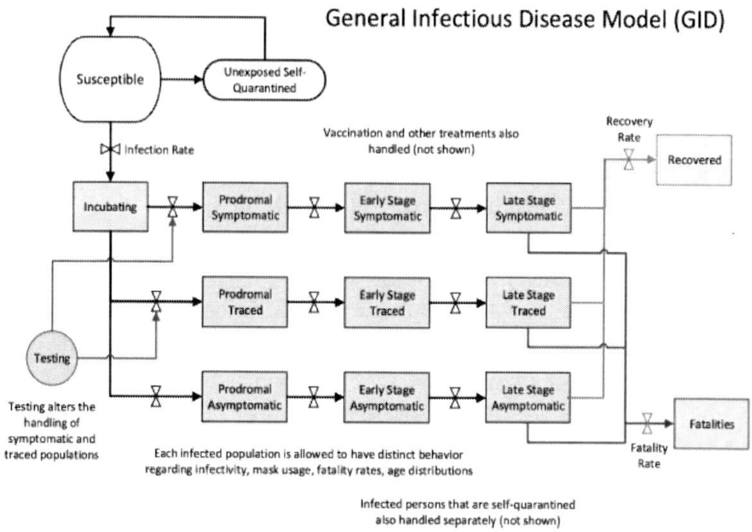

Figure 4. Multi-stage SEIR generalized infectious pandemic disease model (Jeanne et al. (2021).

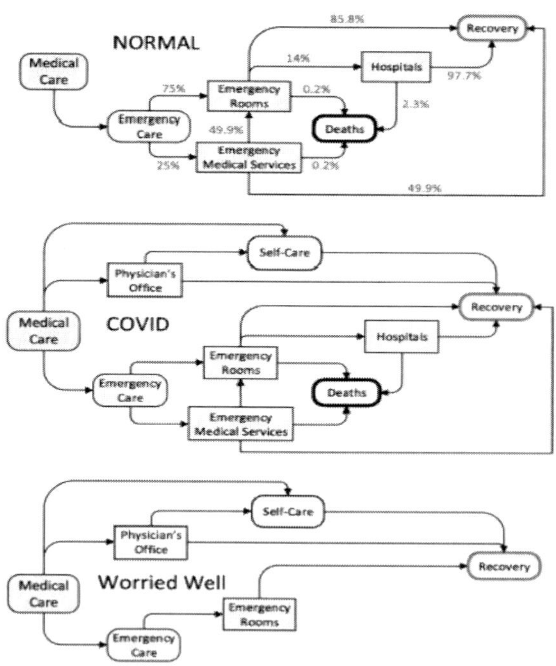

Figure 5. Flow process diagram for emergency care with normal, pandemic COVID-19 patients and worried-well patients in the public health model. (Jeanne et al. (2021).

The above Figures 3, 4, and 5 are investigated by (Jeanne et al. (2021)) by considering the demographic groups such as young, young adults, adults, older adults, elderly, and responders. Further, the sensitivity analysis was conducted to determine the significant interaction between the factors and model validation. Multiple sub-systems systems dynamics modeling can be a flexible and quick way to explain the behavior of epidemics and pandemics. The uncertainty of the system can be better understood when combined with computer-based simulation of the design of experiments using orthogonal Latin sampling, and the sensitivity of mitigations can be readily assessed using correlation analysis. More simulations are simulated and analyzed quickly using the systems dynamics approach.

Conclusion

Unprecedented levels of uncertainty and variability characterize the present COVID-19 pandemic, necessitating a critical knowledge of the diversity recorded in policy, social, biological, and infrastructure outcomes during an epidemic to inform decisions at various levels. With the virus spreading asymptomatically and no quick vaccine or medications available, the best possible diagnosis, tests, a trace of contact, and a quarantine procedure must be optimized. Infected people are not enrolled in trace of contact programs and thus cannot be quarantined if false-negative test results are standard. Asymptomatic people are not recognized and isolated without comprehensive testing. Integrated system dynamics models result in optimizing pandemic decision support and mitigation measures. The discussed mathematical models are significant in predicting psychological and mental illness during the post COVID and the spread rate of COVID.

References

Alharbi, HY, Alharthi, SS, Alzahrani, AS, Dakhel, MKA & Alawaji, ZH. Increased psychological distress after lifting COVID-19 lockdown in the Saudi population : a cross-sectional study. *Middle East Curr Psychiatry* 29, 1 (2022). https://doi.org/10.1186/s43045-021-00167-9.

Anand V, Verma L, Aggarwal A, Nanjundappa P, Rai H (2021) COVID-19 and psychological distress: Lessons for India. *PLoS ONE* 16(8) : e0255683. https://doi.org/10.1371/journal.pone.0255683.

Cassidy, R., Singh, N.S., Schiratti, PR., Semwanga, A, Binyaruka, P, Sachingongu, N, Chama-Chiliba, CM, Chalabi, Za, Borghi, J, Blanchet, K. Mathematical modeling for health systems research: a systematic review of system dynamics and agent-based models. *BMC Health Serv Res* 19, 845 (2019). https://doi.org/10.1186/s12913-019-4627-7.

Daugherty, Darryl, Tairi Roque-Urrea, John Urrea-Roque, Jessica Troyer, Stephen Wirkus, Mason A. Porter, *Mathematical models of bipolar disorder, Communications in Nonlinear Science and Numerical Simulation*, Volume 14, Issue 7, 2009, Pages 2897-2908, ISSN 1007-5704, https://doi.org/10.1016/j. cnsns.2008.10.027.

Fair, Jeanne M., Rene J LeClaire, Lori R Dauelsberg, Mary Ewers, Donatella Pasqualini, Tim Cleland, William Rosenberger (2021), *Systems dynamics and the uncertainties of diagnostics, testing, and contact tracing for COVID-19, Methods*, Volume 195, 2021, Pages 77-91, ISSN 1046-2023, https://doi.org/10.1016/j.ymeth.2021.03.008.

Gallagher, Matthew & Zvolensky, Michael & Long, Laura & Rogers, Andrew & Garey, Lorra. (2020). The Impact of Covid-19 Experiences and Associated Stress on Anxiety, Depression, and Functional Impairment in American Adults. *Cognitive Therapy and Research.* 44. 10.1007/s10608-020-10143-y.

Hueniken, K., Somé, N. H., Abdelhack, M., Taylor, G., Elton Marshall, T., Wickens, C. M., Hamilton, H. A., Wells, S., & Felsky, D. (2021). Machine Learning-Based Predictive Modeling of Anxiety and Depressive Symptoms During 8 Months of the COVID-19 Global Pandemic: Repeated Cross-sectional Survey Study. *JMIR mental health*, 8(11), e32876. https://doi.org/10.2196/32876.

Jiaqi Xiong, Orly Lipsitz, Flora Nasri, Leanna MW, Lui, Hartej Gill, Lee Phan, David Chen-Li, Michelle Iacobucci, Roger Ho, Amna Majeed, Roger S. McIntyre, Impact of COVID-19 pandemic on mental health in the general population : A systematic review, *Journal of Affective Disorders*, Volume 277, 2020, Pages 55-64.

Liang, L, Ren, H, Cao, R, Hu, Y, Qin, Z, Li, C, & Mei, S. The Effect of COVID-19 on Youth Mental Health. *Psychiatr Q* 91, 841–852 (2020). https://doi.org/10.1007/s11126-020-09744-3.

Mansell Warren, Huddy Vyv (2020), Why Do We Need Computational Models of Psychological Change and Recovery, and How Should They Be Designed and Tested?, *Frontiers in Psychiatry*, 11, DOI=10.3389/fpsyt.2020.00624.

Matsumoto, K., Hamatani, S., Shimizu, E., Käll, A., & Andersson, G. Impact of post-COVID conditions on mental health: a cross-sectional study in Japan and Sweden. *BMC Psychiatry* 22, 237 (2022). https://doi.org/10.1186/s12888-022-03874-7.

Mohamadou, Y., Halidou, A. & Kapen, P.T. A review of mathematical modeling, artificial intelligence, and datasets used in the study, prediction, and management of COVID-19. *Appl Intell 50*, 3913–3925 (2020). https://doi.org/10.1007/s10489-020-01770-9.

Murch, BJ, Cooper, JA, Hodgett, TJ, Gara, EL, Walker, JS, Wood, RM. (2021), Modelling the effect of first-wave COVID-19 on mental health services, *Operations Research for Health Care*, Volume 30, 100311 https://doi.org/10.1016/j.orhc. 2021.100311.

Oppenauer Claudia, Burghardt Juliane, Kaiser Elmar, Riffer Friedrich, Sprung Manuel (2021), *Psychological Distress During the COVID-19 Pandemic in Patients with Mental or Physical Diseases, Frontiers in Psychology* 12., DOI=10.3389/fpsyg.2021.703488 https://doi.org/10.3389/fpsyg.2021.703488.

Patric Glynn, Sathya D. Unudurthi, Thomas J. Hund (2014), Mathematical modeling of physiological systems: An essential tool for discovery, *Life Sciences*, Volume 111, Issues 1–2, 2014, Pages 1-5, ISSN 0024-3205, https://doi.org/10.1016/j.lfs. 2014.07.005.

Qu Z, Wang CW, Zhang X, Ho AH, Wang X. Prevalence and determinants of depression among survivors 8 months after the Wenchuan earthquake. *J Nerv Ment Dis*. 2014 ; 202 :275–9.

Ramjeet Singh Yadav, *Mathematical Modeling and Simulation of SIR Model for COVID-2019 Epidemic Outbreak: A Case Study of India,* https://doi.org/10.1101/2020.05.15.2010307.

Richard Twum Ampofo, Eric Nimako Aidoo (2022), Structural equation modeling of COVID-19 knowledge and attitude as determinants of preventive practices among university students in Ghana, *Scientific African*, Volume 16, 2022, e01182, ISSN 2468-2276, https://doi.org/10.1016/j.sciaf.2022.e01182.

Rogers, JP, Chesney, E, Oliver, D, Pollak, TA, McGuire, P, Fusar-Poli, P, Zandi, MS, Lewis, G, & David, AS. Psychiatric and neuropsychiatric presentations associated with severe coronavirus infections : a systematic review and meta-analysis compared to the COVID-19 pandemic. *Lancet Psychiatry*. (2020) 7 :611–27. DOI : 10.1016/S2215-0366(20)30203-0.

Saad Awadh Alanazi, M. M. Kamruzzaman, Madallah Alruwaili, Nasser Alshammari, Salman Ali Alqahtani, Ali Karime, "Measuring and Preventing COVID-19 Using the SIR Model and Machine Learning in Smart Health Care," *Journal of Healthcare Engineering,* vol. 2020, Article, ID 8857346, 12 pages, 2020. https://doi.org/10.1155/2020/8857346.

Shamil, Md. S, Farheen, F, Ibtehaz, N, Khan, IM, & Rahman, MS. An Agent-Based Modeling of COVID-19 : Validation, Analysis, and Recommendations. *Cogn Comput* (2021). https://doi.org/10.1007/s12559-020-09801-w.

Shanbehzadeh S, Tavahomi M, Zanjari N, Ebrahimi-Takamjani I, Amiri-Arimi S. Physical and mental health complications post-COVID-19 : Scoping review. *J Psychosom Res.* 2021 Aug; 147 :110525. DOI : 10.1016/j.jpsychores.2021.110525. Epub 2021 May 20. PMID : 34051516 ; PMCID : PMC8133797.

Subit K. Jain, Swati Tyagi, Neeraj Dhiman, Jehad Alzabut, Study of the dynamic behavior of psychological stress during COVID-19 in India: A mathematical approach, *Results in Physics*, Volume 29, 2021, 104661, ISSN 2211-3797, https://doi.org/10.1016/j.rinp.2021.104661.

Thenral, M, and Arunkumar Annamalai. "Telepsychiatry and the Role of Artificial Intelligence in Mental Health in Post-COVID-19 India: A Scoping Review on Opportunities." *Indian journal of psychological medicine* vol. 42,5 428-434. 8 Sep. 2020, DOI :10.1177/0253717620952160.

Van den Ende, Maarten WJ, Sacha Epskamp, Michael H. Lees, Han L.J. van der Maas, Reinout W. Wiers, Peter MA. Sloot (2022), A review of mathematical modeling of addiction regarding both (neuro-) psychological processes and the social contagion perspectives, *Addictive Behaviors*, Volume 127, 2022, 107201, ISSN 0306-4603, https://doi.org/10.1016/j.addbeh.2021.107201.

Wangari, Isaac Mwangi, Stanley Sewe, George Kimathi, Mary Wainaina, Virginia Kitetu, Winnie Kaluki, "Mathematical Modelling of COVID-19 Transmission in Kenya : A Model with Reinfection Transmission Mechanism," *Computational and Mathematical Methods in Medicine*, vol. 2021, Article ID 5384481, 18 pages, 2021. https://doi.org/10.1155/2021/5384481.

Xu, Zhaobin, Hongmei Zhang, and Zuyi Huang. 2022. "A Continuous Markov-Chain Model for the Simulation of COVID-19 Epidemic Dynamics" *Biology* 11, no. 2 : 190. https://doi.org/10.3390/biology11020190.

Yao H, Chen JH, Xu YF. Patients with mental health disorders in the COVID-19 epidemic. *The Lancet Psychiatry*. 2020 ;7(4) : e21. DOI : 10.1016/S2215-0366(20) 30090-0.

Chapter 9

Impact of Post-COVID-19 on the Elderly-Emotional Stress and Effects: A Data Science Approach

Parimi Shiva Kalyan[1,*], B. Sree Keerthi Meghana[2] and Sriman Naini[3]

[1]Accenture, Hyderabad Telangana, India

[2]Chaitanya Bharathi Institute of Technology, Gandipet, Hyderabad, Telangana, India

[3]Rosenheim Technical University of Applied Science, Germany

Abstract

Considering the current level of the majority of people affected by the COVID-19 pandemic in public, there seem to be lengthy financial and psychiatric consequences. Depression is a significant psychological condition among the aged, affecting their well-being. The goal of this research is to investigate the levels of tension and related variables in older adults. These could result in severe emotional and physiological abnormalities, including PTSD (post-traumatic stress disorder), stress, nervousness, suicidal tendencies, and behavioral issues. Isolation, disinformation on social networking sites, financial instability, and discrimination are all possible causes. Because medical practitioners are at significantly higher risk of getting PTSD and exhaustion, it is critical to study and investigate the effects and drivers to avoid, recognize, and control these disorders. Providing customer service for nervous people, videoconferencing, internet networking & assistance communities, promoting relaxation, investigating psychiatric repercussions, and

*Corresponding Author's Email: pskalyan070@gmail.com.

In: Data Science Applications of Post-COVID-19 Psychological Disorders
Editor: Vijayalakshmi Kakulapati
ISBN: 979-8-88697-165-1

designing and implementing appropriate therapies are relevant diagnoses.

Keywords: aged, panic, psychological, PTSD, consequences, coronavirus, risk, loneliness, misinformation, social media, socio-economic status

Introduction

The coronavirus spread in the United States in early 2020, and older persons were disproportionately affected by the pandemic, even with more severe consequences and increased morbidity. Elderly individuals with psychological stress and more profound behavioral control are better than youngsters. Initial statistics point to a much more complicated scenario. However, during the early phases of the pandemic, elderly adults are more resistive to the anxiousness, sadness, and psychiatric tension problems that plague youth [1].

A small study has viewed prolonged emotional stimuli of people healed from COVID-19; a medicine used to treat colorectal cancer [2]. Unique variables influence a victim's chance of acquiring psychotic disorders and how people deal with reality, and emotional well-being and approaches may be affected. Disposition relates to initial variances in behavioral reaction; it is consistent over the lifetime and has substantial genetic bases [3].

Effective and efficient attitudes may alter feelings systems, with the recurrent depressive attitude that has been linked to panic disorder providing proof [4]. Mood instability is characterized by problems in various aspects, such as the capacity to comprehend and comprehend intense emotions, adjust their intensity or length, and handle emotions. The objective was to collect information that could be used to forecast potential mental disorders, either positively or negatively. It has been demonstrated that distress can reduce psychiatric suffering [5].

This chapter discusses the emotional effects of the COVID-19 pandemic on the older adult community after the outbreak in several nations. The majority thought that the catastrophe had significantly influenced people's everyday lives, particularly disruptions in behaviors and the cancellation of essential tasks. Approximately 40% of the individuals experienced impairment consequences, 25% indicated a risk for severe anxiousness, 40% reported emotional distress, and 40% expressed tension. Women, youngsters, and others who lost their employment throughout the catastrophe revealed significant adverse pain. What scared people the most was the possibility of a financial disaster caused by the epidemic. Investigators discovered characteristics related to more effective mental illnesses, including satisfaction with medical emergency information, participation in entertainment, and the feeling of being in a healthy condition.

The COVID-19 pandemic's self-isolation and self-quarantine procedures are associated with social and medical expertise gained from prior outbreaks [6]. Separation and confinement have been found to enhance suicidal behavior [7]. Increases fatigue, raises worries about transmitting relatives, disrupts vital commodities deliveries, and causes frustration. Quarantine is the isolation and restriction of movement of persons who may have been infected to a compromised immune system to determine if they get ill and thus mitigate the possibility of transmission to others [8], rationing, rage, and lawsuit, as well as stigmatizing afflicted persons.

In this chapter, the general adult public's emotional stability in Worldwide during the initial phases of the COVID-19 epidemic, such as the emotional aspects of the epidemic such as interference, avoidance, emotional dysregulation signs, nervousness, melancholy, and tension. And to investigate the intensity to which the factors, anxiousness, pressure, and uncertainty, are related to emotional effect, which contains demographic factors such as age, gender, income level, and ecological factors throughout isolation.

The remaining chapter describes the proposed study as a background, followed by related works. Section 3 discusses the different contexts of older people's emotional stress. Section 4 discusses implementation analysis followed by discussion, in section 6 concluding remarks followed by future enhancement.

Background

The epidemic of COVID-19 has had a severe influence on societal emotional stability. As a result, surveillance and inspection of the public's emotional wellness throughout a catastrophic situation is an important priority. Although during disease outbreaks, a wide range of psychological impacts were documented at the personal, societal, regional, and worldwide levels. People are more susceptible to being afraid of becoming sick or dying, feeling stressed, and also being stigmatized by everyone [9]. Rapid evaluation of patients in the initial phases of a psychiatric condition improves the effectiveness of therapeutic efforts. Healthcare emergencies, including the COVID-19 epidemic, cause adverse alterations in both clinical professionals and civilians, and these emotional alterations are triggered by dread, panic, melancholy, or uncertainty [10].

Older people confined or locked up with relatives, friends, or carers may be more vulnerable to maltreatment and neglect. Older adults in disadvantaged settings, including refugee homes, underserved areas, and jails, are more susceptible. It is especially suitable for older caretakers, many of whom are women and provide care for the elderly. The transfer might harm our mental health. The hazards are more significant for older people who live separately and should be more technologically connected than others [11].

According to the CDC (US Centers for Disease Control and Prevention), over one-third of US individuals suffered mood swings as of June 2020 [12]. Emerging adults, a generation that's already witnessed significant growth in the number of psychiatric problems over the last age, had nearly twice the incidences [13]. The surge in melancholy and the disturbance of daily existence generated by stay-at-home restrictions, the university shut down, and interpersonal separation techniques [14].

Health professionals and caretakers must evaluate data quality and examine how a specific patient and daughter's lack of resources might be managed. This can involve available funds, such as inaccessibility to advanced technologies, societal influences (an absence of relatives), or intellectual or genetic factors. Technologies have been recognized as crucial in sustaining connectedness and gaining access and quality.

Throughout an epidemic, the maturity level of 21–40 years had much more significant psychological distress, sadness, and emotional turmoil than the entire society. The fundamental cause for this appears to have been that peer group worries about the pandemic's potential consequences and financial crises. This is because they are major functional operational elements in societal structure and are influenced by layoffs and layoffs [15].

Related Works

The epidemic has considerably improved melancholy and harmed the emotional well-being of seniors. Psychological depression is hindered by lacking a confidante or a deep emotional connection [16]. Well-being is defined as lacking social/psychological alienation and unaided psychological wellness. Anxiety, depression, sadness, and a lack of calm and happiness are mental health issues [17].

In aged people, society has been linked to enhanced quality of life, increased muscular strength, stability, cognitively, and decreased morbidity and impairment [18]. Activities associated with communal gatherings and events increase physical fitness, while engagement with other elderly adults stimulates sensations [19]. Communities have stopped as a security precaution during the COVID-19 outbreak. Social distancing may reduce social gathering, negatively influencing emotional well-being [20].

Detached older people engage with much less strength training and more sedentary behavior than non-isolated elderly adults [21]. Performance has been defined as any range of motion that generates an energy expenditure of more than 1.5 metabolic equivalents of work (MET). Fit and healthy behavior is any awake behavior performed while sitting, lounging, or laying. Because, there is a clear relationship between immobility every time spending quality in the aged [22]. Suggestions must be established to minimize psychological effects on those experiencing isolation and loneliness due to the epidemic.

Although teenage folks have the most significant level of COVID-19-related psychological anguish [23], older people are also impacted. Research that followed 776 persons for one week on daily hassles throughout the first epidemic discovered that, although there were identical dimensions of psychological distress, older adults aged 60–91 experienced fewer adverse effects than teenagers [24]. Surprisingly, we discovered a one-year rise in loneliness exclusively among respondents in their 60s, which contradicts the previous UCL COVI-19 research study [25].

About Elder People Emotional Stress

Post-COVID issues are various potential, reoccurring, or persistent illness issues that can arise four or maybe more months after becoming contaminated with the pathogen that affects COVID-19. Such diseases might manifest as various sorts and permutations of medical issues. Even those who did not exhibit signs in the weeks or months following their infection can develop post-COVID problems.

Specific post-COVID symptoms might be prolonged COVID, lengthy COVID, post-acute COVID-19, protracted COVID consequences, or severe COVID. The CDC and scientists worldwide strive to understand more about the objectives and long health implications of COVID-19 [26].

Cognitive difficulties seem to be more likely in those recuperating from comparable disorders. A case analysis of healthcare data in the United States, for instance, found that the probability of acquiring behavioral disease after COVID-19 was more significant than in patients recovering from persons other physical conditions like flu [27].

Following a severe COVID-19 outbreak, emotional dysregulation (anxiety, melancholy, and PTSD) is widespread, with anxiousness being the most frequent. Emotional problems often gradually improve, but they may last longer than six months for a fraction of patients. Those hospitalized are more prone to experience chronic psychiatric issues [28].

Older people and those with various severe clinical illnesses are more likely to have prolonged COVID-19 signs. Instead of better and healthier individuals, even teenagers may feel ill for long periods of infected patients. The following are possible long-term indications and manifestations:

- Tiredness
- Breathing difficulty
- Congestion
- Musculoskeletal discomfort
- Acute coronary syndrome
- Cognition, concentrate,
- insomnia
- Joint stiffness
- migraine
- The rapid or throbbing pulse
- Lack of taste and smell
- Clinical depression
- Temperature
- Standing discomfort
- Deteriorated effects after neurological activity [29].
- 38 percent of patients have feelings of stress;
- Thirty-two percent have psychological distress.
- PTSD – 34 percent

Tiredness and Mood Swings

Patients who experience COVID-19, a novel infection that can create dangers related to pulmonary difficulties, may later suffer PTSD, sadness, and anxiety.

SARS survivors have developed severe tiredness disorder, a complicated illness characterized by an intense weariness that intensifies with real or perceived exertion but does not better with relaxation.

In contrast to the cognitive burden of loneliness, limiting or discontinuing regular exercise harms health. Consequently, the solitary older people in an unsatisfactory situation of socially supportive, intellectual, and sensory activation may aggravate medical conditions and result in a melancholy and unfortunate death. [30].

Complications arise in negligence with preventative efforts, including interpersonal separation, absence of sanitation, and suspension of proper therapy without the aim of obtaining expert support [31]. Loneliness is a psychological problem even for people that do not have a mental disease. If preventive actions are not done, it is anticipated that one-third to the majority of the people are acquiring psychobiological signs.

The aged people are more prone to self-isolation or consciousness, and hence tend to develop anxiousness and discomfort effects. In the meantime, seniors might be less digitally aware, relying on newspaper articles, radios, and tv for news content. News items in the media should provide unpleasant information about the infection and more good news regarding recovery, with little emphasis on "fake news," which promotes anxiety and worry. Assurances concerning employment and wealth throughout self-isolation and self-quarantine may decrease anxiety about money and financial hardship and dissuadc pcrsons.

When many individuals must come together to accomplish a common goal, negative stereotypes such as ageism and the demonization of the elderly are inevitable. It concerns that insults and offensive language directed towards elderly adults have surfaced in ongoing opinion and digital networking. The elderly is incredibly varied, with genetic factors only weakly tied to maturity level. Initiatives and messages must present a particular, unobscured image of the pandemic's influence on elderly adults and their involvement in the responses [32].

Some older people worldwide are impoverished and socially excluded. In certain underdeveloped nations, the proportion of older people living in poverty might reach 80% [33]. Because older women have less accessibility to financial opportunities –through work, commodities like farmland, or retirement protection – than males, the economic recession would most probably affect them.

Inadequate sleep, nervousness, frustration, panic disorder, night terrors, blankness, afraid of contracting coronavirus, fear of disseminating the infectious disease to others, well-being fear, the experience of confinement, anxiousness associated with unpredictability, fatality fear, and death in abnormal conditions without connectivity to other relatives are among some of the emotional problems that can occur in elderly persons.

People with mobility limitations and poor prognosis of physical and psychiatric illnesses, older people, are at an elevated risk of confusion or return of dementia. There are very few specific obstacles in older people before cognitive problems. Behavioral issues are common in elderly people with intellectual disabilities. They are trying to understand better the COVID-19 pandemic's preventative actions and related information. It is challenging for caretakers to limit movement in dementia patients. It is also problematic for elderly affected individuals to comply with routine washing hands and feelings of loneliness through a preventative surgical mask.

Coronavirus in care facilities and hospitals is wreaking effects on the lives of the elderly, with disturbing allegations revealing incidences of negligence or maltreatment. Older people confined or confined with their relatives or carers may be more susceptible to harm, mistreatment, and abuse. Older people in insecure settings, including refugee camps, poor neighborhoods, and monasteries, are especially vulnerable. They're frequently among some caretakers reacting to the epidemic, elevating their risk of contamination.

Lengthy periods of loneliness may negatively impact the well-being of older people since they are more inclined to be digitized and integrated. The earnings and employability consequences are significant, considering that the number of older people in the workforce has grown by over 10% globally during the last 3 decades [34]. Welfare benefits can offer a security net, but distribution shortages are significant in certain emerging regions, with fewer than 20% of older people of retirement age getting a pension.

Methodology and Implementation Analysis

Perceived stress level to the level of risk, with results of 14 and more significant, indicating solid levels of perceived emotional turmoil [35]. The Basic Anxiousness Disorder-7 element measure (GAD-7) [36] was used to assess anxiety, with scores of ten or higher indicating likely Generalized Anxiety Disorder (GAD), and the Health Status scale with scores of ten or higher indicating possible Disruptive Mood Dysregulation [37].

Specific catastrophe research demonstrates that the aged are more susceptible to the adverse affective consequences of significant events, including PTSD [38]. Nevertheless, numerous research has discovered that aging has a neuroprotective effect. Elderly catastrophe patients often exhibit tension, anxiousness, and emotional distress more than young adults, which may be accounted for by their extensive experience, past crisis risk, or fewer lifestyle obligations.

It can be observed from Avg_PSS10_UCLA VS Dem_Age that the stress levels tend to decline in elders as their age progresses. This can be because of various isolation methods used by the government and constant health monitoring for elders, ensuring that they are safe and sound. We can see a steep drop between 90 and 100 as life expectancy becomes too low, leading to missing data for that tenure. The Loneliness VS Age spike tends to increase or be in a steady state; as a result, we can see consistent spikes from 70 to 90 years old. Then there's a steep decline which might be because of them dying or losing their loved ones at the age > 90 years.

The elderly tend to show moderate/appropriate confidence in their respective country measures. As we can observe, the maximum rating goes for 5.0, which stands for appropriate, and the second highest is 4.0, which shows trust issues. However, most Elderly populations stand by Government regulations and practices. All the elderly tend to comply with prevention guidelines, i.e., isolate themselves and limit their outer world contact. We can see a steady increase in the Loneliness VS Stress graph, which makes sense as Stress increases when a person is lonely because of multiple factors. According to the Dem Isolation VS Dem Age graph, most persons over the age of 55 are isolated in medical institutions or other settings, which puts them in danger, or their lives go normal for them.

This research aims to traverse through a data set of 125306 rows and 119 unique column/data variables. Which point towards various levels of stress, isolation, confidence in preventive measures against COVID spread, dependency, job status, etcetera has been considered to have an in-depth understanding of how the pandemic affected lifestyles of individuals above 40. This consists of distinct visualizations in the form of catplots, bar plots, relplots, violin plots, and scatter plots graphs that map across 4-5 unique dimensions, giving a high level and a deep dive into the metric values taken on the Likert scale.

The data set contains variables like
Dem_age, Dem_gender,
Dem_edu, Dem_edu_mom, Dem_employment,Country,Dem_Expat,
Dem_state,

Dem_maritalstatus,
Dem_dependents, Dem_riskgroup, Dem_isolation
Dem_isolation_adults.

Table 1. The sample of data set variables

	ID	answered_all	Duration..in.seconds.	RecordedDate	UserLanguage	Dem_age	Dem_gender	Dem_edu	Dem_edu_mom	Dem_employment	...
2	3	No	127	5/30/2020 22:40	SAR	47	Female	Some College, short continuing education or eq...	Some College or equivalent	Self-employed	...
3	4	No	1710	5/29/2020 22:47	BG	79	Male	College degree, bachelor, master	College degree	Not employed	...
4	5	No	2239	5/29/2020 22:42	SAR	61	Female	Some College, short continuing education or eq...	Up to 12 years of school	Retired	...
5	6	Yes	1221	5/29/2020 21:25	IT	68	Male	College degree, bachelor, master	College degree	Retired	...
10	11	No	656	5/30/2020 20:14	SAR	42	Female	College degree, bachelor, master	Up to 12 years of school	Full time employed	...

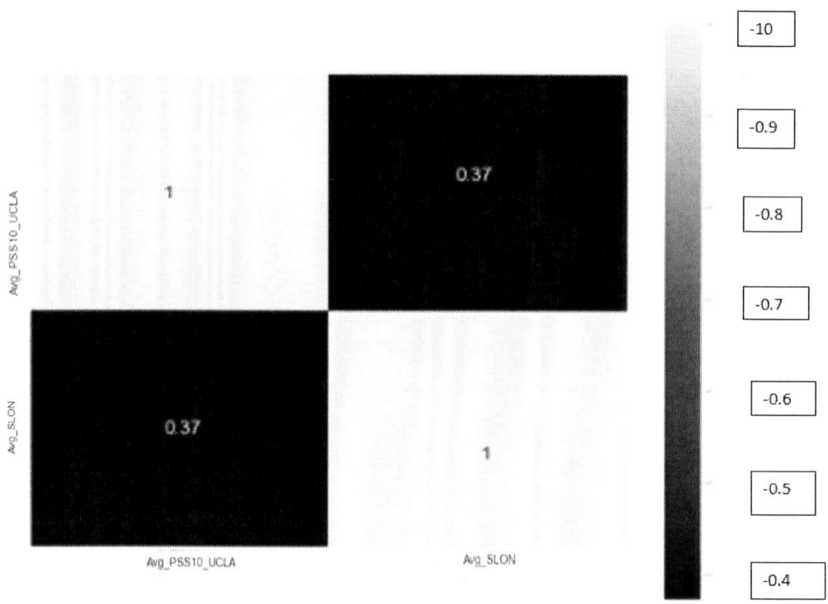

Figure 1. Different variables which have highly related using the heat map as evidence.

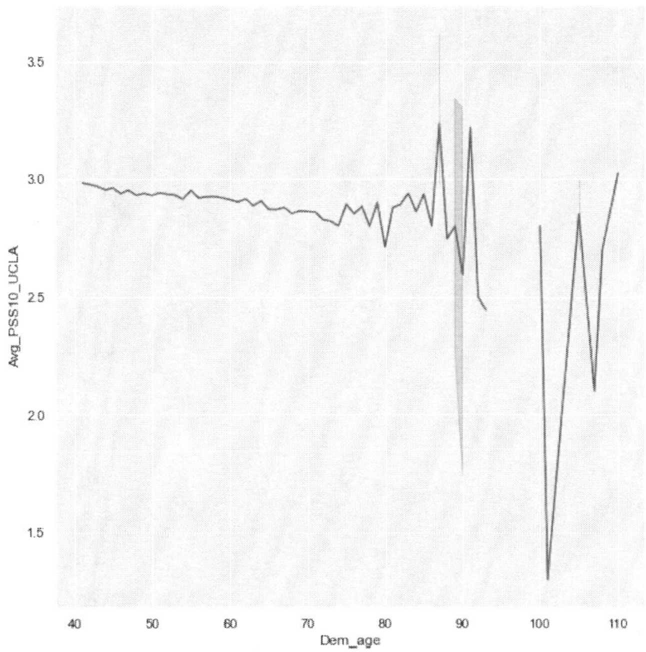

Figure 2. Perceived stress vs. age graph.

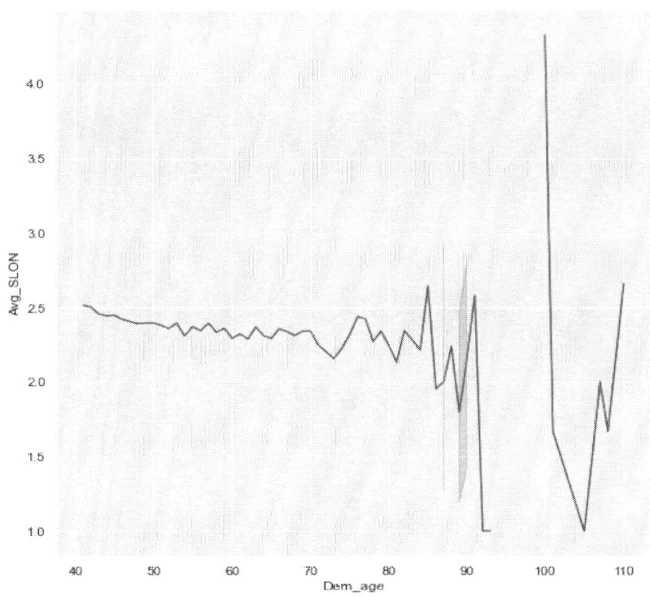

Figure 3. Loneliness vs. age graph.

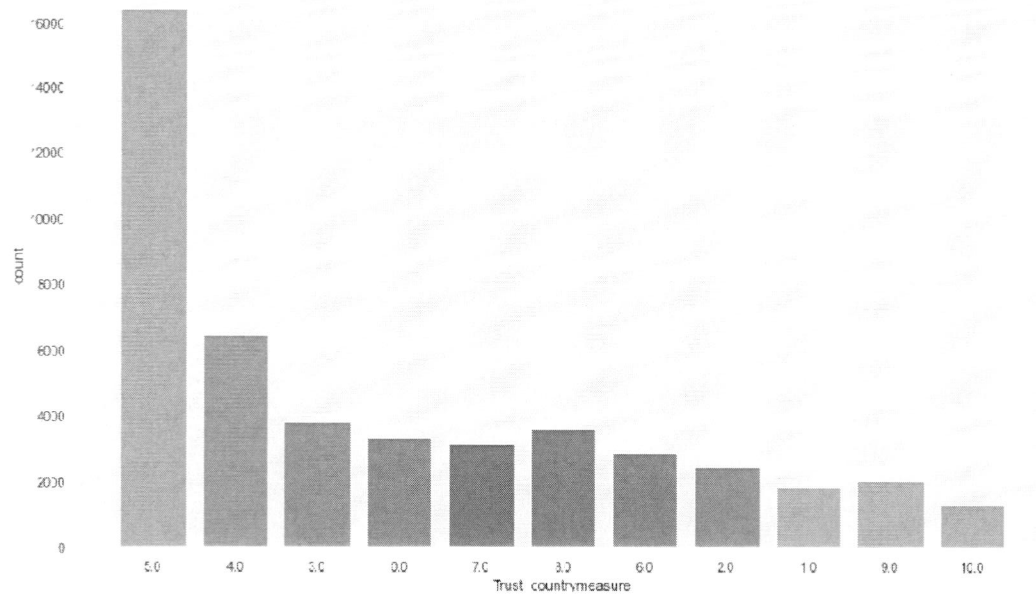

Figure 4. Trust_countrymeasure vs. count.

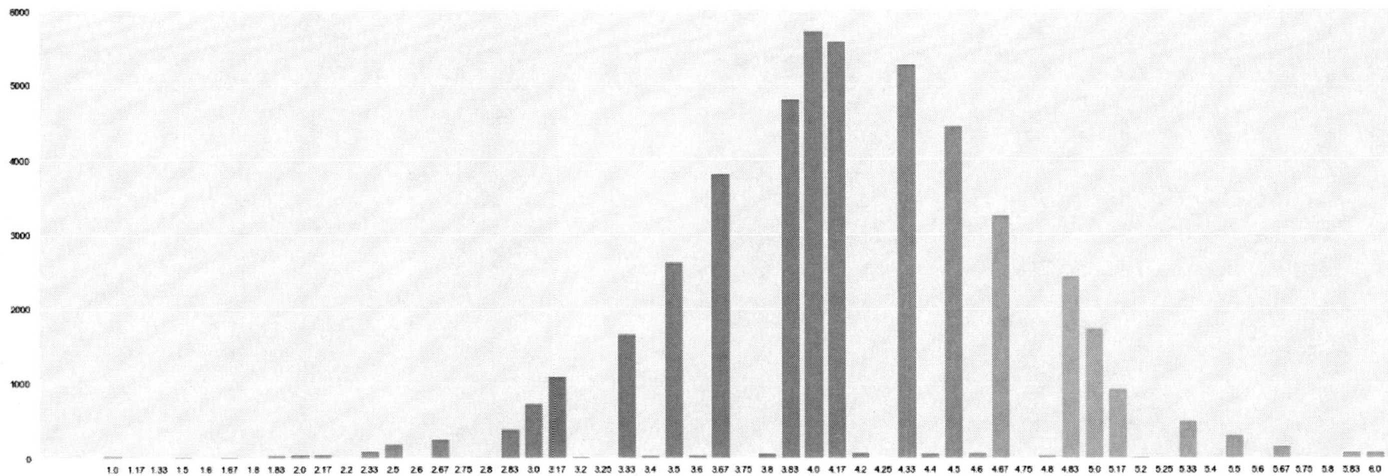

Figure 5. Average compliance vs. count.

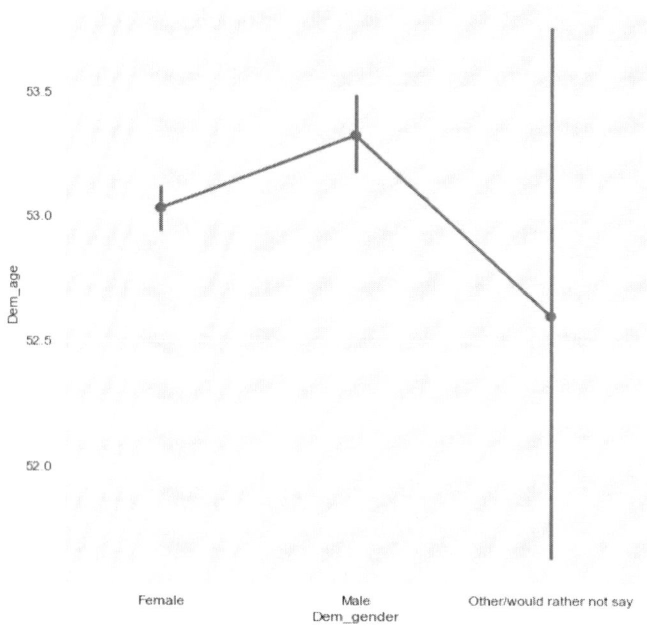

Figure 6. Demographic factors age vs. gender.

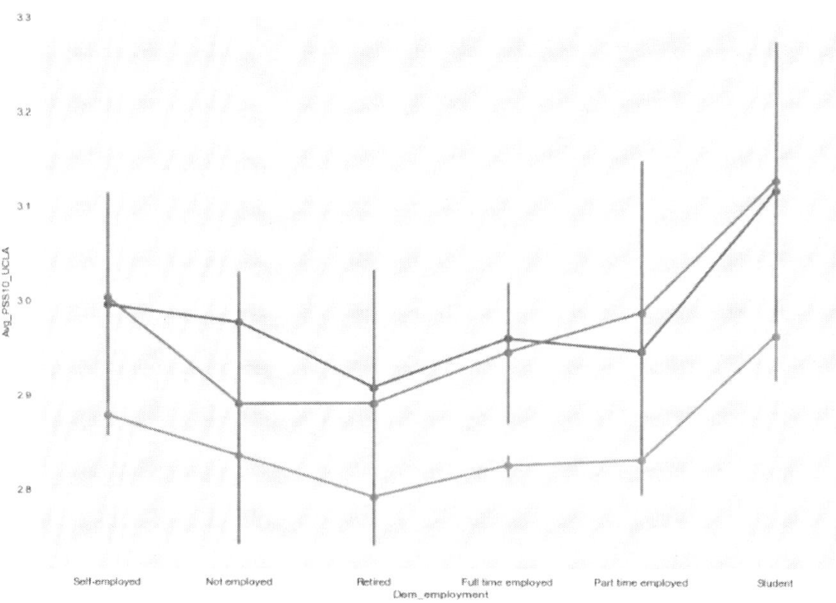

Figure 7. Gender vs. Dem_employment.

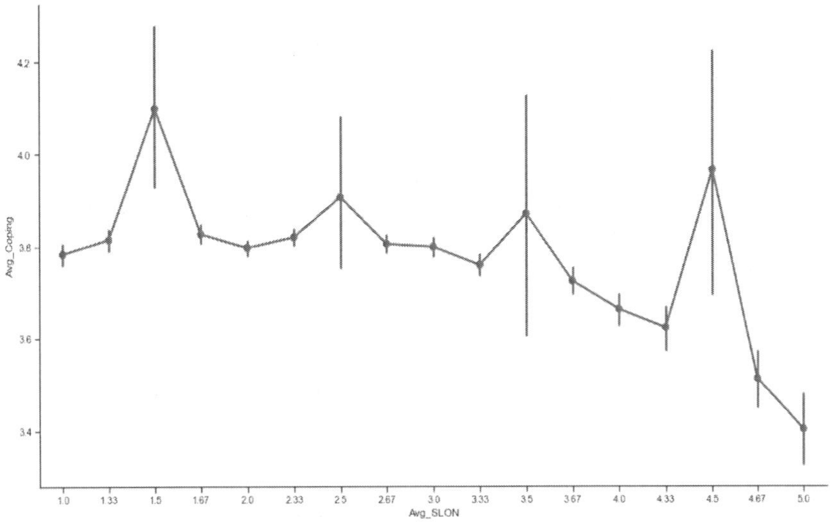

Figure 8. Age coping vs. severe loneliness.

The conclusion from the plot is as below;

- From the data points, it can be observed that as age increases, we can see a sharp incline w.r.t perceived stress in individuals. This can be an outcome because the virus attacks individuals with lower immune systems, i.e., elderly people, in most cases.
- The perceived loneliness Vs. Age shows spikes for age ranges 70-80 years and 80-90 years post which we can see an incomplete section which speaks about missing data points of people aged 100 or above years, proving the point of home isolation for elders and their feedback on the Likert scale.
- Most individuals above 40 (considered elderly) tend to have mixed reactions toward their country's measures to curb the virus. Where the highest votes (> 16,000) on the Likert scale were for 5.0 (Satisfactory) out of 10.0 (Extremely good)
- Loneliness Vs. Perceived stress tends to showcase a directly proportional relationship, i.e., as stress increases, loneliness tends to increase too, which supports the research belief on loneliness vs. stress parameter during isolation.

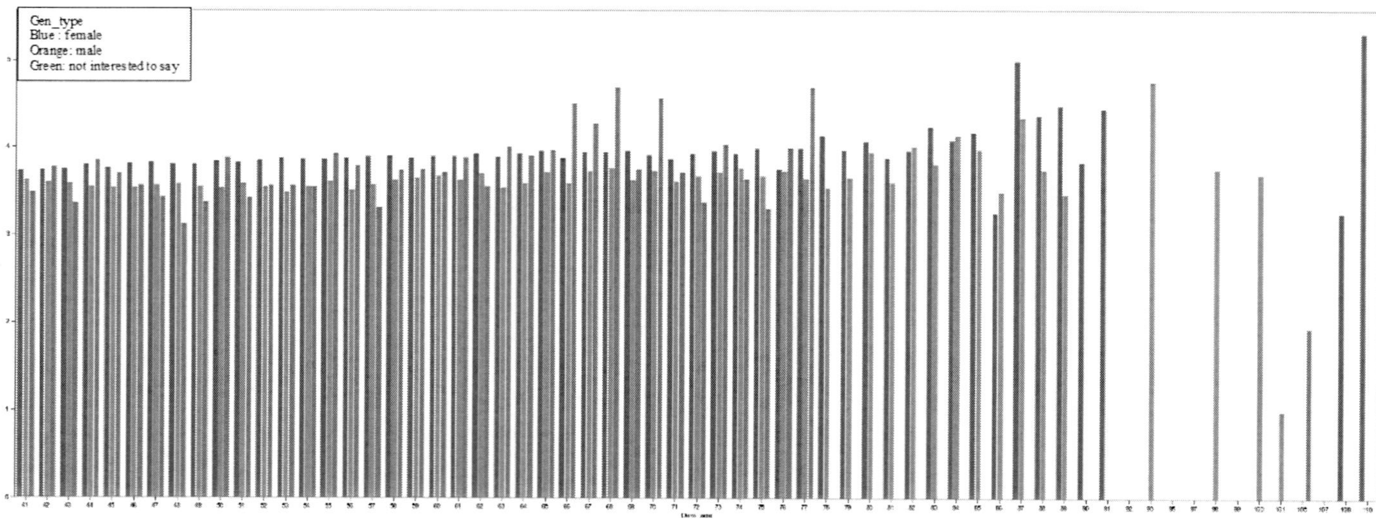

Figure 9. Demographic characters' age vs. Avg_coping vs. gender.

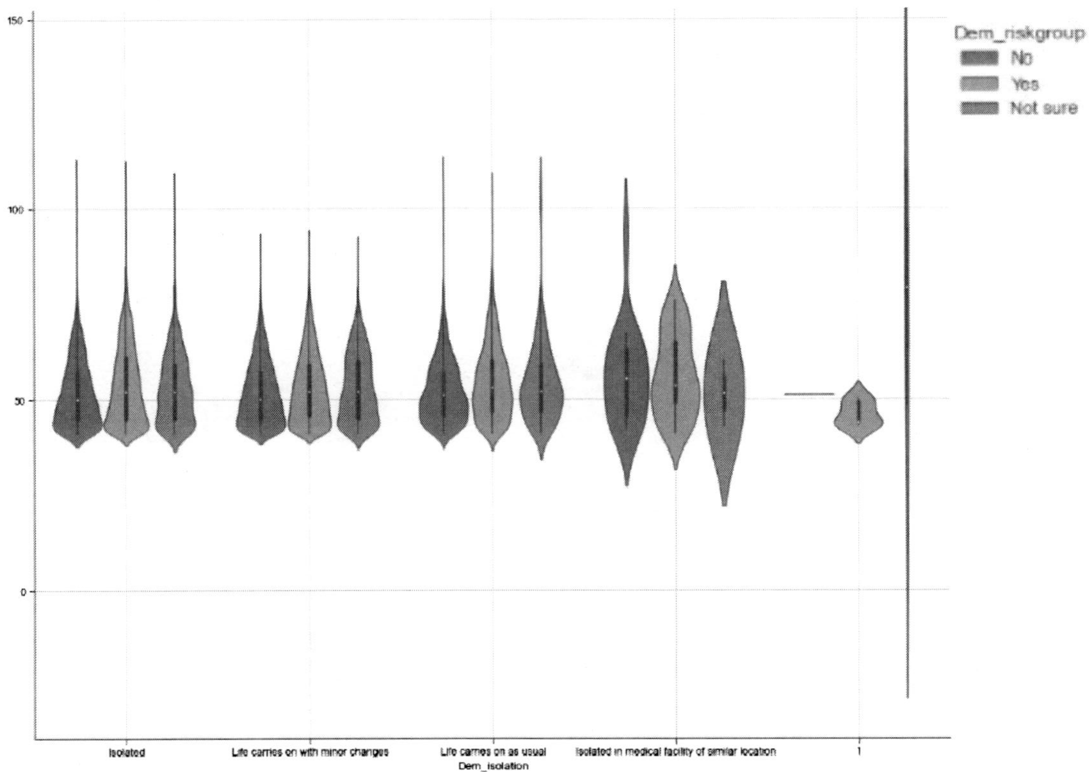

Figure 10. High-Risk groups vs. Dem_age vs. Dem_Isolation.

- It can also be concluded from the bar graph that the loneliness factor tends to be more inclined to individuals who have retired across all age ranges or people who weren't employed.
- It can be observed that elderly individuals who aren't a part of the risk group tend to isolate themselves in homes or similar places. This backs up our research as it's a precaution suggested by most government bodies instructing elders to isolate themselves in a bubble.

Discussion

Scientific advances must educate the elderly on mobile gadgets such as cell phones. The bad news about the illness should be matched with more good information about healing in media pieces. Financial and economic worry may be relieved by assurances about work and riches across consciousness and self-quarantine.

This study aimed to describe the acute psychosocial situation throughout older people and analyze its relationship with prolonged exposure to the broad COVID-19 context during this critical acute phase of illness. It assessed the incidence of clinically significant signs of generalized high anxiety levels and their relationships with other current tragedies, seriousness, and effect on employee performance, economy, and cognitive relationships.

In this epidemic, melancholy among society's elderly persons doubled two months after physical isolation methods were employed, whereas psychological state remained stable. Researchers found no evidence that the intensity of interpersonal communication was relevant in interpreting the increase in well-being. Interpersonal tragedies, epidemic fears, and a drop in faith in society organizations were linked to increased psychiatric problems and emotional alienation. These findings imply that the most successful strategies to ensure detachment and well-being among elderly persons are connected to advancing interpersonal connections, particularly engagement with communal organizations. Economic and political organizations might concentrate on boosting interpersonal interactions with kids and relatives, assuring assistance for requirements such as personal tragedies, and minimizing the overall perception of community vulnerability. Although the findings offer insight into the relatively brief impacts of isolation techniques, the lengthy implications of separation on well-being must be adequately examined.

Conclusion

Separation might harm emotions. The hazards are more significant for older people who live independently or are more connected than others. The epidemic might drastically reduce the earnings and lifestyle changes of the elderly. Consequently, below 20% of people of retirement age receive compensation. Senior citizens are not simply victims. They, too, are reacting. These are health care professionals, caregivers, and caregivers of various essential services. The death rate is five times greater than the worldwide average. Approximately 66% of people aged 40 and up have had at least one chronic medical issue.

The present investigation shows COVID-19's systemic inflammatory influence on the elderly group's psychological disorders. The conclusions are troubling, indicating significantly higher levels of emotional stress in those with no current diagnosis. This deterioration in emotional stability may have worsened the previous harsh wildfire period in the weeks preceding the epidemic. However, the conflagration experience was accounted for. Consequently, the analysis shows that efforts to counterbalance the cultural, economic, and professional difficulties caused by COVID-19 are likely to significantly affect behavioral health and well-being, especially among persons with pre-existing chronic problems.

Future Work

We investigate and explore the link between psychological disorders, anxiousness, stress, adaptability, and loneliness in the future. Researchers can analyze people's lifestyles at various periods of the Age or track changes in the interactions among these elements through age. Then it would be helpful to investigate more into the lack of a link between isolation and quality of life. In the future, the long-term impact of the COVID-19 epidemic on a larger sample of senior people and whether different ages of individuals heal substantially from the COVID-19 emotional effects.

References

[1] https://jamanetwork.com/journals/jama/fullarticle/2773479.

[2] Carfì A, Bernabei R, Landi F. Gemelli against COVID-19 post-acute care study group. persistent symptoms in patients after acute COVID-19. *JAMA*. (2020) 9 : e2012603. DOI : 10.1001/jama.2020.12603.

[3] Akiskal HS, Akiskal K, Allilaire JF, Azorin JM, Bourgeois ML, Sechter D, et al. Validating affective temperaments in their sub affective and socially positive attributes: psychometric, clinical and familial data from a French national study. *J. Affect Disord*. (2005) 85 :29–36. DOI : 10.1016/j.jad.2003.12.009.

[4] Pisano S, Senese VP, Bravaccio C, Santangelo P, Milone A, Masi G, et al. Cyclothymic-hypersensitive temperament in youths: Refining the structure, the way of assessment and the clinical significance in the youth population. *J. Affect. Disord.* (2020) 271 :272–8. DOI : 10.1016/j.jad.2020.03.155.

[5] Laghi F, Pompili S, Bianchi D, Lonigro A, Baiocco R. Exploring the association between psychological distress and drunkorexia behaviors in non-clinical adolescents: the moderating role of emotional dysregulation. *Eat Weight Disord.* (2020). DOI : 10.1007/s40519-020-00912-9.

[6] Taha S, Matheson K, Cronin T, Anisman H. Intolerance of uncertainty, appraisals, coping and anxiety: the case of the 2009 HINI Pandemic. *Br. J. Health Psychol.* (2014) 19 :592–605. DOI : 10.1111/bjhp.12058.

[7] Miles SH. *Kaci Hickox. Public Health and the Politics of Fear*. At : http://www.bioethics.net/2014/11/kaci-hickox-public-health-and-thepolitics-of-fear/.

[8] Centers for Disease Control and Prevention. *Quarantine and Isolation*. (2017). Available online

[9] Hall R C, Hall R C, Chapman M J. The 1995 Kikwit Ebola outbreak: lessons hospitals and physicians can apply to future viral epidemics. *Gen. Hosp. Psychiatry*. 2008 ;30(5) :446–52.

[10] Zhang, J., Lu, H., Zeng, H., Zhang, S., Du, Q., Jiang, T., & Du, B. (2020). The differential psychological distress of populations affected by the COVID-19 pandemic. *Brain, Behavior, and Immunity*, 87, 49–50.

[11] https://unsdg.un.org/sites/default/files/2020-05/Policy-Brief-The-Impact-of-CO VID-19-on- Older-Persons.pdf.

[12] Czeisler, M. É., Lane, R. I., Petrosky, E., Wiley, J. F., Christensen, A., Njai, R., Weaver, M. D., Robbins, R., Facer-Childs, E. R., Barger, L. K., Czeisler, C. A., Howard, M. E., & Rajaratnam, S. M. W. (2020). Mental health, substance use, and suicidal ideation during the covid-19 pandemic—United states, june 24–30, 2020. MMWR. *Morbidity and Mortality Weekly Report*, 69(32), 1049–1057.

[13] J. M. Twenge, A. B. Cooper, T. E. Joiner, M. E. Duffy, S. G. Binau, Age, period, and cohort trends in mood disorder indicators and suicide-related outcomes in a nationally.

[14] American College Health Association, "National college health assessment" (American College Health Association, 2018).

[15] Moghanibashi-Mansourieh A. Assessing the anxiety level of Iranian general population during COVID-19 outbreak. *Asian J. Psychiatr*. 2020 ; 51 :102076.

[16] Berwick, D M, Murphy J M, Goldman P A Ware, J E Jr, Barsky, A J, & Weinstein, M C. (1991). Performance of a five-item mental health screening test. *Medical Care*, 29 (2), 169–176. DOI :10.1097/00005650-199102000-00008.

[17] Weiss, R S. (1973). *Loneliness: The experience of emotional and social isolation*. MIT Press. Perlman, D, & Peplau, L A. (1981). Toward a social psychology of loneliness. In R Gilmour & S W Duck (Eds.), *Personal relationships in disorder* (pp. 31–56). Academic Press.

[18] Douglas H, Georgiou A, Westbrook J. Social participation as an indicator of successful aging: An overview of concepts and their associations with health. *Aust. Heal. Rev.* 2017 ;41(4) :455–462. DOI : 10.1071/AH16038.

[19] Tomioka K, Kurumatani N, Hosoi H. Social Participation and the Prevention of Decline in Effectance among Community-Dwelling Elderly: A Population-Based Cohort Study. *PLoS One.* 2015 ;10(9) : e0139065.

[20] Morley J E, Vellas B. COVID-19, and Older Adults. *J. Nutr. Health Aging.* 2020 ;24(4) :364–365.

[21] Reed S, Crespo C, Harvey W, Andersen R. Social isolation and physical inactivity in older US adults: Results from the Third National Health and Nutrition Examination Survey. *Eur. J. Sport Sci.* 2011 ;11(5) :347–353. DOI: 10.1080/17461391.2010.521585.

[22] Jansen F M, Prins RG, Etman A, et al. Physical activity in non-frail and frail older adults. *PLoS One.* 2015 ;10(4). DOI : 10.1371/journal. Pone.0123168.

[23] Xiong, J. ; Lipsitz, O. ; Nasri, F. ; Lui, L.M. ; Gill, H. ; Phan, L. ; Chen-Li, D. ; Iacobucci, M. ; Ho, R. ; Majeed, A. ; et al. Impact of COVID-19 pandemic on mental health in the general population : A systematic review. *J. Affect. Disord.* 2020, *277*, 55–64.

[24] Klaiber, P. ; Wen, J.H. ; DeLongis, A. ; Sin, N.L. The Ups and Downs of Daily Life During COVID-19 : Age Differences in effect, Stress, and Positive Events. *J. Gerontol. Ser. B* 2020, *76*, e30–e37.

[25] Bu, F. ; Steptoe, A. ; Fancourt, D. Loneliness during a strict lockdown: Trajectories and predictors during the COVID-19 pandemic in 38,217 United Kingdom adults. *Soc. Sci. Med.* 2020, *265*, 113521.

[26] https://www.cdc.gov/coronavirus/2019-ncov/long-term-effects/index.html.

[27] Taquet M, Luciano S, Geddes J R, Harrison P J. Bidirectional associations between COVID-19 and psychiatric disorder: retrospective cohort studies of 62 354 COVID-19 cases in the USA. *Lancet Psychiatry* 2021; 8:130.

[28] Taquet M, Geddes J R, Husain M, et al. 6-month neurological and psychiatric outcomes in 236 379 survivors of COVID-19: a retrospective cohort study using electronic health records. *Lancet Psychiatry* 2021; 8:416.

[29] https://www.mayoclinic.org/diseases-conditions/coronavirus/in-depth/coronavirus-long-term- effects/art-20490351.

[30] 30 Plagg B, Engl A, Piccoliori G, Eisendle K (2020) Prolonged social isolation of the elderly during COVID-19 : between benefit and damage. *Arch. Gerontol. Geriatr.* 89 :104086. 10.1016%2Fj.archger.2020.104086.

[31] Kavoor A R (2020) COVID-19 in people with mental illness: challenges and vulnerabilities. *Asian J. Psychiatr.* 51:102051. 10.1016%2Fj.ajp.2020.102051.

[32] https://unsdg.un.org/sites/default/files/2020-05/Policy-Brief-The-Impact-of-COV. ID-19-on- Older-Persons.pdf.

[33] https://www.un.org/esa/socdev/ageing/documents/PovertyIssuePaperAgeing. pdf.

[34] ILO Spotlight on work statistics, May 2018, https://www.ilo.org/stat/Publications/ WCMS_629567/lang--en/index.htm.

[35] Cohen S, Kamarck T, Mermelstein R. A global measure of perceived stress. *J. Health Soc. Behav.* (1983) 24 :385–96. DOI : 10.2307/2136404.

[36] Spitzer R L, Kroenke K, Williams J B, Löwe B. A brief measure for assessing generalized anxiety disorder: the GAD-7. *Arch. Intern. Med.* (2006) 166 :1092–7. DOI : 10.1001/archinte.166.10.1092.

[37] Kroenke K, Spitzer R L, Williams J B. The PHQ-9 : validity of a brief depression severity measure. *J. Gen. Intern. Med.* (2001) 16 :606–13. DOI : 10.1046/j.1525-1497.2001.016009606. x.

[38] Liu N, Zhang F, Wei C, Jia Y, Shang Z, Sun L, et al. Prevalence and predictors of PTSS during COVID-19 outbreak in China hardest-hit areas : gender differences matter. *Psychiatry Res.* (2020) 287 :112921. DOI : 10.1016/j.psychres.2020.112921.

Chapter 10

Work from Home-Related Depression Analysis

R. Vasuki*

Selaiyur, Chennai, India

Abstract

The pandemic has turned the world upside down, disrupting the working environment of the whole working community and significantly impacting millions of individuals' bodily and emotional health. According to the American Psychiatric Association, around one out of every fifteen persons suffers from depression each year (APA). The researchers sought studies that included people who were routinely employed from home and reported explicitly on medical or psychiatric implications. WFH workers reported feeling very lonely and isolated 19 percent of the time. Loneliness may become chronic and harm one's emotional and physical well-being. Working from home may cause worry, stress and loneliness, contributing to or aggravating depression. Furthermore, it is clear that long-distance jobs commonly lead to loneliness. This paper examines work-from-home (WFH)-related depression in both men and women and ways to overcome this present scenario to restore humanity's natural thinking.

Keywords: pandemic, WFH, depression, COVID, mental health, stress, environment, yoga, meditation

---

*Corresponding Author's Email: hod.bme@bharathuniv.ac.in.

In: Data Science Applications of Post-COVID-19 Psychological Disorders
Editor: Vijayalakshmi Kakulapati
ISBN: 979-8-88697-165-1

Introduction

In December 2019, the Coronavirus produced unexpected instances of pneumonia in the Chinese city of Wuhan [1] and the virus spread swiftly became a worldwide health problem [2]. The COVID-19induced worldwide epidemic has produced an once-in-a-lifetime scenario with far-reaching health and economic ramifications [3]. Thousands of jobs have been lost, with women bearing the brunt of the hardship [4, 5].

Job patterns have shifted due to new technology, with many people being able to work from home [6]. As telecommuting technology developed in the early 2000s, work from home (WFH) grew more popular, enabling employees to save money on transportation and ease to work [7,8].

Work From Home allows individuals to work when they are most productive and may help employees avoid distractions from coworkers, which is especially useful in open-plan workplaces [9]. Finally, employees in WFH may have greater control over their working environment, including lighting, temperature, humidity, air quality, noise, and ergonomics [10]. IEQ factors, for example, influence a worker's convenience, which influences contentment [11].

Workers have total control and responsibility for configuring their workstations from home, allowing them to work in a more IEQ-friendly workplace than a static cubicle or enterprise environment [9]. Employees have entire responsibility and authority for establishing their workstations from home, in contrast to traditional organizations where managers commonly organize workstation's ability to work in a workplace with better IEQ conditions than a static workstation or enterprise environment [9]. Furthermore, investigations have shown that the temperature and air quality at home is better than in a typical office environment.

Employees who work from home cannot communicate with colleagues and are thus likely to participate in less physical activity, such as traveling between meeting locations [1]. Long-term computer usage may also cause weariness, lethargy, headaches, and vision problems [12].

In other cases, seniors may choose to work at night to concentrate on their professional job rather than household responsibilities. Emotional exhaustion might result from work-life conflict [11]. Due to a lack of social and behavioral components, the quick transition to WFH has emotionally and physically befuddled individuals.

The forced confinement at home during the pandemic may cause sadness and anxiety, leading to frequent changes in routines and eating patterns [16].

Other types of stress associated with WFH may interact with many of these effects on cognitive activities and nutrient intake, leading to an immediate impact on mental and physical well-being [17, 18].

Work-related stress, poor body mechanics due to an adequate therapeutic working space, and prolonged sitting activity can result in increased pain and exhaustion [21]. Working in an improper setting may result in poor IEQ, affecting physical and mental well-being and total job performance [22].

Individually, it provides greater variety and authority in managing work responsibilities, such as the ability to alter and maintain a schedule in adapting to shifting requirements and preferences [23]. Additionally, saving time traveling between home and work is immeasurable. Employees prefer telework, including lower transportation expenses and less commute-induced stress [24].

Because a new coronavirus variant has been linked to various symptoms that can range from respiratory illness to more chronic conditions such as SARS and MERS [25], COVID-19 can impair people's emotional health as well as their physical health [26].

Patients are more likely to be anxious about being unwell or death, helpless, and stigmatized by others [27]. The epidemic has harmed public mental health, culminating in emotional disorders [28]. As a result of health crises such as COVID-19, health care workers and the general public-facing psychological changes, which are prompted by emotions such as fear, concern, sadness or uncertainty [29]. Improved family and work integration, less weariness, and increased productivity are just a few of the benefits of teleworking [30].

The Benefits and Drawbacks of Working from Home

- Pro: Remote employees have less stress and are more focused.
- Working from home has the downside of isolating you.
- The benefit is that you don't have to commute every day.
- Collaboration and communication may be challenging.
- Pro: Remote employees have more flexibility in their schedules.

Longer hours, a lack of or ambiguous distinction between work and home and insufficient organizational support, on the other hand, may harm an individual's mental and physical health [31]. According to epidemiological research, women are more likely than males to suffer depression [32]. Stress and post-traumatic stress disorder are more common in women than men [33]. During the epidemic, women were more likely than men to experience worry, depression and stress [34, 35, 36].

Literature Review

Other highly contagious illnesses have appeared in the last two decades, including SARS in 2003, infectious diseases with the H1N1 genotype in 2009, Middle East Respiratory Syndrome (MERS) in 2012 and Ebola virus in 2014 [37, 38]. Research indicates a link between education attainment and increased anxiety and melancholy during the COVID-19 epidemic [15]. As per Chinese studies, the increasing prevalence of major depressive symptoms among people with higher education is due to this group's increased self-awareness of their wellness [39]. Furthermore, those with at least one COVID-19 disease-affected family member, relative or acquaintance reported significantly greater anxiety levels [40].

Issues regarding the predicted return to traditional corporate environments and employee implications grow when businesses begin to recover and some conventional operations restart [41]. Adjustments to their organizational contexts that are relevant to COVID-19 should be avoided. Many firms require working from home (WAH) [42]. Work patterns have changed due to new technologies, with many workers being able to work remotely [43].

People's physical connection with other relatives, acquaintances and colleagues was prohibited throughout the notification period, which may have led to isolation, loneliness and depressive symptoms. [44].

Furthermore, depressive symptoms have been linked to physical inactivity induced by remaining at home [45, 46]. Because of the outbreak, many people were forced to take time off work or lost their jobs and rapid changes in employment status may be a risk factor for depressive symptoms [47-49]. According to one research, people who were unable to work due to the epidemic had worse psychological well-being than those who worked in an office or from home [50]. Additionally, the move to work-from-home (WFH) may be detrimental to workers' mental health [50]. WFH might help alleviate suffering during a pandemic by facilitating travel and assisting employees in maintaining social connections with colleagues [51].

In contrast, other research shows that WFH blurs work and home-based life barriers, leading to longer working hours [52] and overlapping childcare commitments [53], which might exacerbate discontent.

Methodology

The review study contained citations to data from numerous research articles published in reputable journals as determined by Scopus, Web of Science and the internet.

Social isolation, in particular, has been linked to poor mental health, with higher anxiety and depressive symptoms [56]. Telework's negative emotional effect is a contributing cause since teleworkers report more significant degrees of isolation and loneliness than office workers [57].

Sleep quality has been shown to deteriorate during SARS-CoV-2 pandemics, linked to gloomy mood, stress and anxiety in recent studies [58]. However, our group's incidence of sleep problems is much greater than reported in the literature for the present COVID-19 outbreak [59]. On the other hand, physically active individuals were shown to have reduced levels of anxiety and depression in studies done during the COVID-19 lockdown. However, further study is required to examine the impact on sleep quality [60].

Depressive symptoms and sleeplessness are connected to nighttime light exposure and screen usage [61, 62]. As a consequence of the absence of a clear difference between the workplace and the worker's home and family environment, working hours are prolonged into the night, stress is increased and regular social and professional routines are lost, resulting in sleep cycle dysregulation and poor sleep quality [63].

A Single Occurrence or Temporary Circumstances May Cause Types of Stress

This is referred to as acute stress. Stressful situations, such as taking an extensive exam or suffering an acute injury, such as a broken bone, create instant stress.

- Furthermore, stress might linger for an extended period without feeling relieved. Other times, events or diseases may produce constant tension, or the source of your stress may be unknown. Chronic stress is the term for this. Chronic stress is usually brought on by persistent personal, lifestyle, or health problems. Chronic stress may be caused by a variety of factors, including:

- having financial troubles
- working in a high-pressure job
- dealing with personal or interpersonal issues at home
- don't feel like you have enough support from family or friends.

Depression and the Effects of Stress

While stress is bad for your physical and mental health, it's worse if you have depression.

Stress may impair your ability to sustain healthy routines or coping mechanisms, which are essential for depression treatment. This may exacerbate depressive symptoms. When a healthy habit is broken, it may lead to unhealthy coping behaviors like binge drinking or social isolation. These activities might add to your stress level, worsening the symptoms of sadness.

Anxiety and irritability are two frequent stress reactions that may affect your mood. Even if the stressor is temporary, anxiety might increase unpleasant feelings and irritation.

The various disadvantages of remote working, such as associated conflict, professional life immobility and feelings of loneliness, may explain these findings [64]. In terms of economic growth, it's worth noting that poor sleep quality is frequently associated with poorer levels of efficiency among employees across a wide range of vocations [66]. The effect of insufficient sleep on perceived cognitive problems, which has a detrimental impact on job performance [67], is the most likely explanation for this link.

The body's response to physical or emotional difficulties is called stress. Mental anguish can be a source or a consequence of melancholy. A stressful situation may cause sentiments of hopelessness, making tension tasks more effective. The body's response to physical or psychological difficulties is known as stress. Emotional stress may be the cause of depression or a symptom of it.

- Life Unpleasant life events, such as job loss or the termination of a long-term relationship, may lead to depression and make dealing with stress more difficult. Not everyone who is exposed to these circumstances develops depression. Biological reasons may explain why one individual experiences depression while another does not exist in a stressful situation.

- getting enough sleep
- eating a well-balanced diet
- exercising frequently
- taking vacations or frequent breaks from work
- having a relaxing hobby, such as gardening or carpentry
- breathing exercises to help you lower your heart rate

Mindfulness and Yoga

If your personal or professional life gives you stress, you may want to reconsider your lifestyle choices.

There are a few things you may do to reduce this kind of stress:

- Placing yourself under less pressure to achieve at work or school, for example, by reducing your standards to a level that you still consider appropriate
- Sharing duties or delegating chores to people in your environment
- Surrounding oneself with helpful and optimistic friends and family members
- Distancing oneself from stressful circumstances or settings

Yoga, meditation, and religious rituals may also be beneficial in reducing stress. A combination of these approaches might be much more effective. Finding out what works best for you is crucial. And regardless of what you choose, having close friends and family members who are prepared to support you is essential.

Stress and depression may also be helped by talking to a counselor, therapist, or other mental health professional. Talk therapy has been demonstrated to help treat depression and chronic stress, either alone or with cognitive-behavioral therapy (CBT) or medication. The following medications are used to treat depression:

To help cope with stress and sorrow, talk to a counselor, therapist, or other mental health professionals. Whether used alone or combined with cognitive-behavioral therapy (CBT) or medication, talk therapy is a well-established treatment for depression and chronic stress. Antidepressants include the following:

Set reasonable objectives for yourself along the road to help you finish the project. Throughout the hour or day, carry out modest, timed actions until the job is accomplished. This will assist the patient in better managing stress and channeling their energy.

Depression is a common but hazardous mental health condition that interferes with one's capacity to feel, think and behave appropriately.

Depression causes sadness and a lack of interest in previously enjoyed activities in those who suffer from it. Their ability to function may be harmed as a result of this. According to the American Psychological Association, one out of every six people will experience depression at some time.

Depression is characterized by a lack of energy, a gloomy mood, difficulty sleeping or oversleeping and changes in eating. A diagnosis is usually made when symptoms have been present for at least two weeks.

Depression is treated with a variety of therapies and medications. Each situation is unique. If you experience depression, you'll probably discover that a mix of therapies works best rather than just one. A mental health expert can assist you in determining what is most effective for you.

Stress was thought to affect men and women differently at home, experiencing more stress because they perceive work from home to be more difficult. She required them to see both professional and domestic work simultaneously and intervention, coercion, consideration and other factors. The study articles were graded based on men's and women's labor force participation and age groups.

Results and Discussion

According to polls, just 25% of office-based employees report higher stress levels. Depression has been proven to be influenced by psychological stress. Nonetheless, there is little evidence linking remote work to depression. Indeed, according to some studies, people intentionally seek employment that allows them to work from home to alleviate tension. As shown in 2018 research performed by Mental Health America in cooperation with Flex Jobs, approximately 71% of participants would prefer to work from home in order to alleviate commute-related tension.

According to over 75% of research participants, the working distance might help them minimize stress caused by daily interruptions. Isolation, loneliness and difficulties leaving work at the end of the day are all reported as negative mental health implications for those who work from home. Early in the pandemic, research established a link between the number of COVID-19-related workplace measures, such as encouraging workers to start WFH, and employee psychological distress [69].

WFH, on the other hand, expanded quickly due to broad travel restrictions. According to a nationwide poll, 34.6 percent of workers worked from home during the pandemic, with 30.0 percent of men and 19.1 percent of women shifting their primary workplace to their homes in the current research. WFH may help relieve some of the stress of commuting [70]. Meanwhile, some people who started performing WFH may devote considerable time to training or other tasks, while others may blur the lines between work and home life and longer hours [71]. According to one study, those who started WFH during the COVID-19 outbreak increased their sedentary and screen time [72].

Working from home has various drawbacks in contrast to its benefits, such as

- Increased isolation.
- The expenses of maintaining a workspace.
- There's a chance you'll work too much.
- There is a threat to production.
- At-home distractions.
- Disconnect from work.
- An unbalanced work-life balance.
- Less face time.

How can I keep my mental health in check while working from home?

These easy steps may help you feel productive and inspired when working from home and taking care of a patient's mental health.

1. Establish and keep to a schedule
2. Create a separate workstation
3. Take a break
4. Keep in touch
5. Draw lines in the sand
6. Consider the long term
7. Be kind to automatically

Numerous people like the flexibility to work long hours, but it's essential to understand that it is not for everyone. The patient could soon learn that you work better in a social situation with your colleagues. It is entirely up to you to decide what is best for your mental health. Keep in mind that there's little to no evidence that remote work causes depression. A medical professional can help you determine if you are suffering from sadness or depression and how to get the help you need. Keep in mind that getting help is beneficial: many people receiving depression therapy live long and healthy lives. While WFH is simple and convenient, being alone all of the time might be lonely. According to recent surveys, the most challenging aspect of working with faraway personnel is loneliness. One may be experiencing depression if your mood starts to influence your everyday life. A mental health professional can help you get a proper diagnosis and consider your treatment choices.

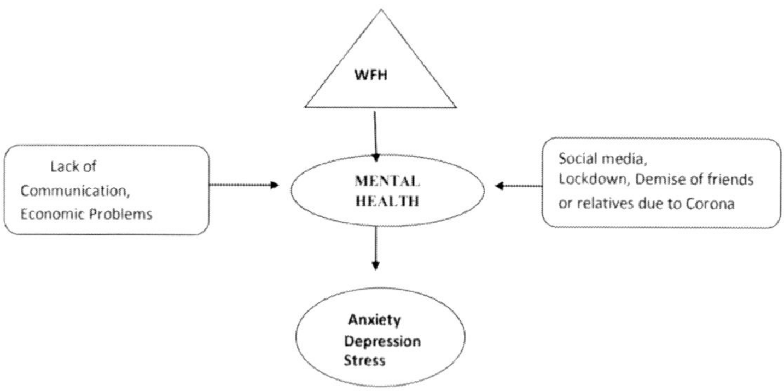

Figure 1. Effect of various factors on mental health.

Our data revealed that working longer hours was linked to an increase in depressive symptoms, potentially negating the advantages of WFH. Furthermore, the negative impacts of sedentary behavior on one's health have been documented [73]. Respect your emotions and take care of yourself. Physical and mental well-being needs a balance of healthy eating, exercise and leisure activities. Make time for these essential aspects of self-care in your daily routine. Consider attending a group fitness class or signing up for newsletters or periodicals that include healthy living suggestions, such as recipes, to make it simpler to practice self-care.

Maintain solid friendships and family ties with people you can trust. Joining an online or in-person support group to exchange advice with others going through similar situations is a good idea.

One of the key reasons why so many people are concerned about their job performance, according to Gemma Leigh Roberts, organizational psychologist and creator of The Resilience Edge, is a lack of 'informal' feedback. Furthermore, there seems to be no description of teleworking at the moment. Telework is defined by the International Labor Organization (ILO) as using Information and Communication Technology (ICTs), including cellphones, iPad, laptops, or personal computers, for work performed away from the company's location.

Conclusion

According to this comprehensive study, the COVID-19 pandemic impacts the mental health of men and women of all ages. Yoga, meditation, spending time with family, friends and pets, as well as setting priorities and goals, becoming self-motivated, eating healthy and nutritious food without skipping meals, focusing on what is around you, and making time for yourself, can all help WFH participants improve their mental health. The health-work connection is complex and optimizing WFH's impact on an individual's health necessitates considering broader system challenges. For the conceivable future, organizations need to adopt defined WFH policies that consider work-home trade facilitation, job clarity, responsibility, quality measures, technical help, peer networking facilitation and professional training. The ultimate objective is to realize that life is valuable and should be enjoyed.

References

[1] Bai Y, Yao L, Wei T, Tian F, Jin D-Y, Chen L. (2020).Presumed asymptomatic carrier transmission of COVID-19. *JAMA*, 323(14):1406-7.

[2] Wang C, Horby PW, Hayden FG, Gao GF. (2020)A novel coronavirus outbreak of global health concern. *Lancet*, 395(10223):470–3.

[3] Douglas M, Katikireddi SV, Taulbut M, McKee M, McCartney G.(2020).Mitigating the wider health effects of covid-19 pandemic response. *BMJ*, 369:1557.

[4] Wenham C, Smith J, Morgan R. (2020). COVID-19: the gendered impacts of the outbreak. *Lancet*, 395(10227):846–8.

[5] Alon TM, Doepke M, Olmstead-Rumsey J, Tertilt M. (2020).*The impact of COVID-19 on gender equality: National Bureau of Economic Research*, 0898–2937.

[6] Henke RM, Benevent R, Schulte P, Rinehart C, Crighton K, Corcoran M. (2016). The effects of telecommuting intensity on employee health. *Am. J. Health Promot.*, 30(8):604–12.

[7] Tavares AI. (2017).Telework and health effects review.*Int. J. Healthc*, 3:30.

[8] Bouziri H, Smith DRM, Descatha A, Dab W, Jean K. (2020).Working from home in the time of COVID-19: how to best preserve occupational health? *Occup. Environ. Med.*, 77:509–510.

[9] Kim J, de Dear R. (2013) Workspace satisfaction: the privacy-communication trade-off inopen-plan offices.*J. Environ. Psychol.*, 36:18–26.

[10] Samani SA. (2015).The impact of personal control over office workspace on environmental satisfaction and performance.*J. Soc. Sci. Humanit.*, 1:163–172.

[11] Abdulaali HS. (2020).Impact of poor indoor environmental quality (IEQ) to inhabitants' health, wellbeing and satisfaction.*Int. J. Adv. Sci. Technol.*, 29:1284–1296.

[12] Majumdar P, Biswas A, Sahu S. (2020).COVID-19 pandemic and lockdown: cause of sleep disruption, depression, somatic pain, and increased screen exposure of office workers and students of India.*Chronobiol. Int.*, 37:1–10.

[13] Mann S, Holdsworth L. (2003). The psychological impact of teleworking: stress, emotions and health.*New Technol Work Employ*, 18:196–211.

[14] Vander Elst T, Verhoogen R, Sercu M, Van den Broeck A, Baillien E, Godderis L. (2017). Not extent of telecommuting, but job characteristics as proximal predictors of work-related well-being.*J. Occup. Environ. Med.*, 59:180–186.

[15] Evanoff BA, Strickland JR, Dale AM, Lisa Hayibor, Emily Page, Jennifer G Duncan, Thomas Kannampallil, Diana L Gray (2020).Work-related and personal factors associated with mental well-being during COVID-19 response: a survey of health care and other workers (preprint).*J. Med. Internet Res.*, 22:21366.

[16] Di Renzo L, Gualtieri P, Cinelli G, Giulia Bigioni, Laura Soldati, Alda Attinà, Francesca Fabiola Bianco, Giovanna Caparello, Vanessa Camodeca, Elena Carrano, Simona Ferraro, Silvia Giannattasio, Claudia Leggeri, Tiziana Rampello, Laura Lo Presti, Maria Grazia Tarsitano, Antonino De Lorenzo. (2020). Psychological aspects and eating habits during COVID-19 home confinement: results of EHLC-COVID-19 Italian Online Survey.*Nutrients*, 12:2152.

[17] Schnitzer M, Schöttl SE, Kopp M, Barth M. (2020).COVID-19 stay-at-home order in Tyrol, Austria: sports and exercise behaviour in change?*Public Health*,185:218–220.

[18] Ricci F, Izzicupo P, Moscucci F, Susanna Sciomer,Silvia Maffei,Angela Di Baldassarre,Anna Vittoria Mattioli,Sabina Gallina (2020).Recommendations for physical inactivity and sedentary behavior during the coronavirus disease (COVID-19) pandemic.*Front Public Heal*,8:8–11.

[19] Arntz M, Ben S, Francesco Y. (2020).*Working from Home and COVID-19: The Chances and Risks for Gender Gaps,* Available at:https://www.zew.de/PU82032-1.

[20] Kaur T, Sharma P. (2020). A study on working women and work from home amid coronavirus pandemic.*J. Xi'an Univ. Archit. Technol*, XII:1400–1408.

[21] Baradaran Mahdavi S, Kelishadi R. (2020).Impact of sedentary behavior on bodily pain while staying at home in COVID-19 pandemic and potential preventive strategies.*Asian J. Sports Med.*,11:103511.

[22] Mahbob NS, Kamaruzzaman SN, Salleh N, Sulaiman R. (2011).A correlation studies of indoor environmental quality (IEQ) towards productive workplace.*2nd Int. Conf. Environ. Sci. Technol. (ICEST 2011)*, 6:434–438.

[23] GajendranRS, HarrisonDA. (2007).The good, the bad, and the unknown about telecommuting: meta-analysis of psychological mediators and individual consequences.*J. Appl. Psychol.*, 92(6):1524–41.

[24] BaileyDE, KurlandNB. (2002).A review of telework research: findings, new directions, and lessons for the study of modern work.*J. Organ. Behav.*, 23(4):383–400.

[25] Ashour HM, Elkhatib WF, Rahman M, Elshabrawy HA. (2020). Insights into the recent 2019 novel coronavirus (SARS-CoV-2) in light of past human coronavirus outbreaks. *Pathogens*, 9(3):186.

[26] Huang Y, Zhao N. (2020).Generalized anxiety disorder, depressive symptoms and sleep quality during COVID-19 epidemic in China: a web-based cross-sectional survey. *MedRxiv*, 288:112954.

[27] Hall RC, Hall RC, Chapman MJ. (2008). The 1995 Kikwit Ebola outbreak: lessons hospitals and physicians can apply to future viral epidemics. *Gen. Hosp. Psychiatry*, 30(5):446–52.

[28] Xiang Y-T, Yang Y, Li W, Zhang L, Zhang Q, Cheung T. (2020). Timely mental health care for the 2019 novel corona virus outbreak is urgently needed. *Lancet* Psychiatry, 7(3):228–9.

[29] Zhang J, Lu H, Zeng H, Zhang S, Du Q, Jiang T. (2020).The differential psychological distress of populations affected by the COVID-19 pandemic. *Brain Behav. Immun.*, 87:49–50.

[30] Gajendran RS, Harrison DA. (2007). The good, the bad, and the unknown about telecommuting: meta-analysis of psychological mediators and individual consequences. *J. Appl. Psychol.*, 92(6):1524–41.

[31] Allen TD, Golden TD, Shockley KM. (2015). How effective is telecommuting? Assessing the status of our scientific findings. *Psychol. Sci. Public Interest*, 16(2):40–68.

[32] Lim GY, Tam WW, Lu Y, Ho CS, Zhang MW, Ho RC. (2018). Prevalence of depression in the community from 30 countries between 1994 and 2014. *Sci. Rep.*, 8(1):1–10.

[33] Sareen J, Erickson J, Medved MI, Asmundson GJ, Enns MW, Stein M. (2013).Risk factors for post-injury mental health problems. *Depress Anxiety*, 30(4):321–7.

[34] Moghanibashi-Mansourieh A. (2020). Assessing the anxiety level of Iranian general population during COVID-19 outbreak. *Asian J. Psychiatr.*, 51:102076.

[35] Zhou S-J, Zhang L-G, Wang L-L, Guo Z-C, Wang J-Q, Chen J-C. (2020).Prevalence and socio-demographic correlates of psychological health problems in Chinese adolescents during the outbreak of COVID-19. *Eur. Child Adolesc. Psychiatry*, 29:1–10.

[36] Wang Y, Di Y, Ye J, Wei W. (2020). Study on the public psychological states and its related factors during the outbreak of coronavirus disease 2019 (COVID-19) in some regions of China. *Psychol. Health Med.*, 30:1–10.
[37] Feldmann H, Jones S, Klenk H-D, Schnittler H-J. (2003).Ebola virus: from discovery to vaccine. *Nat. Rev. Immunol.*, 3(8):677–85.
[38] Team N-O, Dawood F, Jain S, Finelli L, Shaw M, Lindstrom S. (2009).Emergence of a novel swine-origin influenza a (H1N1) virus in humans. *N. Engl. J. Med.*, 360(25):2605–15.
[39] Zhang Y, Ma ZF. (2020).Impact of the COVID-19 pandemic on mental health and quality of life among local residents in Liaoning Province, China: a cross-sectional study. *Int. J. Environ. Res. Public Health*, 17(7):2381.
[40] Cao W, Fang Z, Hou G, Han M, Xu X, Dong J. (2020).The psychological impact of the COVID-19 epidemic on college students in China. *Psychiatry Res.*, 287:112934.
[41] Shimazu A, Nakata A, Nagata T, Arakawa Y, Kuroda S, Inamizu N. (2020). Psychosocial impact of COVID-19 for general workers. *J. Occup. Health*, 62(1):12132.
[42] Belzunegui-Eraso A, Erro-Garcés A. (2020). Teleworking in the context of the Covid-19 crisis. *Sustainability*, 12(9):3662.
[43] Henke RM, Benevent R, Schulte P, Rinehart C, Crighton K, Corcoran M. (2016).The effects of telecommuting intensity on employee health. *Am. J. Health Promot.*, 30(8):604–12.
[44] Cacioppo JT, Cacioppo S, Capitanio JP.(2015).The Neuroendocrinology of social isolation.*Annu. Rev. Psychol.*, 66:733–67.
[45] Kandola A, Ashdown-Franks G, Hendrikse J. (2019). Physical activity and depression: towards understanding the antidepressant mechanisms of physical activity. *Neurosci. Biobehav. Rev.*, 107:525-39.
[46] SchuchFB, Vancampfort D, Firth J.(2018). Physical activity and incident depression: a meta-analysis of prospective cohort studies. *Am. J. Psychiatry* 2018;175:631–48.
[47] Yoo K-B, ParkE-C, JangS-Y. (2016). Association between employment status change and depression in Korean adults. *BMJ Open*, 6:570.
[48] Virtanen P, Janlert U, Hammarström A. (2011).Exposure to temporary employment and job insecurity: a longitudinal study of the health effects. *Occup. Environ. Med.*, 68:570.
[49] Burgard SA, Brand JE, House JS. (2020).Toward a better estimation of the effect of job loss on health. *J. Health Soc. Behav.* 2007;48:369–84.
[50] Zhang SX, Wang Y, Rauch A. (2020).Unprecedented disruption of lives and work: health, distress and life satisfaction of working adults in China one month into the COVID-19 outbreak. *Psychiatry Res.* 2020;288:112958.
[51] Bouziri H, Smith DRM, Descatha A. (2020). Working from home in the time of COVID-19: how to best preserve occupational health? *Occup. Environ. Med.*, 77:509–10.
[52] Eurofound and the International Labour Office.*Working Anytime, anywhere: the effects on the world of work.* Geneva Publications Office of the European Union, Luxembourg, and the International Labour Office; 2017.

[53] Standen P, Daniels K, Lamond D. (1999) The home as a workplace: Work–family interaction and psychological well-being in telework. *J. Occup. Health Psychol.*, 4:368–81.

[54] Pandey D, Bansal S, Goyal. (2020). Psychological impact of mass quarantine on population during pandemics—the COVID-19 lock-down (COLD) study. Santana GL, editor. *PLoS One*, 15(10):0240501.

[55] Cerne A, Rifel J, Rotar-Pavlic D. (2013). Quality of life in patients with depression, panic syndrome, other anxiety syndrome, alcoholism and chronic somatic diseases: a longitudinal study in Slovenian primary care patients. *Wien Klin Wochenschr*, 125(1–2):1–7.

[56] Luo M, Guo L, Yu M. (2020). The psychological and mental impact of coronavirus disease 2019 (COVID-19) on medical staff and general public – a systematic review and meta-analysis. *Psychiatry Res.*, 291:113190.

[57] Mann S, Holdsworth L. (2003). The psychological impact of teleworking: stress, emotions and health. *N. Technol. Work Empl.*, 18(3):196–211.

[58] Targa ADS, Benítez ID, Moncusí-Moix A. (2020). Decrease in sleep quality during COVID-19 outbreak. *Sleep Breath*, 10:11325.

[59] Bigalke JA, Greenlund IM, Carter JR. (2020). Sex differences in self-report anxiety and sleep quality during COVID-19 stay-at-home orders. *Biol. Sex Differ.*, 11(1):56.

[60] Ernstsen L, Havnen A. (2020). Mental health and sleep disturbances in physically active adults during the COVID-19 lockdown in Norway: does change in physical activity level matter? *Sleep Med.*, 77:309–12.

[61] Fossum IN, Nordnes LT, Storemark SS. (2014).The association between use of electronic media in bed before going to sleep and insomnia symptoms, daytime sleepiness, morningness, and chronotype. *Behav. Sleep Med.*, 12(5):343–57.

[62] Münch M, Wirz-Justice A, Brown SA. (2020). The role of daylight for humans: gaps in current knowledge.*Clocks Sleep*, 2(1):61–85.

[63] Rohwer E, Kordsmeyer A-C, Harth V. (2020). Boundarylessness and sleep quality among virtual team members – a pilot study from Germany. *J. Occup. Med. Toxicol.*,1 5(1):30.

[64] Baruch Y, Nicholson N. (1997). Home, sweet work: requirements for effective home working. *J. Gen. Manag.*, 23(2):15–30.

[65] Hill EJ, Ferris M, Märtinson V. (2003). Does it matter where you work? A comparison of how three work venues (traditional office, virtual office, and home office) influence aspects of work and personal/family life. *J. Vocat. Behav.*, 63(2):220–41.

[66] Doi Y, Minowa M, Tango T. (2003).Impact and correlates of poor sleep quality in Japanese white-collar employees. *Sleep*, 26(4):467–71.

[67] Lee S, Buxton OM, Ande lR. (2019). Bidirectional associations of sleep with cognitive interference in employees' work days. *Sleep Health*, 5(3):298–308.

[68] World Health Organization. *Impact of Economic Crises on Mental Health*. WHO Regional Office for Europe, 2011.

[69] Sasaki N, Kuroda R, Tsuno K. (2020). Workplace responses to COVID-19 associated with mental health and work performance of employees in Japan. *J. Occup. Health*, 62:12134.

[70] Bouziri H, Smith DRM, Descatha A. (2020). Working from home in the time of COVID-19: how to best preserve occupational health? *Occup. Environ. Med.*, 77:509–10.

[71] Eurofound and the International Labour Office (2017). *Working Anytime, anywhere: the effects on the world of work.* Geneva Publications Office of the European Union, Luxembourg, and the International Labour Office.

[72] McDowell C P, Herring MP, Lansing J. (2020). Working from home and job loss due to the COVID-19 pandemic are associated with greater time in sedentary behaviors. *Front Public Health*, 8:597619.

[73] Young DR, Hivert M-F, Alhassan S, Sarah M. Camhi, Jane F. Ferguson, Peter T. Katzmarzyk, Cora E. Lewis, Neville Owen, Cynthia K. Perry, Juned Siddique, Celina M. Yong. (2016). Sedentary behavior and cardiovascular morbidity and mortality: a science Advisory from the American heart association. *Circulation*, 134:262-79.

Chapter 11

The Effect of Psychological Disorders on Students' Academic Performance

Appiah Prince[1,*], Alexander A. Menschikov[1,†] and Vijayalakshmi Kakulapati[2,‡]
[1]ITMO University, Saint Petersburg, Russia
[2]Sreenidhi Institute of Science and Technology, Yamnampet, Ghatkesar, Hyderabad, Telangana, India

Abstract

Many institutions worldwide, such as education, corporate, and business firms, have concluded that pandemic illness is as critical as climate change. An epidemic sweeps the globe in a few months. COVID-19, an illness that started to form in China in December 2019, could bring a long-term pandemic to the world depending on its spread rate, which also affects the world's educational systems. Many educational institutions had no option but to change the teaching mode and learn to be online or virtual. The main objective of this analysis was to determine the impact of psychiatric issues on learner progress during the COVID-19 epidemic. Furthermore, the effects of quarantine, self-stigma, and loneliness on students' stress and behavioral health will be evaluated. The research was carried out at ITMO University, where a student was asked to complete a questionnaire via an online survey. The current machine learning approach was used to analyze the data gathered. The study found that 59% of the participants could not pass all their courses within the pandemic frame when studying online, while 41% of the participants

*Corresponding Author's Email: Princeappiah35@gmail.com.
†Corresponding Author's Email: menshikov@itmo.ru.
‡Corresponding Author's Email: vldms@yahoo.com.

In: Data Science Applications of Post-COVID-19 Psychological Disorders
Editor: Vijayalakshmi Kakulapati
ISBN: 979-8-88697-165-1

could pass all their courses. The study clearly shows that students from Russia had bad results compared with students already in Russia. This leads to more international students quitting their graduate studies. Due to this, we propose that colleges and universities offer flexible ways to teach and learn to meet the needs of international students during the pandemic.

Keywords: pandemic, COVID-19, academic performance, educational institutions

Introduction

The increased prevalence of the COVID-19 epidemic has triggered widespread attention. The pandemic led many countries to lock down to provide safety measures to control the spread of the disease [1]. This virus outbreak affected all aspects of humankind, such as education, businesses, work, the economy, sporting activities, transportation, entertainment, research work, social gatherings, etc., which has changed the lifestyles of many people. COVID-19 has been among the most devastating outbreaks in prehistory because of its emergence and spread with other infectious complications and fatality rates [1]. Several observations from all regions indicated a regular rise in the percentage of new cases and mortality rate owing to COVID-19 [2]. Furthermore, 394,707,561 probable instances of COVID-19 have been documented, with several fatalities of 5,609,684 since the beginning of Jan 2022 [1, 2].

Worldwide, the academic sector was severely impacted by the epidemic. COVID-19 caused widespread disruption in educational settings. Due to the apparent disease's tricky position, universities adapted to interactive learning settings [3, 4]. Nevertheless, such practices harm pupils' psychological and emotional well-being. Furthermore, the benefits, flaws, possibilities, and problems of web-based learning during the epidemic must be investigated.

Students are becoming a susceptible demographic, with more significant depression, stress, drug misuse, and dietary restraint than the general populace. Therefore, whenever the quality of higher education drastically changes, the impact on the emotional stability of this susceptible demographic increases during a pandemic. The aims of this work are to 1) recognize the wide range of psychiatric effects have on academics, 2) acquire segments to characterize pupils' predicted aspects of perceived effects throughout the disease outbreak, and 3) to recognize possible sociodemographic, attitude, and consciousness contaminated with coronavirus risk factors that could make learners more vulnerable to depression these effects.

The education sector was highly affected during the pandemic and is still finding ways to control this massive disruption. Because of the virus's vulnerability, several standards of academia were forced to transition to digital learning settings [5]. Unfortunately, this negatively affected learners' psychological and emotional well-being. As a result, the importance of intensifying the difficulties, prospects, and problems of digital learning during the COVID-19 epidemic should be addressed.

The alterations brought about by the coronavirus epidemic always seem to influence the educational environment. All institutions have encountered and seek to overcome several obstacles [6]. Online learning has been used in the case of conventional instruction since Mar 2020. The widespread usage of technology necessitated by the need for social separation caused by the epidemic demanded a high level of adaptability from academic faculty and learners. Furthermore, residential restrictions hampered the ability to fully experience university life by influencing higher education and making it more difficult to receive aid from emotional contact, which can be critical to resolving the issues of the higher education institution [7].

This study utilizes the current trend approach of statistical machine learning to determine the psychological disorders of learners during the pandemic. The significant analysis of the study is categorized into two sections. A classification algorithm and inferential statistics were utilized. Information was gathered from a student using an online survey during the study. The study has the following significant contributions: First, to verify the relevance of digital learning and, study the effect of the outbreak on graduate students' psychological health, raise awareness about the pros and cons of online study tools and digital developments. Also, look into how isolation, quarantine, and being cut off from society affect graduate students' emotional and mental health.

The remaining work is classified as follows: The second section describes the history of post-pandemic psychiatric disorders in pupils; the third examines current systems, and the fourth discusses techniques. The fifth part discusses the broad issue before explaining the implementation analysis. Section 7 addresses the work's final observations and suggestions for further improvements.

Background

In December 2019, a novel coronavirus was discovered in Wuhan, China, causing significant fever-related respiratory infection. The WHO named it Novel Coronavirus, associated with the year it came to be, 2019, which was then called COVID-19. The viral illness is transmitted by SARS-CoV-2, a coronavirus that causes SARS-CoV2.

The pandemic has influenced learners, including dangers to their own and their families' healthcare, lockdown and a shift to online training in Mar 2020, a prolonged vacation of physical distance, and the hardship of attending college in Sep 2020. However, devastating as a worldwide pandemic's health repercussions are, much of it has been anticipated as the "second wave" of psychiatric problems, especially for adolescents and young adults.

Most learners are more susceptible to behavioral and medical issues and experience emotional exhaustion due to an increase, including the transition from youth to adolescence and poor academic achievement, affecting learning performance, interaction, and emotional well-being [8]. Nevertheless, the outbreak impacts young adults' bodily and cognitive functioning, posing the consequence of a cognitive disorder in this group [9]. Generally, learners have felt the potential influence of the epidemic as much as those working [10]. During the epidemic, higher education learners had stress levels connected with fundamental issues, effects on everyday living, and worry about intellectual impairments [11]. In scientific studies, the incidence rates of PTSD (post-traumatic stress disorder) and depression during the outbreak in a subset of isolated graduate students were determined to be 2.7 percent and 9 percent, correspondingly. In this kind of analysis, the learners' fear of contamination strongly predicted anxiety and PSTD [12].

On the contrary, [13] discovered that throughout COVID-19 confinement, young adults had poor sleeping patterns and poor sleep hygiene. According to the investigation, there has been a decline in poor sleep associated with tiredness. Some other research found that young individuals are at risk of a psychiatric condition. Further studies found that the epidemic has deteriorated the psychological state of young individuals with a tendency to emotional health problems [14].

It is hazardous and is associated with typical disease symptoms. COVID-19 has been classified as an airborne disease, which can be easily transmitted from one person to another person through contact with the affected person. COVID-19 manifestations include exhaustion, temperature, impairment or alteration in sensory organs or deliciousness, and prolonged dry coughing from the beginning. Due to different immune systems per individual, such individuals may not progress to COVID-19's progressively catastrophic symptoms. Expect anomalies from patient X-rays in pulmonary illness, although pulmonary joint inflammation seemed to be predicted, as is found with other kinds of bacterial pneumonia.

The pandemic led to a total lockdown of many sectors. Last, this research provides new evidence of the effectiveness of psychological disorders on learners' performance. When it comes to online study, COVID-19 has caused schools to close campuses and transform face-to-face courses into online education. Unlike previous studies on MOOCs or mixed systems, whose methods have a problem with a sample selection of students, students can often choose to participate or not in online classes. Students in this study are forced to go home and take online courses.

The emotional wellness of young adults has become a growing problem, with several graduates enduring psychiatric anguish [15]. Cognitive impairments can significantly hinder learners' quality of education and socialization, impacting their subsequent professional and personal chances. The fast growth of coronavirus and social distancing strategies taken throughout the country are projected to harm the consciousness of the people, particularly young adults. Numerous research studies on healthcare providers and elderly people [16] investigated the emotional effects of the epidemic on ordinary people. Such assessments revealed that participants were more aware of the social separation and experienced higher stress, nervousness, and sadness levels.

Surprisingly, research on the Chinese people primarily associated exposure to correct patient data during the pandemic was linked to decreased psychological stress. In contrast, past outbreak research demonstrates that erroneous data, especially in interactive online forums or social networking sites, is connected with panic and dread [17]. Reliable information, understanding, and perceived risks can lead to behavioral adjustments [18], including fear of isolation, which is presently one of the only approaches to reducing COVID-19 transmission. The research results also suggest that implementing recommended preventive steps (e.g., hand cleanliness, mask usage) to avoid the transmission of COVID-19 may lessen adverse effects by creating feelings of safety in people who participate in these protective efforts. In comparison, many higher education institutions offer knowledge about COVID-19 from trustworthy sources [19]. There is a big chance that misinformation and intentionally false information will spread through young people's websites and social networking sites. This could make student groups feel tense, nervous, and hopeless.

Therefore, this study helps improve knowledge of the influence of internet-based learning on learners. Significantly the education sector was highly affected. The usual way of teaching was then changed to virtual. Online teaching was very favorable to some people and was a big problem for others. Many students could not move from their home country to abroad due to the closeness of borders and travel restrictions. COVID-19 generally had a significant impact on student performance. Therefore, it is well needed to assess the psychological disorder of students during the pandemic using machine learning algorithms.

Related Works

There have been a lot of studies on COVID-19 since January 2020. COVID-19 came to draw many people's attention. Many researchers have researched COVID-19, mainly on how to curb and control the spread of the disease. Only a few addressed the effect and impact on the education of literature.

In online study methods and learning models, qualitative and quantitative data are utilized to determine instructors' and students' impressions of teaching. The authors investigate the usage of web-based learning devices such as smartphones and tablets. They discovered how it affects the emotional well-being of both teachers and pupils [20]. These researchers investigate if there is a link between students' longer use of electronic education technologies due to the COVID-19 epidemic and their emotional and physiological well-being. [21]. The COVID-19 epidemic has impacted all levels of education. Academic institutions are locked down by disasters or restricted layoffs worldwide, impacting around 1.9 billion people.

According to [22], pandemics have catastrophic psychological impacts on those affected by the pandemic and future generations. Even pandemics such as influenza, MERS, SARS, and HIV/AIDS, which have previously appeared and threatened people's health, have had negative psychological consequences. Meanwhile, several additional investigations have been conducted to analyze the effects of the epidemic on learners' educational outcomes and their level of confidence and contentment with online education during the pandemic. The impact of a pandemic on Ghanaian schoolchildren was found [23]. It highlighted the main effects of domestic violence, stress and depression, bodily changes, and a decline in academic performance.

Informative technical start-ups [24] were developed during the epidemic to assist academia in dealing with issues associated with online learning. It was then that some schools decided to use other forms of media to provide teaching and learning to students while at home. These researchers [25, 26, 27] investigated the degree of intellectual pressure encountered by learners during college programs, as well as the coping mechanisms they employed throughout the epidemic.

Furthermore, [28] developed several recursive predictive models for the pandemic and its subsequent recovery. Their models were used to evaluate the influence of the environment on COVID-19 dissemination by analyzing the association between the intensity of reported instances and environmental parameters in specific areas.

Furthermore, previous investigations [23, 29] demonstrated favorable impacts on learner success in improving students' academic. These findings could be explained by the fact that the attainment assessment among investigations was conducted several months after the closing of schools and the efficiency probability. Successful anticipatory assessments are introduced by educators, schools, and community decision-makers during that time to compensate for understanding damages, including providing training organizations during a vacation in German cities [24]. Even though the maximum impact on improving students' academics is equivalent when all analyses are averaged, several incorporated research reported diverse impacts for various disciplines.

The fact that "arithmetic is simpler to instruct via virtual classrooms, as it is straightforward to deliver problems and examinations electronically or as workbooks" [30] may explain why there are more intellectual disability impairments in reading than in arithmetic. An additional factor is that many kids may not know the language they have been evaluated at home, resulting in a slight improvement in their speaking ability between closing schools. On the contrary, discovering more intellectual disability reductions in arithmetic than perusing might indicate that pupils spend time learning in education cuts. Assisting children in improving their learning ability was more accessible for parents to ensure children improved their arithmetic competence [31].

This pandemic has changed the paradigm of various education sectors in the world. Therefore, there is a need to look into how this COVID-19 pandemic has affected the student body psychologically and emotionally. Previous studies mainly relied on essential statistical tools to analyze data gathered from participants to conclude. Nevertheless, these investigations lack a few desirable characteristics that might facilitate us in investigating the appropriate challenges of COVID-19 in the teaching process. This research found a new way to use the relevant factors to figure out the educational stress that online learners face and how to lessen its effects.

Pandemic's Affect on Education

The pandemic prompted a greater emphasis on digital or virtual learning, utilizing a new methodology. Suitable educational technology makes resources for students, including digital training, virtual learning environments, remote learning, cooperative learning, and eLearning, more accessible [32]. As a result, the fast growth of educational technology has shifted from an instructor to a communicator model. Students acquire and develop their learning performance using the training resources [33]. Furthermore, learners confront the issue of moving from traditional face-to-face teaching techniques to eLearning. The most important things that affect how well digital learning works are better Internet access, better academic tools, and the ability to afford and use technology [5, 34].

The pandemic led to schools closing down, the eminence of training and learning waning, and learners with particular requirements had reduced physical attention [35]. The new technologies, such as ZOOM, Microsoft Teams, and Skype, will never completely replace the existing method. Moreover, many students cannot afford the cost of learning online—for instance, buying the necessary learning technology tools and the cost of high internet speed. Specifically, African students face many challenges regarding the high internet rate compared with students in Asia and Europe.

The student with particular disabilities was in horrible shape. All special schools around the globe have closed down. It was challenging for teachers in such institutions to manage and control students during the pandemic. COVID-19 has led to the increased development of web pages for hard-of-hearing students. In the western part of the world, it was effortless for them to use technological tools to assist these particular students. On the other hand, students from developing countries don't have the facilities they need to learn and teach.

The average number of students in each was reduced to limit coronavirus spread. In Russia, the class size was reduced drastically in order to practice social distance and free movement of air within the classroom. All classrooms are well ventilated.

Before most institutions moved to online mode, there was a shift system. In Ghana, there was a gold and green track [32]. In Saint Petersburg, Russia, students have morning and afternoon shift systems.

Methodology

The study design involved students from Saint Petersburg, Russia. Saint Petersburg has many public institutions, but only three higher educational institutions were chosen. These institutions are ITMO University, HSE St. Petersburg, and LETI. Of these, three more responses came from ITMO University. A total of 112 were involved during the study. An online survey was utilized to gather biographical profiles, interpersonal interactions, psychiatric disorders, distress levels, and digitization. A machine learning algorithm, descriptive statistics, chi-square, and linear logistic regression were used to look at the answers.

The proposed method for analyzing the study results focused primarily on the student's psychological reactions to COVID-19. A model was designed for how classification would be done. Below shows the predicted model's methods for evaluating the responses. The three main steps are also shown:

1. preprocessing,
2. In the teaching process, and
3. the effective model.

The available dataset is gathered from the best three institutions in Saint Petersburg. All the datasets were collected and pushed into the model. The preprocessing technique was first applied to the dataset to detect missing data and normalize and make feature selections. The dataset was split into two subsets: the testing dataset (30%) and the training dataset (70%). However, the dataset for this study was not enough for the model, where a part of it was used for validation tasks. Therefore, K-folds cross-validation was utilized to separate the data into k sets to test the classification model. The Hyperparameter optimization method was used to enhance the precision of the specific algorithm. The classification algorithm was established using built-in Python libraries such as sci-kit-learn and Keras. And finally, the third stage predicts the student's response.

Implementation Analysis

This section involves the implementation of the anticipated methodology of evaluating the effectiveness of psychological order on students' performance using machine learning algorithms.

Dataset Description

The dissemination of COVID-19 has affected various aspects of a community, including academia, business, and wellness, to highlight a very few. In Russia, every segment was apprehensive, and the government declared an emergency to combat the disease's dissemination. The government implemented several steps to halt infection transmission, including suspending institutes, closing borders, and quarantining. Russia was the only country that closed its borders to students for almost 1.5 years. It was challenging for students, mainly from Africa, to study online. Many petitions were written by students from Afghanistan, Nigeria, and Ghana. Because of the barrier, learners were forced to study digitally, necessitating using online tools such as computers, cellphones, and data access. The dataset investigated the significant effect of coronavirus online learning technological devices on students' performance in Russian universities and colleges.

This study's survey was divided into two categories. The first section gathered demographic details on every learner, including grade, age, nationality, GPA, and place of residence. The second section collects information about students' psychiatric problems during the epidemic, including their mental condition, educational achievement, and interpersonal interactions. The research team communicates with many Russian scholars in public and private institutions to share their online questionnaires. The selected institutions were LETI, ITMO, and HSE-St. Petersburg. The total number received was in 2011. The percentages and frequencies were accounted for in the gathered data based on the Likert scale [36].

Google Form was used to design the questionnaire for the respondents to respond to, and the survey outcomes were stored in CSV files. The questionnaires were designed and written in English and Russian language.

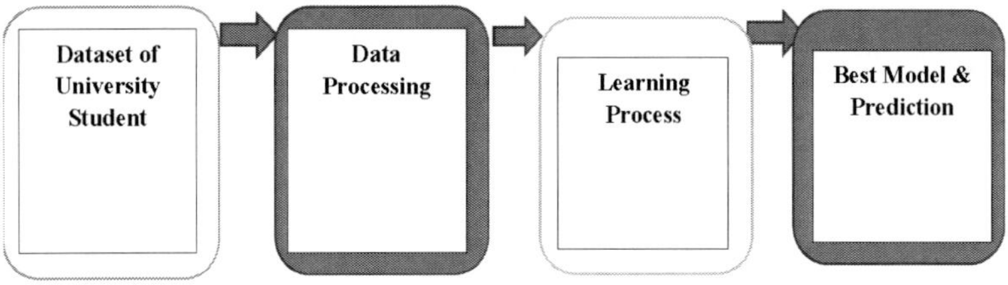

Figure 1. Machine learning analysis steps.

In this work, the ensemble method was utilized to analyze the actual impact of the psychological disorder impact of coronavirus during the pandemic on students' academic performance [37]. The following machine learning algorithms were used: Logistic Regression, SVM, Random Forest, and Decision Tree to forecast the education performance.

The approaches were chosen as they are often employed to address a wide range of real-world issues. Furthermore, approaches were trained with the desired psychological state, academic performance, online learning, social interaction, and quarantine.

Experiment Results and Analysis

The experimental result of the study is discussed here. The significant findings are classified as observational and computational modeling analyses. For improved visualization, these results are given in tables and charts.

Evaluating Multiple-Choice Questionnaires

A measurement model is a basic spreadsheet that displays the covariance between factors. Every column in this table represents the association among factors. An autocorrelation summarizes facts and indicates the existence of a continuous connection among factors [38]. The major orthogonal is Diagonal 1, which runs from the top left to bottom right, indicating that every factor constantly completely corresponds amongst itself. This diagonal is symmetric, and the precise association shows the major diagonally as a reflective surface of the diagonals underneath it. Table 1 depicts the relationship between COVID-19 assessments and student psychiatric illnesses.

Table 1. Student psychological effects heatmap

Before COVID-19	1	0.43	-0.086	-0.061	-0.022
After COVID-19	0.43	1	-0.04	-0.09	0.0012
Before time psychological health	-0086	-0.04	1	0.22	-0.012
After time psychological health	-0.061	-0.09	0.22	1	-0.034
Quizzes and Exams Online	-0.022	-0.012	0.0012	-0.034	1
	Before COVID-19	After COVID-19	After time psychological health	After time psychological health	Quizzes and Exams Online

Descriptive Statistics Results

Students' responses to the questions about the effect of the emotional influence of coronavirus on learner performance were the main objective of using the questionnaires. The questionnaires were distributed utilizing online google forms. As already been said, the questionnaire was based on Likert-type containing 15 items. The students were given the freedom to have the choice to pick responses ranging from "strongly agree" to "strongly disagree." The data was accumulated during the second semester of 2020/2021 from Saint Petersburg, Russia, Universities.

The Outcomes of Models' Effectiveness

In categorization, questionnaire data is frequently divided into two distinct sets: training and testing. The categorization analysis of the chosen training sets implemented is shown in Table 5 underneath. The logistic regression, SVC, Decision Tree, and Deep Learning models performed much better, with specificity, efficiency, recall, and F1 scores of 100 percent, 100 percent, and 100 percent, respectively.

Table 2. The participant's demographic statistics

Variable	Classes	Occurrence	Percentage (%)
Country	Ghana	309	15.36
	Nigeria	902	44.85
	Russian	800	39.78
Continent	Asia	720	35.80
	Africa	1211	60.21
	Europe	80	3.97
Gender	Male	1161	57.73
	Female	850	42.26
Level	Second	1048	52.11
	First	963	47.88
GPA	0-0.2	-	.00
	2.0-2.49	1798	89.40
	2.5-2.99	108	5.37
	3.0-3.49	5	0.25
	3.5-5	0	.00

Table 3. The distribution of participants' responses regarding the psychological disorder's effect on academic performance

	Africa	Asia	Europe
Strong Agree	53.7	49.8	32.1
Agree	20.2	32.2	23.2
Uncertain	14.2	11.4	21.9
Disagree	8.9	4.9	15.4
Strongly Disagree	3.0	1.7	5.9

Table 4. Students' social interaction, psychological state, academic performance

Statement	Strongly Agree	Agree	Normal	Disagree	Strongly Disagree
COVID-19 causes stress, frustration and depression	40.3	22.3	17.1	12.5	7.9
Using e-learning tools leads to boredom, psychologically unhealthy	64.5	26.4	7.0	1.6	0.7
Some students cannot afford the necessary digital tools and bundle	69.4	24.3	6.3	0.0	0.0
COVID-19 has caused students' psychological disorder	51.0	32.2	10.0	5.0	1.8
Online learning leads to students' isolation	45.0	23.5	18.3	9.3	4.0
Face-to-face learning increases academic performance	59.8	28.5	10.2	2.7	1.8

Table 5. The outcomes of algorithms' effectiveness

	Time	Accurateness	Exactness	Recall	F1	ROC_AUC
Logistic Regression	1.0094	1	1	1	1	1
SVC	1.5600	1	1	1	1	1
Deep Learning	193.345	1	1	1	1	1
Random Forest	678.864	0.9923	1	1	1	0.9976

Discussion

This analysis looks into the impact of COVID-19, a psychological condition, on higher education students in Russia and the various frustrations that lead to poor educational effectiveness. As a result, the COVID-19 epidemic has impacted educational activities, increasing psychiatric illnesses among pupils. A few of these problems include learners' lack of learning interests, failure in various courses, and limited access to laboratories. These have resulted in a rise in student debt. The pandemic of COVID-19 cannot be compared to previous centuries. This pandemic affects all sectors, especially in the education system, as it limits the opportunities for many students. The hindrances that prevent many students from joining online learning are poor internet networks, electricity, and inadequate facilities such as advanced technological tools. More than 65% of the participants agreed that physical or face-to-face teaching methods positively impact student academic performance. The study also found out that the pandemic led to the psychological order of students. Almost all the lecturers and students agreed that being isolated and alone with only your computer makes you think differently than a normal human being. This study's results agree with the other studies [37, 39] that the need for traditional education is the best solution. However, the coronavirus pandemic has brought a new face to studying online and will allow people to look at online technologies' fruitful side.

More females had good grades than males during the online studies, indicating that online learning favored females compared with earlier results. The males had better scores than the females.

Every study comes with limitations. There are significant merits to the proposed machine learning model, but it also has several demerits. The sample size used for the analysis was minimal to create an effective machine learning model.

We look forward to providing information on particular topics since we could not do so.

Conclusion

The year 2021 has been challenging for students around the globe. COVID-19 has technically fixed remote learning. This study inquired about the impact of COVID-19 on student psychological disorders during online learning. The survey result has found studying online to be practical and constructive. The lockdown led educational stakeholders to find ways and means to improve teaching and learning through various technology methods. However, most participants agreed that the educational institution should build a robust technological platform for teaching and learning. They can interact with their colleagues and teachers as happens during the standard traditional method of teaching and learning. The study found out that students from Africa suffered the most due to the cost of the internet and technological tools for online learning. Most students from Sub-Saharan Africa had bad results during the online studies compared with the hybrid model.

Moreover, there is a positive relationship between COVID-19 measures and student psychological disorders. Many students clarified that interacting with machines bored them and made them think differently. There was no interaction of sharing ideas with their colleagues as a traditional teaching method involving them. Most African students quit their postgraduate courses due to the cost-effectiveness of affording high-speed internet. Not only some student from places like Afghanistan, Pakistan, and others defer their programs till a hybrid is introduced.

Future Enhancement

In the future, we will focus on applying an efficient predictive model to other countries worldwide to evaluate the effect of COVID-19 on the mental disorder of students in higher institutions. Besides, there should be a solution for eliminating boredom and stress during online learning. Again, researchers may find more flexible artificial neural networking deep learning models based on future extraction achieved by advanced optimization methods. As well as researchers can use this work for further studies.

References

[1] Ahmed, M. Z., Ahmed, O., Aibao, Z., Hanbin, S., Siyu, L., & Ahmad, A. (2020). The epidemic of COVID-19 in China and associated Psychological Problems. *Asian Journal of Psychiatry,* 51. https://doi.org/10.1016/j.ajp.2020.102092.

[2] Abraham A. (2020). *How COVID-19 may increase domestic violence and child abuse.* Retrieved from https://www.apa.org/topics/covid-19/domestic-violence-child-abuse.

[3] World Health Organization (WHO): Pandemic measures, https://www.who.org.

[4] Basilaia, G., Replacing the classic learning form at universities as an immediate response to the COVID-19 virus infection in Georgia *Int. J. Res. Appl. Sci. Eng. Technol.,* 8 (3) (2020), pp. 101-108, 10.22214/ijraset.2020.3021.

[5] Aqeel, M., Shuja, K. H., Abbas, J., Rehna, T., & Ziapour, A. (2020). *The Influence of Illness Perception, Anxiety and Depression Disorders on Students Mental Health during COVID-19 Outbreak in Pakistan: A Web-Based Cross-Sectional Survey.* https://doi.org/10.21203/rs.3.rs-30128/v1.

[6] Sahu P. Closure of universities due to coronavirus disease 2019 (COVID-19): impact on education and mental health of students and academic staff. *Cureus.* 2020;12(4): e7541.

[7] Elmer T, Mepham K, Stadtfeld C. Students under lockdown: Comparisons of students' social networks and mental health before and during the COVID-19 crisis in Switzerland. *PLOS ONE.* 2020;15(7): e0236337.

[8] Regehr C, Glancy D, Pitts A (2013) Interventions to reduce stress in university students: a review and meta-analysis. *J Affect Disord* 148: 1-11. https://doi.org/10.1016/j.jad.2012.11.026.

[9] Grubic N, Badovinac S, Johri AM (2020) Student mental health during the Covid-19 pandemic: a call for further research and immediate solutions. *Int J Soc Psychiatry* 66: 517-518. https://doi.org/10.1177/0020764020925108.

[10] Wang, C., Pan, R., Wan, X., Tan, Y., Xu, L., Ho, C. S., & Ho, R. C. (2020) Immediate psychological responses and associated factors during the initial stage of the 2019 Coronavirus Disease (COVID-19) epidemic among the general population in China. *Int J Environ Res Public Health* 17: 1729. https://doi.org/10.3390/ijerph17051729.

[11] Cao, W., Fang, Z., Hou, G., Han, M., Xu, X., Dong, J., & Zheng, J. (2020) The psychological impact of the COVID-19 epidemic on college students in China. *Psychiatry Res* 287: 112934. https://doi.org/10.1016/j.psychres.2020.112934.

[12] Tang, W., Hu, T., Hu, B., Jin, C., Wang, G., Xie, C., Chen, S., & Xu, J. (2020) Prevalence and correlates of PTSD and depressive symptoms one month after the outbreak of the COVID-19 epidemic in a sample of home-quarantined Chinese university students. *J Affect Disord* 274: 1-7. https://doi.org/10.1016/j.jad.2020.05.009.

[13] Marelli, S., Castelnuovo, A., Somma, A., Castronovo, V., Mombelli, S., Bottoni, D., Leitner, C., Fossati, A., & Ferini-Strambi, L. (2021) Impact of COVID-19 lockdown on sleep quality in university students and administration staff. *J Neurol* 268: 8-15. https://doi.org/10.1007/s00415-020-10056-6.

[14] Young Minds Coronavirus: impact on young people with mental health needs (2020). Available from: https://youngminds.org.uk/media/3708/coronavirus-report_march2020.pdf.

[15] American College Health Association. American College Health Association-National College Health Assessment III: Reference Group Executive Summary Fall 2019. Silver Spring, MD; 2020.

[16] Yang Y, Li W, Zhang Q, Zhang L, Cheung T, Xiang YT. Mental health services for older adults in China during the COVID-19 outbreak. Vol. 7, *The Lancet Psychiatry*. Elsevier Ltd; 2020. p. e19. pmid:32085843.

[17] Song J, Song TM, Seo DC, Jīn DL, Kim JS. Social Big Data Analysis of Information Spread and Perceived Infection Risk during the 2015 Middle East Respiratory Syndrome Outbreak in South Korea. *Cyberpsychology, Behav Soc Netw.* 2017 Jan 1;20(1):22–9.

[18] Janz N. K., Becker M. H. The Health Belief Model: A Decade Later. *Heal Educ Behav.* 1984;11(1):1–47.

[19] Centers for Disease Control and Prevention C. Guidance for Institutes of Higher Education | CDC. 2020 Available from: https://www.cdc.gov/coronavirus/2019-ncov/community/colleges-universities/index.htm.

[20] Bhuiyan, A. K. M. I., Sakib, N., Pakpour, A. H., Griffiths, M. D., & Mamun, M. A. (2020). COVID-19-Related Suicides in Bangladesh Due to Lockdown and Economic Factors: Case Study Evidence from Media Reports. In *International Journal of Mental Health and Addiction.* Springer. https://doi.org/10.1007/s11469-020-00307-y.

[21] Chen, L., & Yuan, X. (2020). China's ongoing battle against the coronavirus: Why did the lockdown strategy work well? *Socio-Ecological Practice Research,* 2(2), 175–180. https://doi.org/10.1007/s42532-020-00048-1.

[22] Dhahri, A. A., Arain, S. Y., Memon, A. M., Rao, A., & Mian, M. A. (2020). "The psychological impact of COVID-19 on medical education of final year students in Pakistan: A cross-sectional study." *Annals of Medicine and Surgery,* 60, 445–450. https://doi.org/10.1016/j.amsu.2020.11.025.

[23] Darko, A. (2020). E-learning: Depression, anxiety, and stress symptomatology among Lebanese university students during COVID-19 quarantine. *Nursing Forum.* https://doi.org/10.1111/nuf.12521.

[24] Bolatov, A. K., Seisembekov, T. Z., Askarova, A. Z., Baikanova, R. K., Smailova, D. S., & Fabbro, E. (2020). Online-Learning due to COVID-19 Improved Mental Health Among Medical Students. *Medical Science Educator,* 1–10. https://doi.org/10.1007/s40670-020-01165-y.

[25] Kim Y. (2003). The impact of the internet on children's daily lives: Physical, Social and Psychological Well-being. Athens, Georgia.

[26] Esnard, A. M., Lai, B. S., Wyczalkowski, C., Malmin, N., & Shah, H. J. (2018). School vulnerability to disaster: an examination of school closure, demographic, and exposure factors in Hurricane Ike's wind swath. *Nat Hazards,* 90(2), 513-535. doi:10.1007/s11069-017-3057-2.

[27] Figlio, D. N., Rush, M., & Yin, L. (2013). Is it live, or is it the internet? Experimental estimates of the effects of online instruction on student learning. *Journal of Labour Economics,* 31(4), 763- 784. doi:10.1086/669930.

[28] Bacher-Hicks, A., Goodman, J., & Mulhern, C. (2021). Inequality in household adaptation to schooling shocks: Covid-induced online learning engagement in real-time. *Journal of public economics,* 193. DOI: 10.1016/j.jpubeco.2020.104345.

[29] Fisher, A. N., & Ryan, M. K. (2021). Gender inequalities during COVID-19. *Group processes & intergroup relations,* 24(2), 237-245. doi:10.1177/1368430220984248.

[30] Almaiah, M. A., Al-Khasawneh, A., & Althunibat, A. (2020). Exploring the critical challenges and factors influencing the E-learning system usage during the COVID-19 pandemic. *Educ Inf Technol* (Dordr), 1-20. doi:10.1007/s10639-020-10219-y.

[31] Andrew, A., Cattan, S., Costa Dias, M., Farquharson, C., Kraftman, L., Krutikova, S., Sevilla, A. (2020). Inequalities in Children's Experiences of Home Learning during the COVID-19 Lockdown in England. *Fisc Stud,* 41(3), 653-683. doi:10.1111/1475-5890.12240.

[32] Baker, M. (2013). Industrial actions in schools: Strikes and student achievement. *Canadian Journal of Economics/Revue canadienne d'économique,* 46(3), 1014-1036. doi:10.1111/caje.12035.

[33] Banerjee, A. V., & Duflo, E. (2014). (Dis)Organization and Success in an Economics MOOC. *American Economic Review,* 104(5), 514-518. doi:10.1257/aer.104.5.514.

[34] Haug, N., Geyrhofer, L., Londei, A., Dervic, E., Desvars-Larrive, A., Loreto, V., Pinior, B., Thurner, S., & Klimek, P. (2020). Ranking the effectiveness of worldwide COVID-19 government interventions. *Nat. Hum. Behav.* 4, 1303–1312. DOI : 10.1038/s41562-020-01009-0.

[35] Kaffenberger, M. (2021). Modelling the long-run learning impact of the Covid- 19 learning shock: actions to (more than) mitigate loss. *Int. J. Educ. Dev.* 81 :102326. DOI : 10.1016/j.ijedudev.2020.102326.

[36] Kuhfeld, M., Soland, J., Tarasawa, B., Johnson, A., Ruzek, E., and Liu, J. (2020a). Projecting the potential impact of COVID-19 school closures on academic achievement. *Educ. Res.* 49, 549–565. DOI : 10.3102/0013189X20965918.

[37] Kuhfeld, M., Tarasawa, B., Johnson, A., Ruzek, E., and Lewis, K. (2020b). Learning during COVID-19: Initial findings on students' reading and math achievement and growth. NWEA. Available online at: https://www.ewa.org/sites/main/files/file-attachments/learning_during_covid-19_brief_nwea_nov2020_final.pdf?1606835922.

[38] Andrew, A., Cattan, S., Dias, M. C., Farquharson, C., Kraftman, L., Krutikova, S., Phimister, A., & Sevilla, A. (2020). Learning During the Lockdown: Real-time data on Children's Experiences During Home Learning. The Institute for Fiscal Studies. Available online at: https://www.ifs.org.uk/publications/14848.

[39] Azevedo, J. P., Hasan, A., Goldemberg, D., Iqbal, S. A., and Geven, K. (2020). *Simulating the Potential Impacts of COVID-19 School Closures on Schooling and Learning Outcomes: A Set of Global Estimates.* Washington, D.C.: The World Bank.

Chapter 12

Psychological Resilience: A Conceptual Framework

Babasaheb Jadhav, PhD
Dr. D. Y. Patil Vidyapeeth's Global Business School and Research Centre, Pune, India

Abstract

Purpose: The significant effect of the COVID-19 pandemic epidemic was unprecedented. Corona Virus (COVID-19) spread across the globe very quickly, and it has caused widespread concern, fear and stress among the people.

Sadness, low mood, poor sleep, hopelessness or aimlessness, isolation, loss of income, low work output, fear, depression, tiredness, stress, and work pressure during work from home are some of the triggering factors of mental health conditions. Pandemics led to mental disorders or complications among the people. The study aims to determine how resilient people overcome challenges using their core strengths and abilities.

Methodology: Psychological Resilience is the mental or emotional ability of humans to cope with a crisis, conflicts, problems, issues, or challenges and return to normal or earlier situations speedily. Psychological Resilience strengthens humanity and supports the system to work for life's goals, overcome negativity, challenges, and adversities, and work through problems. The study has proposed a conceptual framework or model for being more resilient in day-to-day business, which will help individuals develop their strengths and capabilities and achieve desired goals.

Findings: The study has suggested the actions such as regular exercise, yoga & meditation, good relationships with peers, avoiding

In: Data Science Applications of Post-COVID-19 Psychological Disorders
Editor: Vijayalakshmi Kakulapati
ISBN: 979-8-88697-165-1

stress, change management, feasible goals, positivity, relevant actions, searching for opportunities, networking & communication, building confidence, long term stability, self-actualization needs, etc. to be more resilient.

Conclusion: Being resilient is the skills and abilities we can learn, polish, sharpen and develop a never-late-go attitude. Setting SMART goals and continuous motivation helps us become more resilient during distress situations and daily business activities. Last, it is always better to be more resilient for better future results or prospects.

Keywords: psychological disorders, resilience, psychological resilience, model of psychological resilience, mental resilience, theory of psychological emotional resilience, social resilience, framework of psychological resilience, physical resilience, resilience

Introduction

The novel COVID-19 pandemic has primarily affected socio-economic changes and lifestyles of human beings. Health science studies and Government reports stated that the novel Covid 19 pandemic impacts the mental illness and well-being of the general public, resulting in increased levels of nervousness, stress, insecurity, and sadness. The impact of the novel coronavirus pandemic on India and its economy has mainly been troublesome in terms of economic, social, and governance activities, as well as a massive loss of human lives [1].

The novel coronavirus pandemic has spread rapidly throughout the world, instilling fear, anxiety, worry, stress, and concern about life and death in the minds of the general public, including senior citizens, adults, caregivers, and people suffering from major or minor health issues [2].

During the COVID outbreak, one of the most concerning issues was human beings' mental and physical health. This resulted in an increased psychological impact on minds in terms of stress, fear, instability, anxiety, loneliness, depression, alcohol consumption, drug addiction or use, self-harm or suicidal behaviour, and so on.

The COVID pandemic is provoking anxiety among the patients, non-patients, relatives, families, peers, caregivers, and front-line healthcare professionals due to its increased level of infections. The uncertainty of indexes, future predictions, and government restrictions led to discomfort in social, occupational, psychological, familial, economic, and other functional domains. The high level of anxiety in people's minds was created because of unnecessary rumors, wrongly flooded information by media and the internet, changes in daily lifestyle and routine activities, economic instability, discrimination, disgrace, humiliation, feeling of unfriendliness, isolation, distancing and guilt.

In extreme cases, people may suffer through depression characterized by low mood, tiredness, pessimism, poor sleep or sleepless nights, appetite, feeling helpless, guilty, loneliness, hopelessness, work from home pressures with a gradual reduction in work output [3].

The World Health Organization monitored the novel COVID infections outbreak crisis and its impact on people's mental and physical health. It has been reviewed seriously and started monitoring the situation with national authorities by providing necessary information and guidance to local authorities, Governments, and the public.

Psychological Disorders

It refers to stress, mental illness, unstable behavior, and mind abnormalities resulting in relentless behavior that affects our day-to-day business activities.

The symptoms of the psychological disorder include mood patterns, personality forms, personality types, psychotic sicknesses, sexual syndromes, and others.

The causes of psychological illness or syndromes are not known. Still, some of the symptomatic factors may include an imbalance in brain function of the brain, hereditary issues, irritating behavior, childhood know-how, persistent illnesses, parenting issues, loneliness, lifestyle, likely earning, and stress [4].

The symptoms of psychological disorders can be chronic, unending, deterioration and degeneration. The common psychological disorder symptoms include:

- Agitation
- Unfriendliness or alone
- Aggression
- Alcohol addiction
- Drug addiction
- Physical health stamina

- Degradation in body energy level
- Anxiety level
- The confused state of mind
- Disconnectedness behavior
- Unpredictable behavior
- Irritable behavior
- Sudden changes in mood
- Perception thought process
- Contradictions in opinion or thoughts
- Social disconnectedness
- Strange physical and health issues
- Tiredness
- Dissatisfaction
- Loss of sleep
- Weight gain or loss
- Lack of enthusiasm
- Lack motivation
- Change in appetite
- Change in taste and preferences

Psychological and mental health issues among the Indians during post-COVID-19 have been a matter of concern in front of psychologists and scientists. The COVID pandemic has resulted in joblessness and illness at a higher level. In December 2021, the Central Government of India stated in Rajya Sabha that 10.6% of adults in India face psychological and mental disorders.

Adults and children in India sense the impact of post-COVID-19 on their mental health and well-being for many years to come for the long term. COVID-19 pandemic is heading into its third year, and the impact on the mental health of children [5], young people, and senior citizens continue to ponder very severely.

The study has proposed some standard practices to avoid psychological or mental disorders.

The influence of Post COVID-19 on children, youth, adults, and older people's mental health is very high. Special care and precautions are essential to avoid such circumstances. Families must maintain their work-life balance and quality of life and improve their psychological and mental health.

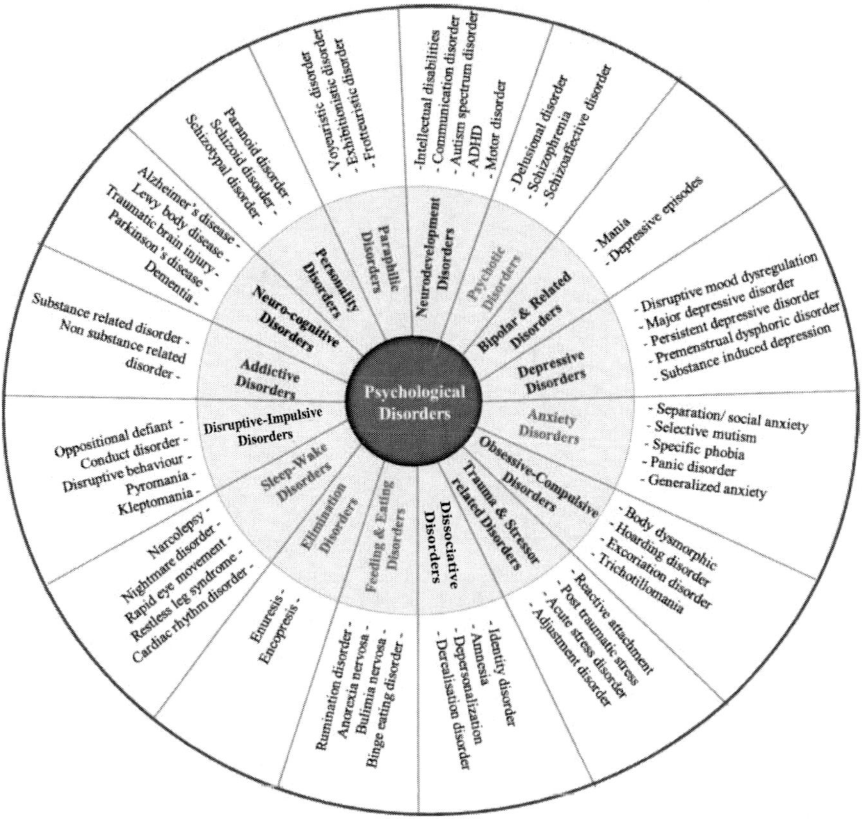
Psychological Disorders
Neurodevelopment Disorders
- Intellectual disabilities
- Communication disorder
- Autism spectrum disorder
- ADHD
- Motor disorder
Psychotic Disorders
- Delusional disorder
- Schizophrenia
- Schizoaffective disorder
Bipolar & Related Disorders
- Mania
- Depressive episodes
Depressive Disorders
- Disruptive mood dysregulation
- Major depressive disorder
- Persistent depressive disorder
- Premenstrual dysphoric disorder
- Substance induced depression
Anxiety Disorders
- Separation/ social anxiety
- Selective mutism
- Specific phobia
- Panic disorder
- Generalized anxiety
Obsessive-Compulsive Disorders
- Body dysmorphic
- Hoarding disorder
- Excoriation disorder
- Trichotillomania
Trauma & Stressor related Disorders
- Reactive attachment
- Post traumatic stress
- Acute stress disorder
- Adjustment disorder
Dissociative Disorders
- Identity disorder
- Amnesia
- Depersonalization
- Derealisation disorder
Feeding & Eating Disorders
Rumination disorder -
Anorexia nervosa -
Bulimia nervosa -
Binge eating disorder -
Elimination Disorders
Enuresis -
Encopresis -
Sleep-Wake Disorders
Narcolepsy -
Nightmare disorder -
Rapid eye movement -
Restless leg syndrome -
Cardiac rhythm disorder -
Disruptive-Impulsive Disorders
Oppositional defiant -
Conduct disorder -
Disruptive behaviour -
Pyromania -
Kleptomania -
Addictive Disorders
Substance related disorder -
Non substance related disorder -
Neuro-cognitive Disorders
Alzheimer's disease -
Lewy body disease -
Traumatic brain injury -
Parkinson's disease -
Dementia -
Personality Disorders
Paranoid disorder -
Schizoid disorder -
Schizotypal disorder -
Paraphilic Disorders
- Voyeuristic disorder
- Exhibitionistic disorder
- Frotteuristic disorder

Figure 1. Psychological disorders.

Everyday actions need to be taken, or a code of conduct has to be followed to overcome psychological disorder-related issues such as:

- Anti-anxiety medications
- Regular exercise
- Antidepressant medications
- Meditation
- Antipsychotic medications
- Regular health check-ups
- Cognitive-behavioral therapy
- Family therapy
- Group therapy
- Yoga

- Hospitalization
- Identification of health conditions
- Individual therapy
- Mood-stabilizing medications
- Psychodynamic therapy
- Talk therapy
- Avoiding the use of alcohol or drugs
- Avoiding the use of caffeine, drugs, or other things
- Eating at regular intervals
- Getting enough sleep
- Keeping appointments with health advisors or family physicians
- Taking medications as suggested

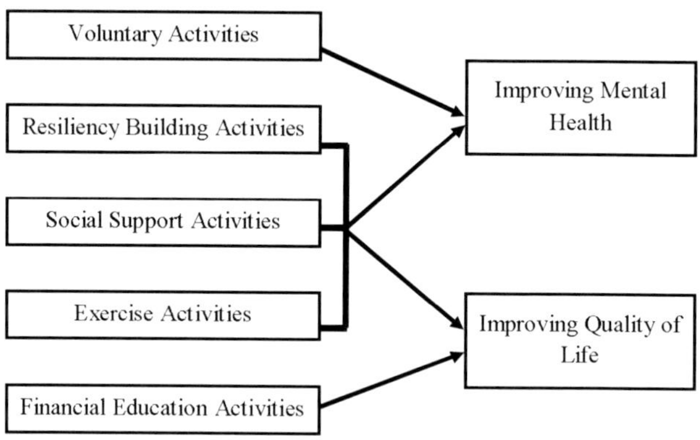

Figure 2. Activities for avoiding psychological disorders.

Psychological Resilience

Human beings can deal with whatever severe challenges or issues in life. A resilient person always overcomes challenges or adversities by using strengths and other core abilities such as hopes, optimism, motivation, and positivity.

Psychological resilience exists in people who have developed behavioral strengths, abilities, competencies, and holistic proficiency that permit them to remain calm and quiet during problems, emergencies, or chaos [6]. Psychological resilience is always studied and often worked out similarly to the Psychological immune system among human beings.

The best example of positive psychological resilience is the actions or efforts taken by Americans to rebuild [7] the lives of their people during the terrorist attacks of September 11, 2001.

One best example of positive psychological resilience is the efforts taken by the Japanese people after the nuclear weapons attack and explosions by the United States on August 06 & 09, 1945, to rebuild a new and vibrant Japan.

Dr. Ginsburg has proposed seven different essential and solid components [8] that build and construct human beings as strong, resilient people, such as confidence, connection, competence, character, coping, contribution, and control.

Competence is the ability to deal with the state of affairs carefully, effectively, and efficiently. To construct and develop competency, individuals need to imbibe a specific set of attitudes, skills, and knowledge that will help them trust their decisions, judgments, and conclusions to make choices.

Confidence: True and correct self-confidence and courage are developed through competency skills. Individuals can gain self-confidence and courage by representing their aptitude and competency skills in real-life business or situations.

Connection: Strong network, social connectedness, and bonding with family members, friends, colleagues, peers, and community service providers give a sense of safety, protectiveness, secureness, and belongingness.

Character: The exemplary character of an individual reflects a shared sense of right or wrong, good or bad, primarily to make wise choices, contribute towards society at significant, social responsibility and experience self-actualization.

Contribution: It is very well said that having an intellectual common sense, purpose, objective, and appetite among the individuals proved to be one of the powerful motivators. People contributing to the community, society, or service providers regain positive and shared relationships.

Coping: Coping is the ability and skills to overcome problems and adversities in day-to-day business. When humans learn how to cope with stress, fear and anxiety efficiently and effectively, they are highly prepared and well set to handle future difficulties, challenges, adversities, and uncertainties.

Control: Building and developing strong self-contentment and internal control function of physique and body assist individuals to act as problem-solvers rather than culprits or victims of any circumstances. As soon as individuals learn that he or they can control the results and outcomes of their decisions, they are most likely to see themselves as deserving, capable, and confident people in their life.

The unique abilities and pillars resilient persons develop are self-awareness, mindfulness, self-care, positive relationships, motivation, and clarity in goals or purpose of life, which will help them in problem solving and self-actualization.

Resilience gives psychological strength to humans to cope with their stress, disorder, challenges, and hardship. Psychological studies observed that resilient individuals are better at handling difficulty and rebuilding their lives.

Resilience is the thought process of positive vibes, confidence, and gut feeling after stressful, unpleasant, or unfavorable activities when a person is flooded with stress, disturbances, imbalances, challenges, or opportunities.

Psychological resilience is built or developed among humanity because of individuals' changing behaviors and thought processes. To develop strong resilience, a person must eliminate negativity, negative talks, loose talks, de-motivation, dissatisfaction, or negative vibes. Such as I can't do this task, it's not my cup of tea, it's beyond my control, or I can't handle this problem, and replace them with positive talks or positive vibes such as I can do this, I can manage this, I can solve this problem, I will succeed, or I can handle this. This small change in management actions, thought processes and behavior facilitates the reduction of psychological stress or mental pressure whenever persons are dealing with complex problems, challenges, or unbeatable life tragedies. Positive thought processes and vibes help keep human beings' intellects at an extraordinary level in their work-life balance. Resilient people are always ready well before to deal with challenges, crises, unforeseen events, difficulties, uncertainties, and emergencies and keep themselves more robust. People's resilience is improved through positive learning and cognitive abilities such as meditation, exercise, yoga, socialization, and self-care activities.

American Psychological Association [9] has suggested ten different ways to bring more resilience among persons, such as:

1. Maintaining healthy relationships with peers, family members, and friends
2. Ignore crises, stressful events, or unbeatable problems
3. Accept the reality
4. Feasibility in goals
5. Take relevant problem-solving actions
6. Looking for alternatives and opportunities

7. Self-confidence
8. Long-term plans and perspective
9. Follow positive approach
10. Pay attention to needs, satisfaction level, and feelings

The term resilience is commonly used to showcase the strengths, capabilities, confidence, and coping skills during a wrong time or difficulties. The components of resilience are categorized into Psychological, Emotional, Physical, and Community.

Psychological resilience is the ability to spiritually and mentally stand with or overcome uncertainties, difficulties, dangers, hard times, challenges, and problems. It is also referred to as 'mental courage or strength.' The person who shows such skills develops successful plans, actions, and abilities that enable persons to remain cool, calm, positive, and motivated during bad times and move on without negativity in the long term.

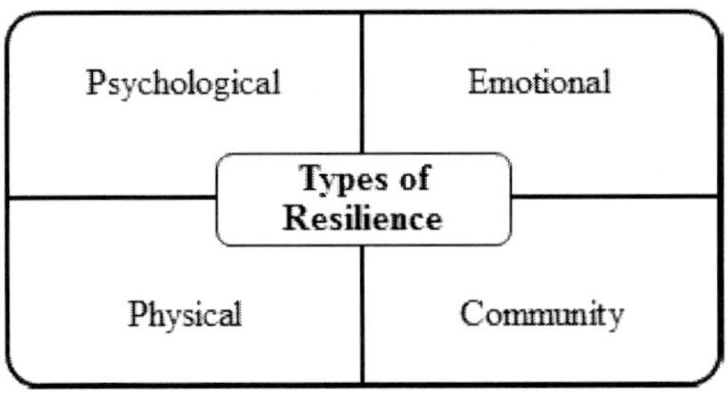

Figure 3. Types of resilience.

Emotional resilience is a person's ability to deal with stress and problems emotionally. Some of the person's traits are strong, weak, emotional, emotionless, sentimental, etc. By nature or personality traits, some people are more, or some are less sensitive to accepting and adapting to new changes [10]. How a person responds to situations or problems can generate or develop more emotions.

Such people understand what they are feeling, what they want to achieve, where they want to be, and why they want to achieve it. They are always optimistic, even when dealing with a crisis and making the best use of available resources. Emotionally resilient people are able to manage stressors from their peer teams as well as their emotions in the right way.

Physical resilience is the ability of human beings to adapt to new challenges, maintain physical stamina and a high level of energy or strength and recover swiftly and efficiently from complex problems. Human beings can work proactively and recover smoothly from illness, accidents, or other physical issues.

It also plays a significant role in solid aging while people encounter health issues and physical stress.

Mind control, change in lifestyle, consumption, preferences, choices, appetite, building relations, bonding, regular exercise, finding sufficient time for rest, medication, overcoming illness, deep breathing, yoga, and engaging themselves in enjoyable activities plays a significant role in building physical resilience [11].

Community resilience is the ability of groups to take action, respond and get better things done from adverse problems such as natural disasters, acts of God, violence, economic slow-down or crisis, and other community-related challenges.

Some real examples include the 9/11 terrorist attacks, hurricanes, wars, terrorism attacks, floods, etc.

During the COVID-19 Pandemic Lockdown, everybody was at home. Schools, Colleges, and Offices were operational from home. While operating work from home, tremendous work, assignments, pressures, deadlines, and stress resulted in conflicts, disputes and inequality in the work-life balance.

For work-life balance, handling stress and keeping resilience at work, we must follow certain practices in our routine lifestyles. The structure above suggests how the ordinary person or human beings can build resilience at work or in offices.

Literature Review

Research studies on resilience need to state the concept of resilience clearly [12].

Over the last two to three decades, resilience has become a prevalent concept in science [13]. It seems that the conceptual framework interprets a positive approach among the individuals to deal with complex, challenging, and even hopeless situations.

Even though many studies on psychological resilience research from health science, some concerns regarding the clarity and utility of the term are still unattempted or unresolved [14].

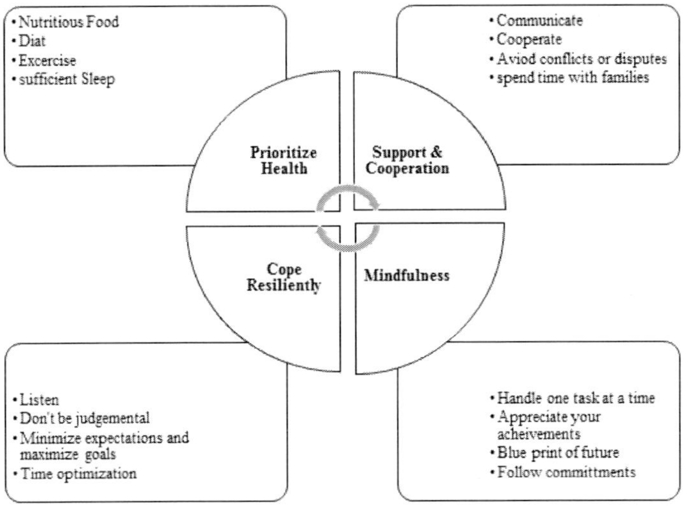

Figure 4. Building resilience at work.

A lack of comprehensive and meaningful ways of measuring resilience adaptability [15].

The pandemic has caused unpredictable threats to the well-being of families, such as anxiety, stress, and depression [16].

Resilience factors are linked with a lower level of anxiety over COVID, stress, negative thoughts of the pandemic, and improved well-being [17].

A cognitive approach to investigating the relationships between adversity, stress, and resilience was propose [18]. Cognitive models provide a theoretical framework resilience process.

A multi-dimensional model evaluated [19] psychological resilience in terms of adverse outcomes such as stress, distress, and health.

A study found a positive relationship between levels of personal resilience and adverse outcomes such as tiredness, stress, or fatigue [20].

A review and critique the variety of definitions, concepts, and theories of psychological resilience. In the end, these narratives are divided into three main sections [21].

Methodology and Framework

Resilience structure or framework is presented as the conceptual model or framework to understand how individuals can bounce back in their career or life after experiencing adverse problems with the help of their strengths and focused approach.

The new, vibrant, disciplined country that is Japan emerged after the nuclear weapons attack, and explosions is the best example.

The Resilience methodology, theory, and framework summarize ideas and practices that build and promote resilience. It is based on a conceptual body of study and practice development called Resilient Therapy.

The study found that the factors influencing people's psychological well-being are perceived mental stress. Every individual experiences stress and work pressures in life by way of life transitions, social change, life events, and environmental change, all of which are surrounded by poverty, hunger, and social violence.

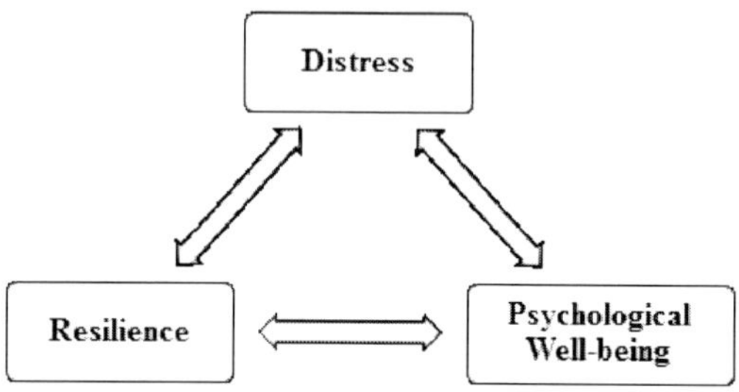

Figure 5. Resilience well-being framework.

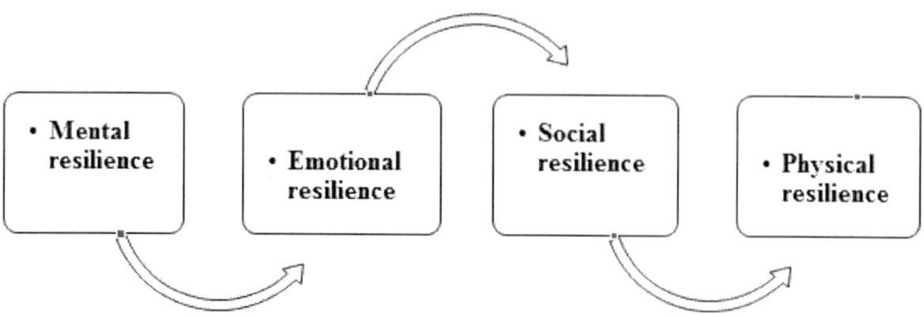

Figure 6. Types of resilience.

Resilience is the positive integration of people's physical, mental and spiritual qualities during good or bad times.

In general, there are four different kinds of resilience observed among human beings:

a) Mental resilience is the ability to strongly adapt to life goals and challenges in highly adverse conditions.

b) Emotional resilience is the skill to adapt to stressful situations or crises. More resilient people always think out of the box whereas less resilient people never come out of their comfort zone.
c) Social resilience is an ability to stand, absorb, cope with & adjust to threats from social entities.
d) Physical resilience is the ability to adapt to challenges, gain energy and develop stamina, determinant approach, and strengths.

Organizational growth is one of the significant factors behind the long-term stability, success, and sustainability of the business. The model below considered optimum available resources, optimistic behavior, time-to-time feedback, and core capabilities for organizational growth and sustainable results.

Psychological resilience is best understood as a continuous process of generating strength through various actions. Whenever persons are facing adverse problems or conditions, there are three common ways to tackle it such as:

a) Annoyance or Anger
b) Negative emotions
c) Upset, disturbances, and disruptive change

The conceptual model found that several common factors help in developing resilience, such as:

a) Abilities
b) Confidence
c) Communication
d) Feelings and satisfaction level

However, these variables may vary among different age groups or person to person in practice? Resilience is positively related to various personality traits such as openness and positive emotions.

A positive emotion serves an important function that helps individuals to overcome stressful events and encounter problems.

Social support doesn't mean good relationships with others. Such relationships may also evolve harmony of trust, bonding, humanism, cohesion, communication, unity, and fruitful dialogues within and outside the group of family and peers.

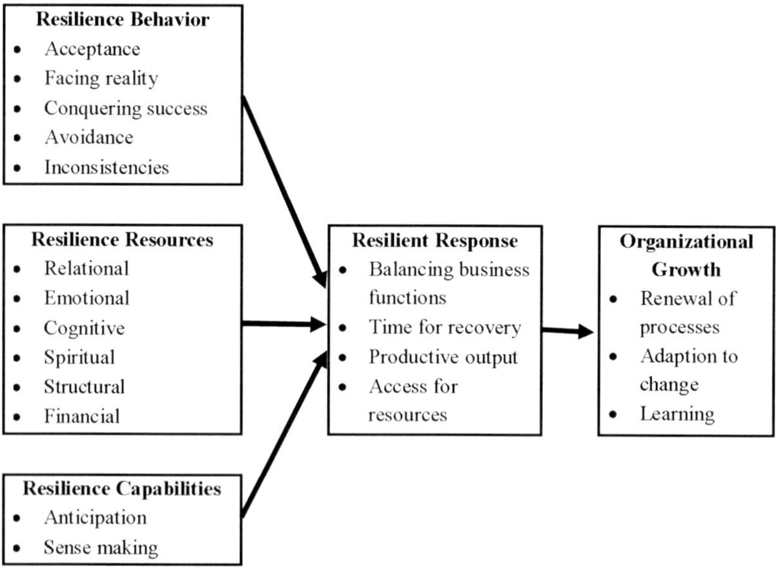

Figure 7. Resilience framework for organizational growth.

Conclusion

Psychological resilience is the ability of a person to handle issues or problems mentally or emotionally. Resilience exists with a person's psychological processes and behaviors in promoting and protecting themselves from stress.

Being resilient skill or quality, we can imbibe into our personality. Setting SMART goals helps us to become more resilient. The study and framework suggest some of the following actions to be more resilient.

Meditation helps relax our body which helps in lowering blood pressure, heart rates, breathing rate, oxygen consumption, and stress.

Reframe conditions or situations and measure the dilemma's positive side rather than the opposing side.

Social networks are the critical stress boosters. We can cope better if we have good people to share thoughts with.

Whenever there are adverse situations or problems, promote and encourage positive thinking among the group or peers.

Laughing and exercising more can decrease stress and boost the immune system.

Look for a positive outcome and not a negative, and be optimistic.

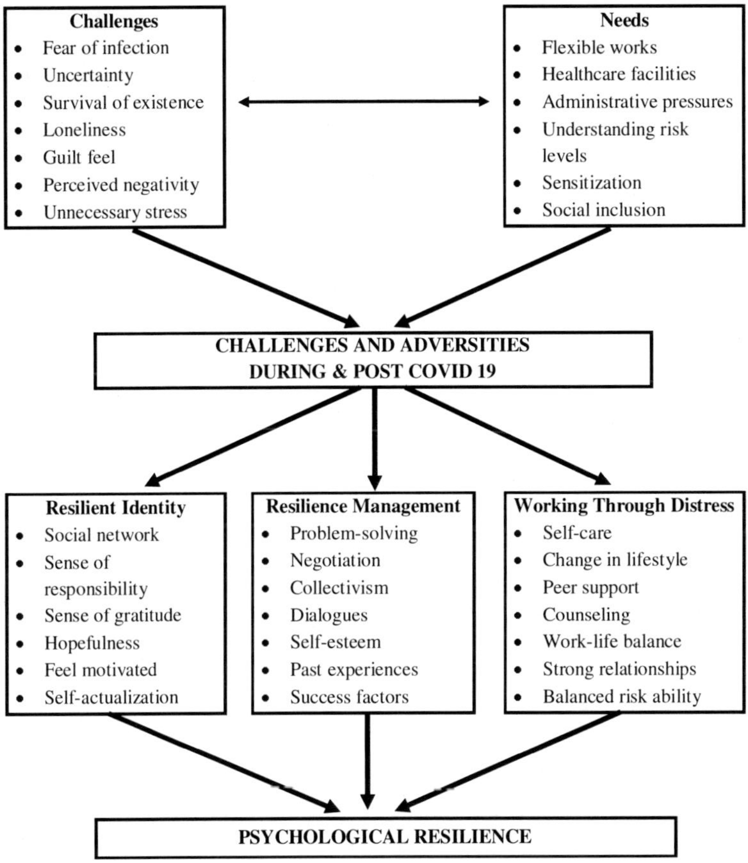

Figure 8. Psychological resilience model.

Lacking Psychological resilience among persons can be met with unhealthy issues. Resilience gives people the strength and courage needed to overcome hardships. Resilient people regularly knock their strengths to defeat their challenges and problems.

References

[1] Wu, Yu, Wenzhou Yu, Xiuyun Wu, Huihui Wan, Ying Wang, and Guohua Lu. Psychological resilience and positive coping styles among Chinese undergraduate students: A cross-sectional study. BMC Psychological 8, 79 (2020). https://doi.org/10.1186/s40359-020-00444-y.

[2] Wu Y, Sang Z, Zhang X C and Margraf J (2020). The Relationship Between Resilience and Mental Health in Chinese College Students: A Longitudinal Cross-Lagged Analysis. Front. Psychological. 11:108. https://doi: 10.3389/fpsyg.2020.00108.

[3] Ayed N, Toner S, Priebe S. Conceptualizing resilience in adult mental health literature: A systematic review and narrative synthesis. Psychological Therapy 2019; 92:299-341.

[4] Davis M C, Luecken L, Lemery Chalfant K. Resilience in ordinary life: Introduction to the special issue. Journal Perspective 2009; 77:1637-44.

[5] Godara, M., Silveira, S., Matthäus, H. et al. The Wither or Thrive Model of Resilience: an Integrative Framework of Dynamic Vulnerability and Resilience in the Face of Repeated Stressors During the COVID-19 Pandemic. ADV RES SCI (2022). https://doi.org/10.1007/s42844-022-00069-7

[6] Hu T, Zhang D, Wang J. A meta-analysis of the trait resilience and mental health. Perspective Individual Difference 2015; 76:18-27.

[7] Klitzman S, Freudenberg N. Implications of the World Trade Center attack for the public health and health care infrastructures. Am J Public Health. 2003 Mar;93(3):400-6. doi: 10.2105/ajph.93.3.400.

[8] https://cbtprofessionals.com.au/the-7-cs-of-resilience

[9] Park, C L, Finkelstein-Fox, L, Russell, B S, Fendrich, M, Hutchison, M, & Becker, J (2021). Psychological resilience early in the COVID-19 pandemic: Stressors, resources, and coping strategies in a national sample of Americans. American Psychologist, 76(5), 715-728. https://doi.org/10.1037/amp0000813.

[10] Pai N, Vella S L. Can one spring back from psychosis? The role of resilience in severe mental illness. August NZJ Psychiatry 2018; 52:1093-4.

[11] Infurna F J, Jayawickreme E. Fixing the growth illusion: New directions for research in resilience and post-traumatic growth. Current Directory of Psychological Science 2019; 28:152-8.

[12] Vella S L C, Pai N B. A theoretical review of psychological resilience: Defining resilience and resilience research over the decades. *Arch. Med. Health Science* 2019; 7:233-9.

[13] Stainton, Alexandra, Katharine Chisholm, Nathalie Kaiser, Marlene Rosen, Rachel Upthegrove, Stephan Ruhrmann, and Stephen J. Wood. Resilience as a multimodal dynamic process. *Early Interventional Psychiatry* 2019; 13:725-32.

[14] Windle, G. (2011). What is resilience? A review and concept analysis. *Reviews in Clinical Gerontology, 21*(2), 152–169. https://doi.org/10.1017/S0959259810000420

[15] Panter-Brick, C. and Leckman, J.F. (2013) Resilience in Child Development: Interconnected Pathways to Wellbeing. Journal of Child Psychology and Psychiatry, 54, 333-336. http://dx.doi.org/10.1111/jcpp.12057

[16] Maria Gayatri, Dian Kristiani Irawaty, Family Resilience during COVID-19 Pandemic: A Literature Review, First Published July 14, 2021 Research Article. https://doi.org/10.1177/10664807211023875

[17] Janusz Surzykiewicz, Karol Konaszewski, Sebastian Skalski, Paweł Piotr Dobrakowski, Jolanta Muszyńska, Resilience and Mental Health in the Polish Population during the COVID-19 Lockdown: A Mediation Analysis, DOI: 10.3390/jcm10214974

[18] Sam Parsons, Anne-Wil Kruijt, Elaine Fox, A Cognitive Model of Psychological Resilience, First Published June 26, 2016, Research Article https://doi.org/10.5127/jep.053415
[19] Ian de Terte, Christine Stephens, Lynne Huddleston, The development of a three part model of psychological resilience, DOI: 10.1002/smi.2625
[20] Clare S Rees, Lauren J Breen, Lynette Cusack, Desley Hegney, Understanding individual resilience in the workplace: the international collaboration of workforce resilience model, DOI: 10.3389/fpsyg.2015.00073
[21] Fletcher D, Sarkar M. Psychological resilience: A review and critique of definitions, concepts, and theory. *European Psychological* 2013; 18:12-23.

Chapter 13

Challenges and Privacy Concerns Related to Mental Health

K. Shirisha*

Department of CSE, Sreenidhi Institute of Science and Technology, Hyderabad, India

Abstract

The outbreak of the COVID-19 pandemic, since time surged across nations, has affected millions of people in several nations. With over 268 million cases and 5.28 million reported deaths, the caseload is rising further in many countries. The stipulated measures are undertaken worldwide to contain the spread of infections through social distancing, quarantine, and lockdown in the regions. The numerous lockdowns imposed across nations in the past several months to contain terrorism have slowed economic growth. Isolation, grief, and loss of income trigger mental health conditions or aggravate existing ones. In the long term, the impacts on the population are wide-ranging from depression, post-traumatic stress syndrome, anxiety, insomnia, domestic and substance abuse, emotional chaos, and behavioral changes. People with pre-existing morbidities face higher chances of acute severe medical outcomes that may eventually be fatal. These factors affect an individual's mental health, leading to economic and social withdrawal. The first global data drawn from the survey of the 130 severely affected countries suggests that symptoms of anxiety, depression, and severe psychological reactions amount to 15 to 30%. Addressing such a population's mental health conditions has become a pressing issue for healthcare providers. The challenges involve the identification of the

*Corresponding Author's Email: shirisha49@yahoo.com.

In: Data Science Applications of Post-COVID-19 Psychological Disorders
Editor: Vijayalakshmi Kakulapati
ISBN: 979-8-88697-165-1

population segment requiring medical services to treat psychological and mental illnesses post-COVID-19 pandemic. At the same time, addressing the privacy concerns of such a large population is also pivotal. The privacy regulatory frameworks adopted by the regional and federal governments are pressing upon procedures to preserve the privacy of people suffering from post-COVID-19 psychological distress syndrome. In this chapter, the privacy mechanisms are detailed, which will provide non-disclosure of personal and sensitive data during treatments. The exchange of health-related data and personal identifiers is subject to territorial privacy rules without revealing personally identifiable information (PII).

Keywords: mental health, COVID-19 post-traumatic distress syndrome, privacy methods, personally identifiable information

Introduction

In December 2019, the widespread outbreak of novel coronavirus pneumonia, COVID-19, an infectious health problem caused by the SARS-CoV-2 virus, hit scores of individuals across continents. Originating from Wuhan province in China, the epidemic has taken the world population by storm, forcing the World Health Organization to declare it a pandemic in March 2020 [1]. Millions affected by acute respiratory illness seek emergency medical help. Acclaimed as a high contagion, SARS-CoV-2 has spread across 220 countries so far. As of Jan 18, 2022, approximately 365 million people worldwide have been infected with SARS-CoV-2, with the cases still rising [2]. Out of this, about 359 million people have recovered, and more than 5.6 million have died due to the coronavirus. These statistics project the recovery and death rates at about 98.3% and 1.53%, respectively.

The precedence, in recent decades, has been the regional outbreaks of contagious and infectious illnesses, namely, Ebola virus (2013) [3, 4, 5], Middle East Respiratory Syndrome Coronavirus (MERS-CoV) (2012) [3, 6], the 2009 H1N1 Pandemic (H1N1pdm09 virus) influenza [7, 8,] the 2002 SARS [9, 10], and the 1968 H3N2 virus pandemic [11]. Previous studies and responses found that acute medical needs must be treated on an emergency basis. Thirty cores of people have been affected when we write this article, and two waves of COVID-19 have been completed [12]. Tens of thousands of healthcare workers (HCWs) are fighting at the front lines, either directly (e.g., physicians, nurses) or indirectly (e.g., aides, laboratory technicians, and medical waste handlers), in delivering care to patients and racing against the clock to resolve the challenges manifested in healthcare systems.

From the preceding times, it is observed that epidemics and pandemic outbreaks vitiate sustainable development as human health is greatly affected. The magnitude of the COVID-19 pandemic has stymied the countries' economic growth and is regarded as one of the most significant public health emergencies in human history [13]. With millions of children left orphaned, eroded civil order, and disrupted social life due to the recent pandemic, there are other bothersome issues to be taken care of.

Scientists worldwide have driven their efforts to provide vaccines via accelerated processes to usher in much-needed antidotes for COVID-19 and provide immunity to the public. Many pharmaceutical industries and drug R & D institutes, including public organizations and private companies, have worked together to make COVID-19 vaccines available to the public. Much-needed success is also achieved with the varying vaccine efficacy by the leading pharmaceutical research bodies. While COVID-19 vaccines were developed rapidly, all steps have been taken to ensure their safety and effectiveness. Right from Initial Development, Clinical Trials, Authorization or Approval, Manufacturing and Distribution, and Tracking Safety Using Vaccine Monitoring Systems, remarkable achievements are garnered in controlling and containing the pandemic.

Although the recovery rate is improving, the isolation and quarantine phases that the person undergoes during the infection and treatment courses are triggering mental health illnesses [14] or exacerbating prevailing co-morbidities. In the reports, many people are said to be facing increased levels of contraband use [15].

Meanwhile, COVID-19 can lead to neurological and mental complications, such as agitation, increased cases of delirium, and emergency hospital admissions due to stroke. When SARS-CoV-2 infects a person, they are more likely to have harmful effects or even die. This is especially true for people with drug or mental or neurological problems [16].

The vital infrastructural unit of the healthcare ecosystem providing services to patients suffering from various mental ailments is the data stores containing the patients' health information. The health department's primary concern was disinfecting the patients and preventing the infection chain from spreading further. COVID-19 patients who had pre-existing psychological ailments or developed similar mental ailments during the treatment stage had to be treated for COVID-19 on priority to contain further spread in the community. The medical agencies, from the diagnostic centers to treatment institutes, maintained the electronic health records (EHRs) of individuals infected with the coronavirus. Many institutions are engaged, such as medical institutes, quarantine centers; isolation wards; diagnostic centers; insurance companies; government authorities such as the health department, and municipal and civic amenity departments.

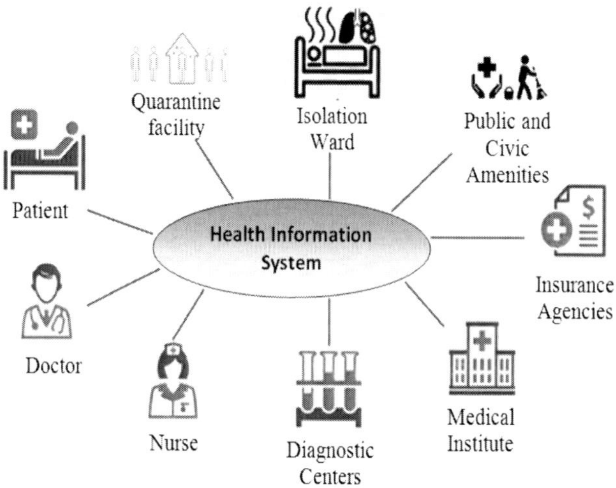

Figure 1. Entities sharing the EHRs of the Health Information System.

The sharing of EHRs is extensive, thereby bringing in security concerns regarding the information shared. As a result, data secrecy and privacy become vulnerable, resulting in threats and, eventually, breaches. This chapter provides an extensive account of the challenges faced while implementing the security mechanisms. A detailed study is being conducted on the measures available to preserve the EHRs' privacy. We present an analysis of using a hybrid model to secure information while maintaining the privacy and anonymity of EHRs shared over the public internet.

The arrangement of the sections in this chapter is as mentioned here. In Section 2, the impacts of quarantine and social distancing in detail. The following section details a discussion on mental health issues after COVID-19 recovery. Sections 4 and 5 explain the psychological impacts suffered by healthcare workers and the interruptions in critical mental health care, respectively. The subsequent section mentions social inequalities suffered by the bereaved individuals affected by the coronavirus. In section 7, the significance of the MHIS is accounted for, and in Section 8, the security challenges in accessing EHRs. In Section 9, popular privacy-preserving mechanisms are detailed. In Section 10, the benefits of both encrypting confidential and sensitive data and keeping it private are laid out. Section 10 ends with some conclusions.

Psychological Impacts of Social Distancing Curbs

One of the main measures to contain the spread of infectious diseases like SARS, MERS, and persisting novel coronavirus, is quarantine and social distancing. These measures are extended further in specific regions where the spread and infected individuals are more. The persons need to undergo a quarantine period and stay in isolation until the individual is free of symptoms, becomes non-contagious, and tests negative for the virus.

Immediately after the quarantine period, the individuals experience a feeling of loneliness, depression, emotional perturbation, job losses, financial difficulty, insomnia, irritability, and post-traumatic stress symptoms. Infected people resort to careful hand washing and alcohol abuse and undergo behavioral changes, including avoiding crowded avenues [17]. In the long run, the effects are aggravated considerably in terms of anger, depression, anxiety, post-traumatic stress, domestic violence, child abuse, and substance abuse. Individuals may suffer from these psychological ailments for a long time, ranging from six months to three years post-COVID-19 quarantine [18]. Hikikomori is a health condition that arises from long-drawn-out social isolation leading to social withdrawal [19], which the socioeconomic crisis of the pandemic may further aggravate. COVID-19-related social distancing and isolation norms often appear the same as those of Hikikomori syndrome. There exists an underlying cause that creates distinct variations between the two. The government's quarantining and isolation related to COVID-19 are self-imposed to ward away infections, whereas the other is the individuals' avoidance behavior [20]. The impacts are amplified for individuals who experienced losing a loved one due to the spread of such contagious and deadly illnesses [21, 22]. Such distressing events pose a potential threat, leading to the downfall of the mental well-being of many.

Mental Health Issues after COVID-19 Recovery

The new norms set by the local and federal governments, like working from home and social distancing, are causing a distressing impact on communities. Income loss aggravates the existing mental illnesses in the individuals of the family. Mounting expenditure for essential goods and services, home-schooling of children due to the closure of the study centers, and lack of physical contact among the members of the family, friends, and colleagues are taking a toll on the emotional stability and mental well-being of an individual.

In some hospitalized patients who had to be treated for COVID-19, their mental health status deteriorated as they developed neurological and mental complications, such as agitation, mental aggression, delirium, and stroke. People with pre-existing mental health co-morbidities or who are addicted to substances are more vulnerable to being infected with SARS-CoV-2 [21], which can cause severe illness and even death. Sufficient data is not available to infer the long-term psychiatric complications of people with severe COVID-19 infection. However, they may be similar to previous epidemics that broke out regionally, such as severe acute respiratory syndrome (SARS) and Middle East Respiratory Syndrome (MERS), exhibiting an increased prevalence of neurological effects like anxiety, depression, and PTSD.

Among the survivors of COVID-19, continual psychiatric impairments are reported after one year of discharge, with significant levels of PTSD, anxiety, and depression [22]. Neurocognitive impairments are reported worldwide, especially among the elderly and patients with pre-existing psychological conditions. From the data available, conditions primarily recorded are reduced mental processing speed and concentration, impaired attention, reduced memory retention, and severe acute respiratory distress syndrome. People hospitalized for a long time in the ICUs and treated with invasive treatments like mechanical ventilators and life-support systems for COVID-19 were found to have a much lower quality of life and overall health than those with the same treatments in-patients for other illnesses [23].

Psychological Impacts on Frontline Healthcare Professionals

Previous epidemic outbreak studies [24] provide an excellent record of the long-term implications for frontline healthcare workers (HCWs). The well-being of the healthcare team treating a multitude of patients suffering from infectious diseases is reported as being hindered, leading to persistent psychopathological consequences. In handling the recent coronavirus pandemic, the healthcare fraternity faced a compounded global crisis in terms of medical infrastructure available, insufficient staff, and other potential mediating factors in handling scores of patients admitted to hospitals with acute medical needs. This has caused massive burnout among frontline healthcare workers. The medical professionals played a vital role in discharging their duties diligently in a challenging and bitter fight against COVID-19. The repercussions are compounded for individuals who have lost loved ones in the battle against such a virulent and highly infectious disease. Because of the sudden rise in demand for healthcare services, healthcare workers have been forced to work longer hours. Poorer sleep quality while wearing personal protective equipment (PPE), limiting their ability to move freely, and because of their fear of spreading infections to their families and coworkers, all of which have contributed to an increase in psychosomatic problems among them.

Unlike the preceding epidemics, which were eventually contained for a shorter time than the prevailing coronavirus pandemic, some specific features heightened its potential to negatively impact the mental health of healthcare providers (HCPs) [25].

In light of the massive number of individuals impacted by the epidemic and the widespread dissemination of information via the media, many believe that "being ill sooner or later" is an unavoidable part of life. The health bulletins have been doing the rounds, informing us about the alarming rise in the number of infected people and the rise in deaths due to COVID-19. This, in turn, is creating emotional panic among the people of the HCP group, causing further distress in their psychological health in negative ways.

Secondly, many HCWs' usual workplaces have been changed by healthcare demand. They are put in high-risk frontline jobs in places like intensive care units where there are a lot of viruses. The medical students are also being sent to help stop the infections from spreading further and worsening.

Thirdly, the doctors and other assisting staff must be in their protective equipment (PPE), which forbids free bodily mobility and raises the absolute risk of transmission during the discharge of the healthcare services. As a result of COVID-19, HCWs' mental well-being has been negatively impacted by the uncertainty about the PPE supply and quality and diminished social events. Kits' respiratory discomfort and difficulties prove to be aggravating factors for HCWs' psychological symptoms when using the continuous PPE system.

Unlike other services, which pose a reduced threat of getting infected while performing duties, the HCWs see a potential danger while being in service. The British Medical Association found that 45 percent of UK medical practitioners suffer from mental health issues such as depression, anxiety, stress, and exhaustion. This has been exacerbated by the COVID-19 situation in their survey conducted in May 2020 [26].

As the pandemic continues, HCWs play a critical role in our response to the COVID-19 infection. Among the medical fraternity, it is a well-known fact that HCWs exhibit high rates of pre-existing mental health disorders worldwide, which may negatively impact the quality of patient care [27]. In the aftermath, healthcare givers are also more prone to experiencing long-term mental health issues. During the COVID-19 pandemic, reported cases among frontline healthcare workers and medical residents increased by 60% [28] and are expected to continue for years. An HCP who worked in the ward for respiratory medicine during the SARS outbreak in 2003 is reported to have suffered from comparatively higher levels of psychological distress a year later [29]. PTSD during epidemic or pandemic outbreaks was up by 11%–73% among health care professionals, lasting up to 10–40% after 1–3 years [30].

In several other studies, issues relating to the mental health of the HCWs have been reported worldwide, with anxiety, depression, and insomnia being the most common [31]. For the betterment of the medical field, changes are needed to provide better psychosocial support and more accurate information about diseases.

Interruptions to Critical Services of Mental Healthcare

During the third quarter of 2020, a survey of 130 countries was carried out throughout the six WHO regions to evaluate how COVID-19 has altered patient care. This survey evaluated the services in place for treating mental, neurological, and substance abuse patients. Countries' responses to interrupted services and their obstacles were also examined in the research. Several types of vital mental health services were noted to be lacking by nations in the WHO study [32].

- More than 60% of healthcare services for addressing the mental health conditions of vulnerable people were reported to be disrupted, with children and adolescents making up 72% and senior citizens amounting to 70%. Out of all, 30% reported disruptions to access to medications for mental, neurological, and substance use disorders.

- Over 35% of people reported disruptions in emergency medical care for experiencing prolonged seizures, including cases with severe withdrawal syndromes and delirium, which is often considered a sign of a serious underlying medical issue.
- More than 65% had to face cancellation disruptions to psychotherapy and counseling sessions, critical harm reduction services amounted to 65%, and 45% received treatment to eliminate opioid dependence.
- Partial disruptions of the mental healthcare services offered at school and workplace were reported to be over 75% and 78% in the countries surveyed.
- More than half of the countries looked at treating people with mental health problems through telemedicine or teletherapy. However, technological impediments are significant bottlenecks in reaping the benefits of these interventions. This is viable in countries where medical aid patients have good internet and telecommunications facilities. When it comes to filling in the gaps in mental health treatment, high-income nations are more than twice as likely as low-income countries to have used technology like telemedicine and teletherapy.

In the majority of countries, cases remain unreported unless and until they become an emergency. Most of the time, patients don't use mental health services because they don't know enough about mental health they don't know about mental health services, they are afraid of being stigmatized, don't have enough money, culture rejects them, or they can't get there.

Only 17% of the 110 countries surveyed could initiate activities covering services relating to mental health and psychosocial support by utilizing the allocated total supplementary funding. Although the governmental support was endorsed as a part of their national COVID-19 response plans, the implementation is glitched with technical challenges and financial slowdown.

The prevalence of these conditions focuses on the need for more funding to provide mental healthcare as good as that available for other ailments. With the pandemic continuing and other discouraging factors such as a financial slowdown, joblessness, and grief over the loss of loved ones, the number of mental health issues is increasing globally.

Mental healthcare programs, nationally and internationally, have seen underfunding in the past many years. Only 2% of the national health budget is allocated to mental healthcare schemes, which is insufficient. An agency catering to mental health issues receives far below 1% of the international aid earmarked for health.

Social Inequalities and Decline in Psychological Healthcare Post COVID-19

The immune-compromised are the most impacted group with mental health issues. The COVID-19 infected face humiliation, and survivors of the infection face harassment, discrimination, and non-acceptance in the family due to the fear of infection. The HCWs experience social stigma, stereotyping, and social isolation, with few cases of physical violence [33] surfaced. Stigmatized individuals become the vulnerable sub-group experiencing mental health troubles which may lead to anxiety, disturbance, and depression.

The economic slowdown is the other factor that induced mental health issues among infected and vulnerable groups. According to a WHO assessment [32], the post-COVID-9 pandemic may lead to a worldwide recession and economic collapse. People from all strata were affected during the pandemic with the rising unemployment, financial constraints, and recession that further triggered levels of anxiety, psychological grief, feeling despair, developing substance abuse disorders, increased suicidal tendencies, and suicides. In the post-COVID-19 times, lowered socioeconomic status, insecurity looming large over restoring the pre-existing financial condition within the family, and bereavement have put the issue of dealing with mental healthcare at the forefront [34].

Following the economic recession, one of the factors seen as the primary reason for the increased numbers of suicides in 2008 was the unemployment caused. Taking precedence, the potential threat post-COVID-19 remains to be tackled.

Mental Health Information System Access and Management

The potential sources of data in the mental health Information system (MHIS) are patient-doctor consultations, treatment records, intelligent and portable devices, specialist referrals and self-filled checklists, medical and insurance policy information and claims, drug intake details, family history and personal information like occupation, residential details, and income. The information can be stored in medical health information systems and is accessible to patients and the other stakeholders in the corresponding medical fraternity treating the patient through mobile phones, computers, or the cloud.

The patient is the owner of his mental health-related data and is of use to consulting, knowing the course of treatment, its timelines, and in case, referring to other health care teams, if required. In the case of the health care team, the data records are of immense use to decide upon the further course of action as a part of treatment and illness history [35]. The researchers can use the data to determine the factors affecting mental health, progression, and decline with varying interventions. The outcomes of analysis and research provide measures for controlling psychiatric disorders in individuals and infer effective treatments to be used on a wide scale. Insurance companies, government agencies, pharmaceutical companies, and the engineering sector use electronic health records to settle claims, monitor the demand for medicines and supply in the healthcare market, and develop wearable devices for monitoring vitals. Critical health determinants usher in practical and new-age treatment equipment. The stakeholders have different purposes and goals for accessing the volume of mental health care data.

Security Challenges of MHIS

One of the critical factors in maintaining the sanctity of the mental health information system (MHIS) is the correctness of the patient's stored and exchanged data. The updates must only be incorporated by the authorized and authenticated stakeholders. Confidentiality is the key to maintaining the correctness of the electronic records of health information systems shared across stakeholders. In turn, confidentiality is crucial in maintaining the integrity and the ethical standards levied by the healthcare industry and the demographic laws. During the access of the e-health records by the authorized stakeholders, utmost care is exercised to contain the secrecy and correctness of the information. The right to update and add to the patient's records lies with the patient, medical care team, diagnostic centers whose services were used by the patient, and a subset of the authorized access group. In this section, the security measures are detailed for restoring the secrecy of the data exchanged between the stakeholders:

- *Authenticated Logging:* Post COVID-19, there has been a surge in the cases of mental ill-health among individuals due to either pre-existing conditions or complemented pandemic woes. Due consideration is required for the data stored in MHIS due to its sensitivity level of higher-order. The stakeholders of the MHIS must be identified for authenticated logging and categorized further into different groups. Auto-logout must be enabled in the systems to prevent data hacks.
- *Access control policies:* The people and systems for accessing the patient's health records are classified to view and update data operations with varying degrees of sensitivity. This popular mechanism prevents over-privileged access to the EHRs of the MHIS. Besides, the log records give a peek at the information being accessed by the other unprivileged entities.
- *Encryption of sensitive fields of the patient data*: A number of the information systems holding the sensitive data rely on the encryption of the same to anonymize the record. Data encryption procedures help safeguard the confidentiality of the EHRs during transmission and access by the stakeholders [37]. The sensitive fields of the EHRs in the MIHS are hidden from the unwarranted entities, which may pose a potential risk of revealing the patient's identity. The additional leverage is the advantage of maintaining the secrecy of the mental health information of an individual in the advent of breaches. The challenges in implementing the cryptic procedures are the low computational cost, robustness, muscular cipher strength, withstand the security attacks, forward secrecy, and backward secrecy.
- *Security Protocols of the MHIS:* The other security features must be in place while sharing the data over the social media platforms to ensure end-to-end secrecy. Specific guidelines must be practiced to communicate the healthcare details between the patient and the care providers. Post pandemics, teleconsultation, and tele-prescriptions gained momentum in the healthcare industry, especially among patients suffering from mental health issues. The tele-conversations between the patient and the care team must maintain privacy.

More and more disruptive technologies are paving the way in the healthcare industry. With the introduction of edge computing, fog computing, and the internet of things for providing services effectively addressing critical healthcare and mental health disorders, more thrust is on the security of the e-health data transmitted between nodes connected and the MHIS. Continuous electronic health data transmission between the patient and the care team's connected medical things raises concerns about its privacy. The other central challenge of mental health information is privacy restoration. Because of the inherent distributed architecture and the enormous amount of live health information streaming, conventional security procedures and privacy mechanisms do not sufficiently foolproof MHIS. The resource-constrained nodes and edge entities used in the transmission of the EHRs pose security and privacy challenges in the wake of insufficient processing power and less memory to meet the high computational complexity of the conventional robust encryption mechanisms. Alternatively, the critical bunch matrix block ciphers [38, 39] and the other lightweight block ciphers [40] promise to address requirements in resource-constrained devices.

Popular privacy preservation mechanisms are enlisted and widely used where processing and storage capacities are resourceful.

Existing Privacy-Preserving Mechanisms

This section details the available and researched privacy-preserving mechanisms used for sensitive data present in the mental health datasets. There must be some safeguard in place to protect sensitive information like the data owner's financial condition or their medical history from being leaked through the open internet channels accessible to everybody. The procedures widely used for preserving the privacy of the sensitive information of the entities [36] are as under:

- T-closeness
- *k-anonymity*
- Randomization
- *L-diversity*

T-closeness: The procedures adopted to ensure the threshold difference between the contents of the T^* with that of the $T_i^* \mid 1 \leq i \leq n$ to obtain $T^*_{t-close}$ Thus, an equivalence class has/calculated as the dissimilarity between the distribution of the attribute in the whole table and the distribution of a sensitive attribute in this class and found to be not more than a threshold t.

A table is inferred to have $t-closeness$ if all equivalence classes have $t-closeness$.

K-anonymity: A dataset version is said to observe the k - anonymity property [8][9] in case a tuple is indistinguishable from at least $(k-1)$ similar tuples existing in the same dataset. *The k-anonymization* technique mainly handles the quasi-identifiers (QI) of the dataset. The equation was governing *k-anonymity* property within a given arbitrary dataset T where $\forall t \in T, \exists(\text{t}_{\text{i}_1}, \text{t}_{\text{i}_2}, \ldots t_{i_{k-1}}) \in T$ such that $t[C] = t_{i_1}[C] \cup t_{i_2}[C] \cup \ldots \cup t_{i_{k-1}}[C], \forall \text{C} \in QI$. The application of *k-anonymization* can be performed in either of the two techniques, namely Suppression and Generalization. In the suppression technique, specific values of the attributes are replaced by a unique character. All or some values of the attribute are affected accordingly to conceal an individual's identity. In the latter, individual values of the attributes are replaced with a broader category, *aka* range or bin representation, to get the anonymized table T^*, with $T_1 \cup T_2 \cup \cdots \cup T_n = T^*$, for communicating with the other stakeholders.

Randomization: One of the well-known techniques to preserve an individual's privacy is to introduce a certain amount of noise in the dataset. The nature, position, and type of noise to be introduced in the raw data are discretionary to the beholder of the data. The original aggregate can be reconstructed by removing the noise introduced from the inferences drawn.

L-diversity: Unlike the former, the *L-diversity* technique handles sensitive attributes of the dataset, namely, disease and financial status. The dataset obtained after *k-anonymization* would contain the same values under each of the QIs in $\forall T_i \,|\, 1 \leq \text{i} \leq \text{n}$. However, to introduce more privacy, the L-diversity technique ensures to re-distribute the tuples in T^*, such a way that in each T_i^*, the order under each sensitive attribute would be at least $(l-1)$ distinct. The governing equation followed by each $T_i^* \,|\, 1 \leq i \leq n$ to be diverse is given by the following:

$$-\sum_{s \in S} p(T_i^*, s) \log(p(T_i^*, s)) \geq \log(l)$$

where $p(T_i^*, s) = \frac{n(T_i^*, s)}{\sum_{s' \in S} n(T_i^*, s')}$ indicates the ratio of the records in the T_i^* with sensitive attributes.

Privacy Preservation of the Encrypted Dataset Using K-Anonymization

One of the promising techniques to safeguard the electronic health records of patients suffering from mental health issues is encryption techniques and privacy mechanisms. The challenges remain to devise a stealthy procedure to work on the edge nodes and provide stiff resistance to the attacks on confidentiality. Subsequently, the cryptic data must undergo the privacy-preserving mechanism after the records are anonymized to prevent its identification. In this regard, it is essential to sanitize the valuable information resulting from the quasi-identifier before making it public, so de-identification is impossible. $K-\text{anonymization}$ is the privacy preservation algorithm designed which anonymize the quasi-identifiers and will lead to K-indistinguishable records on any attempt to the identification. Quasi-identifiers (QI) are the attributes that can be associated together or with other background information for re-identifying a particular individual in the table. Examples of QI are age, gender, 6-digit zip-code, date of birth, place of birth, parents', siblings' and children's names, work status, company name, etc. These QIs can be handled with generalization and suppression techniques. As per the k-anonymity principle, every record must be indistinguishable from at least k-1 records to specific identifying attributes, illustrated in Table 1.

Table 1. Patient EHRs before Anonymization under the Qis

Patient_Id	Age	Gender	Zip-Code	Place of Birth	Disease
M1001	32	F	110001	New Delhi	Anxiety
M1102	48	M	230523	Mumbai	ADHD
M1003	28	M	230045	Pune	Insomnia
M2343	35	M	232201	Nagpur	Insomnia
M1212	21	F	230532	Mumbai	Bipolar Disrider
M4321	34	F	799002	Agartala	Addiction/Substance Abuse
M2002	56	M	600013	Chennai	Schizophrenia
M2051	65	F	600203	Chennai	ADHD
M2021	29	M	500031	Hyderabad	Schizophrenia

K-anonymization is applied with k value as 3 to Table 2, thus ensuring that at least three indistinguishable records emerge during any attempt to decipher the anonymized EHR data. In this illustration, K anonymity is applied to the two quasi-identifiers: age and zip code. The other quasi-identifiers: a place of birth is suppressed with the higher concept hierarchy, as shown in Table 2.

Table 2. Patients EHRs after K-Anonymization

Patient_Id	Age	Zip-Code	Place of Birth	Disease
M1001	3*	11****	Delhi	Anxiety
M1102	>45	23****	Maharashtra	ADHD
M1003	2*	23****	Maharashtra	Insomnia
M2343	3*	23****	Maharashtra	Insomnia
M1212	2*	23****	Maharashtra	Bipolar Disrider
M4321	3*	799***	Tripura	Addiction/Substance Abuse
M2002	>45	600***	Tamilnadu	Schizophrenia
M2051	>45	600***	Tamilnadu	ADHD
M2021	2*	500***	Telangana	Schizophrenia

Conclusion

The mental health impacts are seen in the post-COVID-19 times in the years and months much later in the post-infection phase. More and more cases are surging in the post coronavirus affected individuals with the medical complaints ranging from heart, liver, stomach, lungs, and mental ill-health. During the post-pandemic months, reports of the surge of common psychiatric disorders and suicide are predominant. Besides enhancing access to mental healthcare services, it is essential to safeguard the anonymity of the individual when electronic health records are shared during treatment. And because the COVID-19 virus infection is highly contagious, the medication and therapy in the post-infection phase are challenging. The medical conditions juxtapose their revelation among the care team professionals, family, and dear ones for treatment. Better procedures must be adopted for the treatment, safeguarding the affected individuals' secrecy and privacy, including early assessment, screening, telepsychiatry, and support through psychosocial groups. These would help mitigate for a long time the ill effects the COVID-19 has borne on the infected, bereaved ones, dependents, and orphaned children on mental well-being and address the stigma prevalent in the society, which is paramount in addressing the problem.

References

[1] World Health Organization. Statement on the second meeting of the International Health Regulations (2005) Emergency Committee regarding the outbreak of novel coronavirus (2019-nCoV) 2020. [Last accessed on 2020 Feb 12]. Available from: https://wwwwhoint/news-room/detail/30-01-2020-statement-on-the-second-meeting-of-the-international-health-regulations-(2005)-emergency-committee-regarding-the-outbreak-of-novel-coronavirus-(2019-ncov)

[2] World Health Organization. Weekly epidemiological update on COVID-19 - Jan 18, 2022, Edition 75, Jan 18, 2022, Emergency Situational Updates. [Last accessed on 2022 Janurary 19]. Available from https://www.who.int/publications/m/item/weekly-epidemiological-update-on-COVID-19---18-january-2022.

[3] WHO Ebola Response Team Ebola virus disease in West Africa – The first 9 months of the epidemic and forward projections. *N Engl J Med* 2014;371;1481–95.

[4] Hsu CH, Champaloux SW, Keïta S, Martel L, Bilivogui P, Knust B, and McCollum AM. Sensitivity and specificity of suspected case definition used during West Africa Ebola epidemic. *Emerg Infect Dis* 2018; 24 :9–14.

[5] Fähnrich C, Denecke K, Adeoye OO, Benzler J, Claus H, Kirchner G, Mall S, Richter R, Schapranow MP, Schwarz N, Tom-Aba D, L'Acker M, Poggensee G, & Krause G. Surveillance and outbreak response management system (SORMAS) to support the control of the Ebola virus disease outbreak in West Africa. *Euro Surveill* 2015; 20 :21071.

[6] World Health Organization. Middle East respiratory syndrome coronavirus (MERS-CoV), Mar 11, 2019. [Last Accessed on Jan 12, 2022]. Available from https://www.who.int/news-room/fact-sheets/detail/middle-east-respiratory-syndrome-corona virus-(mers-cov).

[7] Howden KJ, Brockhoff EJ, Caya FD, McLeod LJ, Lavoie M, Ing JD, Bystrom JM, Alexandersen S, Pasick JM, Berhane Y, Morrison ME, Keenliside JM, Laurendeau S, Rohonczy EB. An investigation into human pandemic influenza virus (H1N1) 2009 on an Alberta swine farm. *Can Vet J.* 2009; 50 :1153–61.

[8] Britton AP, Sojonky KR, Scouras AP, Bidulka JJ. Pandemic (H1N1) 2009 in skunks, Canada. *Emerg Infect Dis*. 2010; 16 :1043–5. 10.3201/eid1606.100352.

[9] Tsai LK, Hsieh ST, Chang YC. Neurological manifestations in severe acute respiratory syndrome, *Acta Neurol. Taiwan*, 14 (3) (2005), pp. 113-119.

[10] Cheung YT, Chau PH, Yip PS. A revisit on older adults' suicides and severe acute respiratory syndrome (SARS) epidemic in Hong Kong. *Int J Geriatr Psychiatry*. 2008 Dec;23(12) :1231-8. DOI : 10.1002/gps.2056. PMID : 18500689.

[11] Rogers, Kara. 1968 flu pandemic, *Encyclopedia Britannica*, Mar 25. 2020, [Accessed on Jan 7, 2022.] Available from https://www.britannica.com/event/1968-flu-pandemic.

[12] Harris Phil, and Danny Moss. "Managing through the Covid second wave: Public affairs and the challenge of Covid vaccination." *Journal of Public Affairs* 21.1 (2021).

[13] Szmigiera M. Impact of the coronavirus pandemic on the global economy - Statistics & Facts, Feb 21, 2022, [Last Accessed on Feb 22, 2022] Available from https://www.statista.com/topics/6139/COVID-19-impact-on-the-global-economy/#topicHeader__wrapper

[14] Xiong J, Lipsitz O, Nasri F, Lui LMW, Gill H, Phan L, Chen-Li D, Iacobucci M, Ho R, Majeed A, & McIntyre RS. Impact of COVID-19 pandemic on mental health in the general population : A systematic review, *Journal of affective disorders* vol. 277 (2020) : 55-64. DOI : 10.1016/j.jad.2020.08.001.

[15] Ahmed MZ, Ahmed O, Zhou A, Sang H, Liu S, Ahmad A. Epidemic of COVID-19 in China and associated psychological problems. *Asian Journal of Psychiatry.* 2020; 51 DOI 10.1016/j.ajp.2020.102092.

[16] Cao W, Fang Z, Hou G, Han M, Xu X, Dong J, Zheng J. The psychological impact of the COVID-19 epidemic on college students in China. *Psychiatry Res.* 2020;287.

[17] Saladino Valeria, Algeri Davide, Auriemma Vincenzo, The Psychological and Social Impact of COVID-19 : New Perspectives of Well-Being, *Frontiers in Psychology,* Vol. 11, 2020. Available from https://www.frontiersin.org/article/10.3389/fpsyg.2020.577684. doi=10.3389/fpsyg.2020.577684. ISSN=1664-1078.

[18] Alvarez F, Argente D, and Lippi F. (2020). A simple planning problem for COVID-19 lockdown. *Covid Econ.* 14, 1–33. Doi: 10.3386/w26981.

[19] Teo AR, Gaw AC. Hikikomori, a Japanese culture-bound syndrome of social withdrawal? A proposal for DSM-5. *J Nerv Ment Dis.* 2010;198(6) :444-449. DOI :10.1097/NMD.0b013e3181e086b1.

[20] Gao J, Zheng P, Jia Y, Chen H, Mao Y, Chen S, Wang Y, Fu H, Dai J. Mental health problems and social media exposure during COVID-19 outbreak. *PLoS ONE.* 2020;15(4).

[21] Ho CSH, Chee CY, Ho RCM. Mental health strategies to combat the psychological impact of coronavirus disease (COVID-19) beyond paranoia and panic. *Ann. Acad. Med. Singapore.* 2020;49(3) :155–160.

[22] Lei L, Huang X, Zhang S, Yang J, Yang L, Xu M. Comparison of prevalence and associated factors of anxiety and depression among people affected by versus people unaffected by quarantine during the COVID-19 epidemic in southwestern China. *Med. Sci. Monit.* 2020;26.

[23] Rogers JP, Chesney E, Oliver D, Pollak TA, McGuire P, Fusar-Poli P, Zandi MS, Lewis G, David AS. (2020). Psychiatric and neuropsychiatric presentations associated with severe coronavirus infections: a systematic review and meta-analysis with comparison to the COVID-19 pandemic. *Lancet Psychiatry* 7, 611–627. doi: 10.1016/S2215-0366(20)30203-0.

[24] Hwang T., Rabheru K., Peisah C., Reichman W., Ikeda M., 2020. Loneliness and social isolation during COVID-19 pandemic. *Int. Psychogeriatr.* 1–15. https://doi.org/10. 1017/S1041610220000988.

[25] Pisciotta M., Denneson LM, Williams HB, Woods S., Tuepker A., Dobscha SK, 2019. Providing mental health care in the context of online mental health notes :

advice from patients and mental health clinicians. *J. Ment. Health* 28 (1), 64–70. https://doi.org/10.1080/09638237.2018.1521924.

[26] Sønderskov KM, Dinesen PT, Santini ZI, Østergaard SD, 2020. The depressive state of Denmark during the COVID-19 pandemic. *Acta Neuropsychiatr.* 1–3. https://doi.org/10.1017/neu.2020.15.

[27] Li Z, Ge J, Yang M, Feng J, Qiao M, Jiang R, Bi J, Zhan G, Xu X, Wang, L, Zhou Q, Zhou, C, Pan Y, Liu S, Zhang H, Yang J, Zhu B, Hu Y, Hashimoto K, Yang C. 2020. Vicarious traumatization in the general public, members, and nonmembers of medical teams aiding in COVID-19 control. *Brain Behav. Immum.* https://doi.org/10.1016/j.bbi.2020.03.007.

[28] Que J, Shi L, Deng J, Liu J, Zhang L, Wu S, Gong Y, Huang W, Yuan K, Yan W, Sun Y, Ran M, Bao Y, & Lu L. Psychological impact of the COVID-19 pandemic on healthcare workers: à cross-sectional study in China. *Gen Psychiatr*. 2020;33(3) : e100259. Published 2020 Jun 14. DOI : 10.1136/gpsych-2020-100259.

[29] McAlonan GM, Lee AM, Cheung V, Cheung C, Tsang KW, Sham PC, Chua SE, Wong JG. Immediate and sustained psychological impact of an emerging infectious disease outbreak on health care workers. *Can J Psychiatry*. 2007 Apr;52(4) :241-7. doi: 10.1177/070674370705200406. PMID : 17500305.

[30] Preti E, Di Mattei V, Perego G, Ferrari F, Mazzetti M, Taranto P, Di Pierro R, Madeddu F, & Calati R. "The Psychological Impact of Epidemic and Pandemic Outbreaks on Healthcare Workers: Rapid Review of the Evidence." *Current psychiatry reports* vol. 22,8 43. Jul 10. 2020, DOI :10.1007/s11920-020-01166-z.

[31] Cheng HY, Jian SW, Liu DP, Ng TC, Huang WT, Lin HH; Taiwan COVID-19 Outbreak Investigation Team. Contact Tracing Assessment of COVID-19 Transmission Dynamics in Taiwan and Risk at Different Exposure Periods Before and After Symptom Onset. JAMA Intern Med. 2020 Sep 1;180(9) :1156-1163. Doi: 10.1001/jamainternmed.2020.2020. Erratum in : *JAMA Intern Med.* 2020 Sep 1;180(9) :1264. PMID : 32356867; PMCID : PMC7195694.

[32] Brunier A, Drysdale C. COVID-19 disrupting mental health services in most countries, *WHO survey*. World Heal Organ. 2020.

[33] Bagcchi Sanjeet. "Stigma during the COVID-19 pandemic." *The Lancet*. Infectious diseases vol. 20,7 (2020) : 782. DOI : 10.1016/S1473-3099(20)30498-9.

[34] Frasquilho D, Matos MG, Salonna F, Guerreiro D, Storti CC, Gaspar T, & Caldas-de-Almeida JM. "Mental health outcomes in times of economic recession: à systematic literature review" *BMC public health* vol. 16 115. 3 Feb. 2016, DOI: 10.1186/s12889-016-2720-y.

[35] Coventry L, Branley D. Cybersecurity in health care : a narrative review of trends, threats, and ways forward. *Maturitas* 2018; 113 : 48–52.

[36] Shirisha Kakarla, and Geeta Kakarla, D Narsinga Rao, Two-fold Security Model using 2d-Vector Key Bunch and Privacy Preservation of the EHRs in the distributed Network involving Blockchain, *Recent Trends in Blockchain for Information Systems Security and Privacy*, eBook ISBN9781003139737, CRC Press, Taylor and Francis, USA, 1st Ed. Nov-2021, pp. 117-138.

[37] Shirisha Kakarla, Securing large datasets involving fast-performing key bunch matrix block cipher, "Healthcare Data Analytics and Management, *Advances in*

Ubiquitous Sensing Applications for Healthcare," Vol 2. Elsevier Publications, (Paperback ISBN : 9780128153680), https://doi.org/10.1016/C2017-0-03245-7, 2019, pp. 111-132.

[38] Sastry VUK, Shirisha, K. "A Block Cipher Involving à Key Bunch Matrix and an Additional Key Matrix, Supplemented with Modular Arithmetic Addition and supported by Key-based Substitution," *International Journal of Advanced Computer Science and Applications (IJACSA),* Vol. 3, No. 12, 2012, pp. 110-115.

[39] Sastry VUK, Shirisha, K. "A Block Cipher Involving à Key Bunch Matrix and an Additional Key Matrix, Supplemented with XOR Operation and Supported by Key-Based Permutation and Substitution," *International Journal of Advanced Computer Science and Applications (IJACSA),* Vol. 4, No. 1, pp. 187-194, 2013.

[40] Bassam J Mohd, Thaier Hayajneh, and Athanasios V Vasilakos. 2015. A survey on lightweight block ciphers for low-resource devices. *J. Netw. Comput. Appl.* 58, C (December 2015), 73–93. doi: https://doi.org/10.1016/j.jnca.2015.09.001

Chapter 14

Post-COVID Impact on Skin Allergies

Sunil Bhutada*, Vijayalakshmi Kakulapati, Rokkam Krishna Vamsi, Akkenapally Sharanya and Maddineni Mahima Chowdhary

Sreenidhi Institute of Science and Technology,
Yamnampet, Ghatkesar, Hyderabad, Telangana, India

Abstract

The pandemic raises several concerns for medical providers. Speedy screening and therapy, susceptibility categorization, effective utilization of acute medical utilities, proper drugs, observation, and quick release are vital for protecting as many victims as feasible. We discussed several ML (machine learning) classification strategies for analyzing skin-related concerns. This chapter tries to give appropriate skin specialists a strategy plan to comprehend its potential and difficulties. In this study, we employ several classification approaches and multi-model classification methods—design autonomous assessment assistance to reliably detect a specific type of allergic rhinitis ailment for deployment.

Keywords: symptoms, skin, itching, machine learning, classification, diagnosis, predict, allergies, precision, measures, intelligent, COVID-19

*Corresponding Author's Email: sunilb@sreenidhi.edu.in.

In: Data Science Applications of Post-COVID-19 Psychological Disorders
Editor: Vijayalakshmi Kakulapati
ISBN: 979-8-88697-165-1

Introduction

Generally, patients with skin infections aren't more vulnerable to COVID than any other. Various acne disorders might be exacerbated by anxiety and concern. It is vital to treat the skin issue successfully. If the patient is worried regarding their dermatitis or drugs, seek assistance from the Primary care physician or the Dermatological Service. Allergies are relatively frequent in crisis periods, with almost 50% of the population experiencing wrinkles each year. However, many skin disorders have been seen in COVID patients, and others are more common [1].

A preliminary observation from specialists dealing with COVID-19 victims in Italy indicated that approximately 20% of 88 identified infected individuals experience skin symptoms, with less than 50% acquiring dermatitis at the illness start but a bit higher than 50% experiencing one after hospitalization. The most prevalent symptom among the afflicted individuals was an eczematous rash or a widespread red rash. Very few people had urticaria, sometimes known as itching, and one person experienced scarlet fever lesions [2].

Dermal disorders have significantly captivated critical medical care, progressing from basic clinical applications to a scientific research agreement [3]. While the actual occurrence is unclear, it impacts 2% of the people. After curing COVID-19, most patients are now experiencing a variety of skin dermatitis. Dermatologists assisted current studies in establishing a link between skin issues and COVID-19. It has become a complicated process to visually identify skin abnormalities without the assistance of a qualified professional, and therapeutic approaches for this disease or disorder are complex.

Allergies are a substantial cause of fatalities, impacting many lives globally. A clinician checks only 28 percent of dermatological problems because of a scarcity of professionals. Experts play an essential role in diagnosing epidermis disorders and commencing treatments. The diagnostic effectiveness of nonspecialists is predicted to be much lower [4-6].

Itching is more and more associated with Coronavirus outbreaks. Like some of those linked with many other breathing problems, including asthma and syphilis, specific hypersensitivity can manifest in various ways. The most common manifestation is a "maculopapular rash." These allergic reactions are characterized by a small number of red bumps and modest, increasing lesions.

A frequent wound is common in anti-inflammatory patients, and it usually subsides when the treatment is stopped. Adverse rashes and discomfort in the eyelid may occur, necessitating treatment with moisturizers and multivitamins. Fungal infection, a pathogenic illness of the epidermal, is expected in several people. In certain circumstances, detergents and washes in combination with treatments are sufficient. Treatments may benefit just a small number of individuals suffering from long-term skin cancers [7]. Whereas eczema necessitates immediate treatment, diagnosis is determined mainly by healing and diagnosing effects. The symptoms above can be seen in elderly adults and children: Widespread allergic reactions, vast redness, discomfort, eye diseases, and irritation of the eyes, mouth, neck, tooth, face, or other body cells are all dermatological signs.

- Pandemic is consistently related to allergic reactions that can result in blemishes.
- Outbreak skin signs include maculopapular, chilblain-like, urticarial, vesicular, livedoid, and petechial lesions. Furthermore, lesions are frequent in kids with complex multifactorial reactive syndromes, a novel and deadly healthcare illness with Kawasaki disease features, and are most probably connected to COVID-19.
- Skin blisters caused by PPE (personal protective equipment) are a significant issue because disrupted epidermal layers can allow COVID-19 viruses to enter the body.
- Bccause the SARS-CoV-2 infection is still spreading quietly, primarily via infected patients, precise and timely detection of these dermatological signs may be critical for timely recognition. It may result in a better disease outcome in COVID-19 victims [8].

"Redness, psoriatic, and melanoma are common causes that worsen before or after contagion healing. Autoimmunity ailments deteriorate as drugs are delayed in the proportion of individuals during the therapy cycle. Various factors, such as loneliness and anxiety, may also contribute to smoking. A timely restart of current therapy and mental health support is beneficial in treating the condition. Dermatology in lotion usage, good food and hydration, and enough regular exercise are all highly beneficial."

A few children birthed to women with a corona at delivery experienced temporary dermatitis. Two different babies appeared with dermatitis in a study of nine minor samples of patients in Chinese, which comprised a combination of 65 prenatal women who had been contaminated with SARS-CoV-2 in pregnancies and 67 newborns [9]. The rashes were reported as a spreading, maculopapular reaction that cleared in one day, with ulcerations in one kid and a dispersed, red, malaria-like response that recovered in 10 days without therapy [10].

There are multiple cases of COVID-19 people diagnosed with atypical dermatological lesions. For instance, aged women with COVID-19 in France developed dermatitis compatible with Symmetrical Substance Intertriginous and Flexural Exanthema (SDRIFE) 4 days after becoming feverish [11]. Even though SDRIFE is often a drug-induced eruption, the investigators seem unable to pin this instance down to a specific medicine. In contrast, Joob and colleagues [12] described petechial rashes in COVID-19 patients that resembled the dermatological manifestation found in Dengue.

Motivation

Objectives

- Developing robust disease surveillance and monitoring systems.
- Exploiting digital health tools and coordinating mechanisms to support surveillance and monitoring.

Scope

Image processing is becoming widely attractive and is used in various fields. It can help automate multiple operations that need manual intervention, such as pruning, diagnosis of diseases, crop development stage detection, etc. The goal of the investigation is to detect skin disorders that are a consequence of coronavirus. This method has the potential to be a viable model for simplifying the procedure and assisting clinicians in evaluating it. It can make it much easier to utilize, and it is cheaper to construct than a medical method.

Benefits

- Timely identification of dermatitis decreases the adverse influence of the reactions
- Adequate and convenient assessment for the individual caused by environmental interactions

- Improved forecasting of findings
- Relatively inexpensive utilisation from the patients' perspective.

The rest of the research is divided into the following categories: The second portion explains the history of the suggested procedure, and the fourth component digs into the relevant studies of post-COVID-19 skin reactions. Section 5 elaborates on the planned work technique. Section 6 investigates the effectiveness of the recommended technique in several experiments. This is followed by an analysis of the recommended work's topic in part 5, a chapter summarized in section 6, and recommendations for future enhancements in section 7.

Background

The pandemic has resulted in many behavioral changes, including the regular use of hand sanitizers or soap. As a result, numerous people acquire palm itches. Wearing masks and eyeglasses promotes face epidermal blisters, hyperpigmentation, and worsening dermatitis among healthcare practitioners [13].

Whereas this infection is not dromotropic, it has caused various skin lesions, generally due to extended interaction with PPE and frequent utilization of hand sanitizers. Coronavirus-induced stress invasion, urticaria, irritation, dermatitis herpetiformis, and worsening of also before the epidermal conditions like eczema and atopic dermatitis. Mucous membranes, particularly the conjunctiva, were immediately recognized as the most prevalent mechanism of virus transmission, with the optic canal having a lower probability of dissemination. The hyper-hydration impact of PPE mainly causes dermatology abnormalities in coronavirus. These devices can induce impaired skin disruption, contact response, and discomfort, aggravating what is already an existing skin infection. The most prevalent skin adverse effects associated with the continued use of personal protective equipment include papules, scaling, maceration, and erythema. Itching, stinging, and burning are among the symptoms noted. The nasal bridge is the most commonly afflicted skin region, and 83% of such instances are caused by the usage of protective eyewear but not by the hygiene mask. Excessive hand washing with detergents and disinfectants can harm the hydro-lipid mantle of skin surfaces, causing irritation and eventually leading to contact dermatitis [14].

Numerous cases of skin rashes in COVID-19 patients are spreading across the globe. The rashes can take many forms; some appear as tiny red spots, while others are larger flat or raised lesions. Some have a hive-like appearance, while others look like frostbitten feet. According to Spanish research, coronavirus-related skin eruptions are classified into five types: a "maculopapular" rash, or one that is typical of viral infections such as measles, with red bumps on reddish skin; a hives-related "urticaria" rash; a lace-like or fishnet pattern "livedo" rash; a "vesicular eruption" or blistering rash; and frostbite [15].

People may have acute allergies, widespread eczema, and tiny blisters and ulcers that resemble unpredictable irritability. It can remain for many days after the COVID has been cleaned up. Body care treatments and outside antifungal creams can be helpful. An itching triggered by the virus's cure can impact any part of the human body, most notably the heart, though it can also affect the extremities. Erythema is frequently painful, although it depends totally on the severity of the response, and lesions heal fast, appearing in two or three days and dissipating in a week. The most common dermatitis symptoms include acral lesions resembling pseudo-chilblains, multifaceted urticaria, and different skin irritations. Most of these allergy responses might be caused by COVID-19-specific extremely infectious life situations. Specific dermatological symptoms may affect SARS-CoV2 and autoimmune deregulatory activities [16].

The integration of its high mutation rates and lengthy pathological latency stage led to a significant in an infectious disease that affected vast numbers of patients and killed more persons [17]. Whereas it is most commonly associated with autoimmune disorders and pulmonary hypertension, experimental knowledge from throughout the world shows that it also might produce dermatitis issues.

The pulmonary infections caused by SARS-CoV-2 are commonly linked to increased risk consequences. These conditions are frequently classified into five categories: itchy red eczema, epidermal itching, semi, livedo, or mortification, and antidepressant. Communicable propagation eczema is present in paediatric patients with chronic inflammation multifaceted disorder, a severe and rare condition in teenagers. These patches are generated by cutaneous bleeding. However, they do not change colour when touched [18].

Related Works

Allergic sensitization to medicines, meals, or other supplements is becoming increasingly widespread in the United States [19]. One out of every five identified allergies causes skin irritation, ranging from minor blemishes to deadly reactions. Because of the personalized experiences, patients in the therapeutic setting are much more sensitive to allergic responses [20].

The heart has become the most commonly impacted area. Due to the lack of or false information, itching, redness, varioliform infections, and dermatitis symptoms were detected in patients, which disappeared within a few days. Additionally, scientists in Spain discovered that mild itchiness is linked to the erythematous red related to COVID19 in a subset of individuals. The COVID19 contamination is predicted to cause bleeding lesions [21], comparable to Dengue. It is important to remember that around one-third of Dengue patients have itchiness. On the third day of hospitalization, an older lady [22, 23] experienced itching to purpuric, millimetric, aggregation macules in the transverse areas due to coronavirus. There was some pruritions itching noted. Atherosclerosis is widespread, with the illness affecting 20% of COVID19 people who have severe urticaria. Regardless of discomfort, urticaria is a well-known cutaneous condition characterized by intense irritation. Chickenpox-like blisters [24] were detected in 6% of the study individuals. Consequently, there appears to be a lack of research on itchiness in such patients, yet, few doctors who care for COVID19 patients mention that the disorder may be uncomfortable.

Numerous elements of the immunological condition have recently been highlighted in research [25]. One of the most comprehensive Italian analyses revealed that COVID-19 might affect thermal problems. Diagnostic dermatological signs are similar to those seen in common bacterial infections. The most comprehensive hypothesis was that cutaneous signs did not correspond to infection intensity. Based on the most recent shareable statistics, patient complications can occur in 0.2 percent to 21% of COVID-19 patients. As per specialist views, three cases underlined discomfort in affected victims.

Epidermis clinical signs developed 64 percent subsequently or concurrently with some other acute infected indications in a retrospective analysis of persons with coronavirus [26], with several iterations of 8 days in the elderly from the start of contamination of the respiratory problems to cutaneous disorders [27]. After six months of follow-up, around 3% of responders in the post-COVID-19 group reported dermatitis discomfort. Hair loss was the most common retinal disease issue, affecting nearly 20% of all patients. Estrogen levels in intestinal contents, which can occur due to infections or worry, might have catastrophic consequences. The extensive investigation might provide information on abnormal immunological or immunological reactions [28].

About Skin Allergies after Recovering from COVID-19

Apart from rashes produced from other fungal viruses (which include mumps, smallpox, meningitis, and chickenpox), COVID-19 rashes can manifest in a variety of forms.

Once the cutaneous aspects of COVID-19 are crucial to the effective the fingers or fingertips, or even both, the disorder is known as COVID toes, and it can appear as color change (red to violet) and swollen of the palms or toes. It may be accompanied by discomfort, pus development, and irritation in the affected areas.

COVID-19 is a multiple organ systems illness caused by the Coronavirus Middle East Respiratory Syndrome (MERS) that mainly produces breathing problems. Nevertheless, cutaneous indications of coronavirus have recently been recognized as acute viral symptoms. Several patients experience allergies after recovering from COVID-19 [29]. Scientific investigations concluded, with the assistance of dermatology, that there is a linkage between skin reactions and COVID-19. It is challenging to identify skin abnormalities without the aid of a dermatologist correctly, and effective treatments for this type of illness are complicated. Morbilliform rash, maculopapular and purpuric lesions, chilblains, vesicular eruptions, urticaria, acral lesions, millimetric erythematous-purpuric macules on the muscles and tendons at the pivotal role level, erythema itchiness, and other abnormalities have been observed in COVID-19 victims [30]. Several possible skin-related symptoms of coronavirus illness were documented in clinical studies throughout the world in 2019. The incidence and duration of COVID-19 dermatological symptoms are challenging to know. The relationship between various skin symptoms and the intensity of the infection is also uncertain.

Therefore, it cannot be ruled out that the reported skin abnormalities in specific individuals may reflect cutaneous responses to the various COVID-19 therapy. The severity of COVID-19-related cutaneous symptoms is documented thus far, skin issues linked with PPE, and the different cutaneous anti-COVID-19 medication responses. The prevalence of skin lesions was 0.2 percent at the start of the COVID-19 pandemic. However, the categories of lesions or their characteristics were not identified. As the COVID-19 outbreak progressed, dermatological alterations fluctuated between 5% and 20%. As a result, the prevalence of cutaneous symptoms associated with COVID-19 has increased to a high level, coinciding with the vast impact of SARS-CoV-2. Skin disorders are a clinical diagnostic sign that expands the spectrum of observable information regarding COVID-19 [31-33].

The identified features of skin rashes might aid in the earlier stage of illness of acute respiratory syndrome. It also extends the spectrum of diagnostic analyses between highly contagious co-infections or bad reactions to COVID-19 medicines. The dermatological symptoms of COVID-19, although not providing a predictive benefit in the stratified of illness deformation, can provide information that supports the notion of a higher risk of linked disorders [34]. Skin lesions may now be diagnosed, managed, and treated by all phases of care, including healthcare coverage and hospitalization treatment [35]. Furthermore, primary healthcare professionals should collaborate to analyze, inspect, plan for, and treat such skin infections linked with severe acute respiratory disease. In this context, knowledge of the many forms of cutaneous symptoms related to COVID-19 [36] is significant. A few days after the pandemic's inception, various tales and comprehensive investigations on the dermatology symptoms of COVID-19 were documented [37]. Researchers have attempted to investigate all aspects of this severe ailment, trying to identify the distinctive features of SARS-CoV-2 in order to create tests and medications to improve resilience [38]

Dermatological skills became more complicated earlier in occurrence than anticipated because of the potential of SARS-CoV-2 to cause skin lesions. However, much is still mysterious about COVID-19 and even more about the dermatological manifestations noticed in cases affected with SARS-CoV-2. In a few sufferers, the diagnosis of skin lesions could help in communicable measures in order to avoid disease in patients accompanying minor or asymptomatic symptoms, the one present skin manifestations contributing to COVID-19 without a diagnosis by research laboratory tests. Early analysis of skin changes provides satisfactory medication to prevent progression to more extreme stages of COVID-19. Diagnosis of the cutaneous manifestations leads to SARS-CoV-2 infection, and their understanding by health management specialists is essential to evolving an appropriate plan of care [39].

Various skin conditions post COVID are [40]:

Maculopapular Eruptions

These are widespread red bumps called maculopapular eruptions associated with more severe diseases. These eruptions can be seen as multiple flat red patches on the skin.

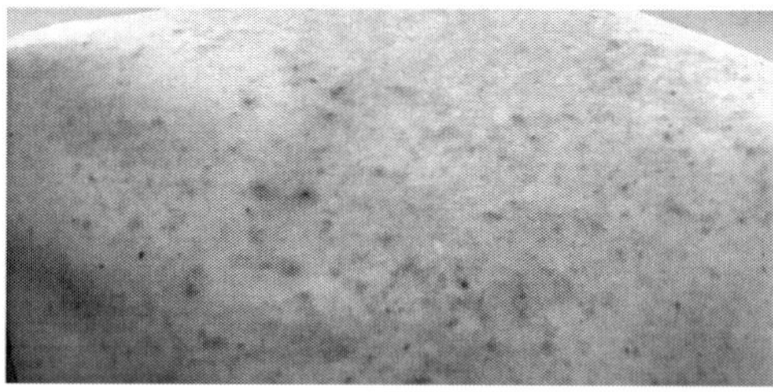

Figure 1. Red bumps on skin.

COVID Toes

Chilblain-like symptoms are also known as "COVID toes." These can affect either the hands, feet or both at once. The reddish-purple discolored skin can be unpleasant and irritating, and tiny blisters or bumps may appear. These chilblain-like lesions are widespread in children and develop late in the disease after other symptoms have faded.

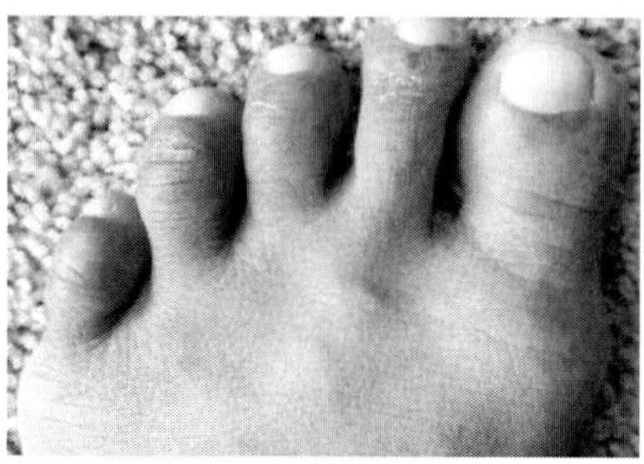

Figure 2. COVID toes.

Hives

Hives, also known as urticaria, are irritating rashes that appear as patches or raised red lumps and are pink or red (wheals). They might be as small as a pinhead or as large as a dinner plate. Swellings in one spot usually go away within minutes to hours, but they can come and go. In most cases, hives disappear after ten days. They appear at the same time as other symptoms in people of all ages and are linked to more severe illnesses.

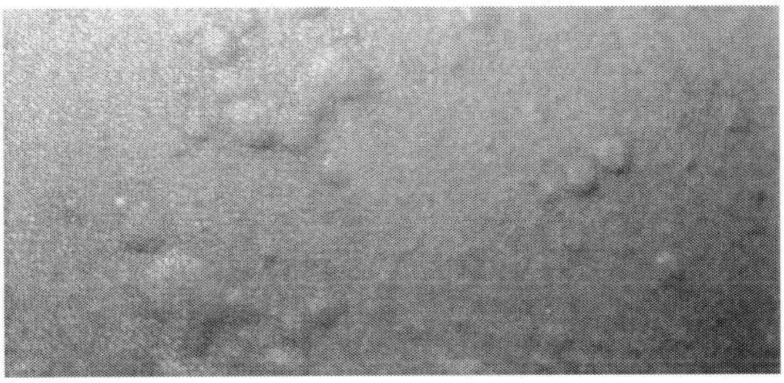

Figure 3. Skin hives.

Water Blisters

Water blisters, also known as vesicular eruptions, are microscopic fluid-filled micro-blisters that can arise at any moment during the disease, most commonly on the hands. Patients in their forties and fifties are more likely to be affected. The blisters are connected with a medium-severity condition and last slightly over ten days.

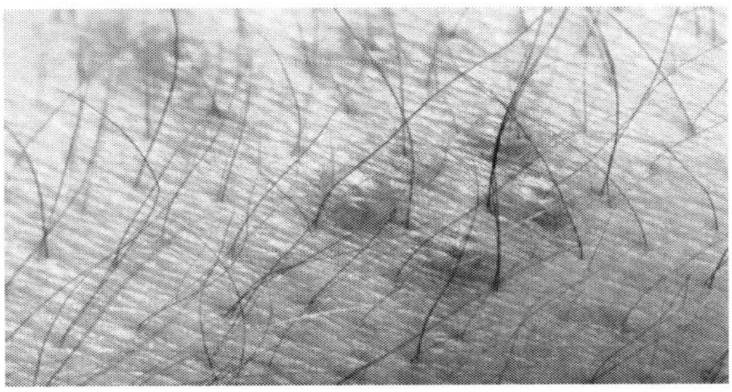

Figure 4. Water blisters.

Livedo

A 'fishing net-like' red-blue pattern on the skin, known as livedo, is linked to more severe diseases and older age groups and can include microscopic bruises (purpura). Blood vessel obstructions cause this pattern during the body's immunological response to the virus.

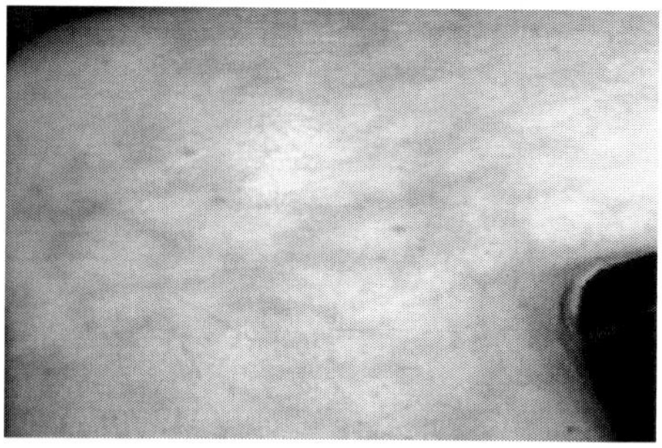

Figure 5. Fishing net-like rashes.

MIS-C

The rash associated with MIS-C, or multisystem inflammatory syndrome in children. This "immune system overdrive" causes heart and blood vessel inflammation, leading to blood clots and shock symptoms. This infrequent side effect can happen up to three months after a child has received COVID-19.

Figure 6. Blood clots.

Methodology and Framework

An allergy does not necessarily imply the existence of an ailment. This terminology includes any irritation or erythema that disrupts the usual smoothness of the epidermis. Frequent infections include post-COVID dermatitis, itchiness, skin issues, hypersensitivity, and athlete's feet. As medications may cause cutaneous diseases, any adverse reaction that lasts more than three days should be evaluated by a dermatologist.

Further, as you advance through the ML model, you would most likely initialize an element until it meets the targets, then move on to the next job. Furthermore, even before the first version is implemented, compile feedback from past deployments and make objectives for the next deployment cycle.

Data Set

Image data sets of dermatitis are acquired from several openly accessible places. Upon collecting the data, use pre-processing methods to remove redundant data and noise components. To model was trained for accurate epidermis diagnoses.

Feature Extraction

Collecting attributes includes reducing the resources required to explain a large number of observations. Numerous ML professionals believe that a well-suited input image is the product of the effective building of the model. The term "feature extraction" refers to creating parameter variants that avoid these difficulties while properly capturing the source [41].

Logistic Regression

The sigmoid activation function is used in regression to anticipate certain events. It examines the input and allocates values ranging from 0 to 1. To determine the approximate value, the input parameters (X1, X2,...Xn) are gradually integrated, and the best values [42] are chosen (Y).

$$Y = \frac{1}{2}\left[\frac{e^{(mX1+c)}}{1+e^{(mX1+c)}} + \frac{e^{(mX2+c)}}{1+e^{(mX2+c)}}\right]$$

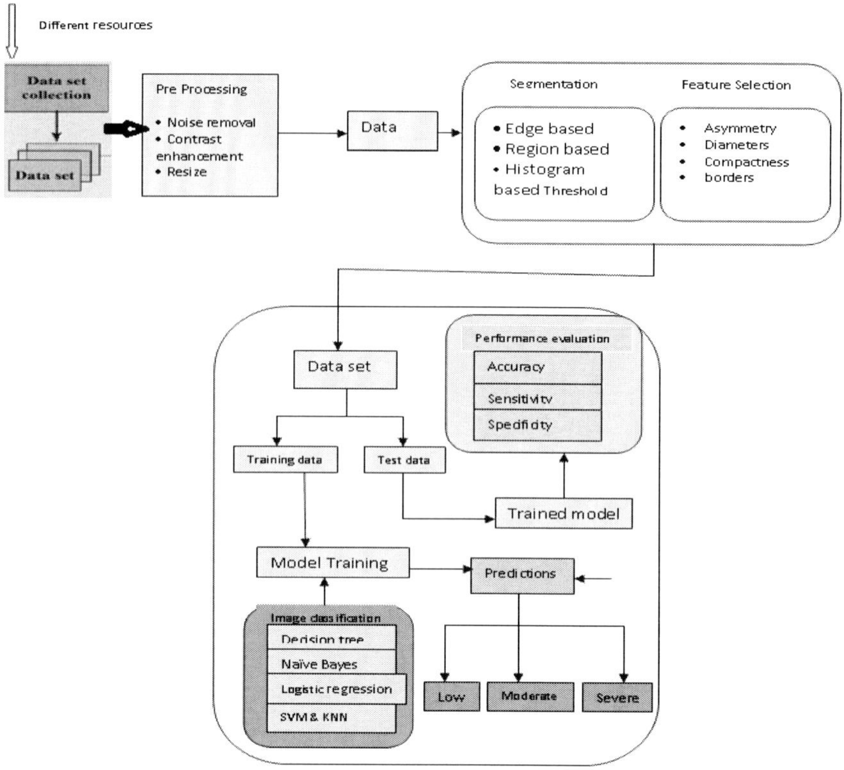

Figure 7. Framework of the proposed system.

'c' is the interceptor and is the provided two independent variables (in our case, X1 and X2 are age and gender). Every input variable must be trained using the classification model by the coefficient of determination (X1, X2). This experiment was performed with a methodology to classify the dying and surviving post COVID19 victims.

Decision Tree (DT)

The DT methodology employs an intelligent strategy for classification problems. A layout is used to represent the DT algorithms. The root node of the tree-like structure is identified, and the input features are partitioned based on a particular characteristic to decide the approximation in the DT (x) [43].

For estimations, the DT classification approach is used to determine the infection proportion of the dendrogram. This research shows that the patients' cutaneous symptoms are categorized as mild, medium, and severe using the post-COVID-19 skin dermatitis data.

$$G = \sum_{i=1}^{n} xk(1 - xk)$$

The proportion of the input image in the specified classes 'k' is referred to as 'x.' The binary logic tree structure of the dataset is part of the approach to keep things as basic as possible.

Support Vector Machines (SVM)

Supervised learning produces support vectors for each learner using upper and lower bounds in the vector space. By appropriately partitioning subspaces, the SVM minimizes loss among classes. Traditional SVM may be utilized for classifiers if the supplied samples are sequentially constrained; if the instance is non-linear, that can be employed [44].

Both linear and non-linear input may be classified using this approach. It starts by converting each data set into an n-dimensional train set, with n the number of characteristics. The hyperplane that separates the data into multiple classes is found, with the minimal closeness for both types maximized and the model's performance reduced.

The Classification technique [45] is defined as (A1, B1,....An, Bn), where (A1,... An) is the number of input variables, (B1,..., Bn) is the result variable, and 'C' is the interception.

$$SVM = \sum_{i=1}^{n} \beta_i - \frac{1}{2}\sum_{i,j=1}^{n} b_i b_j C(a_i, a_j)\, \beta_i \beta_j$$

i = 1,2, 3...n, and C = bii + bjj in the following equation. The SVM algorithm was used to classify cases of post-COVID-19 cutaneous discomfort.

K-Nearest Neighbors (KNN)

The KNN technique is a multivariate approach. The training and forecasting evaluations are conducted using the task or sample given. The number of k closest data points is indicated by the 'K' in KNN. Depending on the value of 'K,' the KNN algorithm determines how to categorize the given samples [46].

The KNN technique effectively categorizes the training samples. It ensures that the new instance's prediction is created by examining the whole learning algorithm for comparing 'K' neighbor examples and classifying them according to the category of maximum occurrences. To discover a comparable situation, the distance measure approach is employed.

$$Euclidean_{i,j} = \sqrt{\sum_{k=1}^{n} (x_{ik} - y_{jk})^2}$$

Gaussian Naïve Bias

The Bayesian hypothesis determines this. This hypothesis can describe the likelihood of an event based on prior knowledge of factors that favor a specific result. Despite the fact that qualities in a category may be interdependent, this categorization means that a given feature in that category isn't closely connected with other aspects.

Gradient Boosting

It's an ML method to predict the dependent variable assessment and classifications that assembles a classifier's effectiveness from various insufficient estimation approaches, the most prominent of which is a decision tree. It combines inadequate characteristics to provide a considerable, stable rate of good prediction efficiency. The error function is a single one that is tailored to the job at hand.

XGB

It has become one of the kinds of boosting in Supervised Machine learning. A supervised technique is a group of predictors utilized to determine the model's dependability. Classifications seek to remedy prior models' faults in the boosting method by raising variables in the modeling methods.

Stochastic Gradient Boosting

Stochastic gradient boosting is a strategy that combines bagging and boosting. SGB is a supervised learning method that combines boosting and decision trees to provide a forecast by analyzing ensemble members from all trees. The new classifier is trained repeatedly using the steepest descent direction of the error function of the previous tree. SGB aims to decrease the prediction error between the classification technique and the actual operation by training the learner.

Performance Metrics

Conventionally, the CM (confusion matrix) and ROC (receiver operating characteristic) curves have been employed to evaluate categorization detection accuracy [37]. In ML techniques study, the CM is also known as the loss or uncertainty matrices. True positives (TP) are occasions on which the categorization is correctly identified. Similarly, TN (true negatives) are negative examples that the classifier accurately identified. False positives (FP) are adverse events that were misclassified as positive by the classifiers, whereas false negatives (FN) are positive events that were misclassified as negative by the classifiers.

Implementation Analysis

ML techniques anticipate data more precisely and train them more efficiently. The image dataset is imported and transformed into labels, then utilized to extract features. During feature extraction from the pictures, classification methods categorize various skin-related disorders following corona recovery. The generated NumPy array is then divided and trained using Machine Learning techniques, with the best-suited model being chosen for examination. It works well with a significant volume of data and practical applications. We study how such a system diagnoses diseases using supervised learning, which significantly improves recognizing skin responses.

- The technology enables users to assess sensitivities quickly.
- Network Users will seek counseling after learning about the illness.
- Different techniques are used to design and construct ml models.

Methodologies get the dataset and analyze the data in this module for pre-processing. While beginning the fundamental analysis, the data should always be thoroughly checked for biases. When data becomes accessible due to an inquiry, the next stage examines the findings to extract useful information. The data output may be excessive, insufficient, or fragmented. Pre-processing records requires classifying data into three categories and evaluating it accordingly. As a result, any pre-processing data approach must include data cleansing, organizing, formatting, and noise modeling.

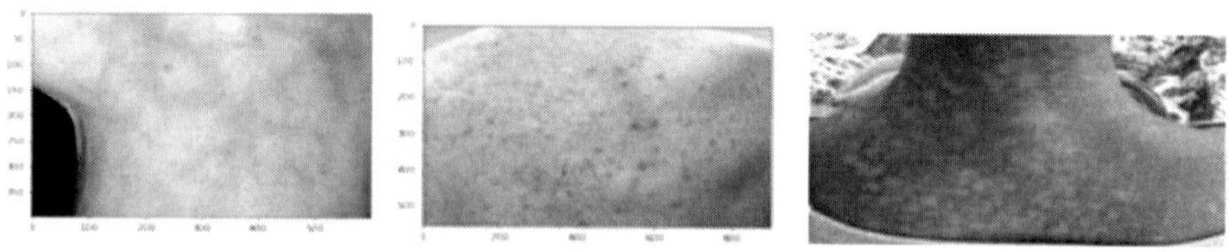

Figure 8. Sample of collected data set images.

Feature Selection Module

Feature selection module is a way for choosing data variables that contribute to the goal variable or performance effectively. The accuracy of data is lowered when hyper parameters are present. The following are some of the benefits of using the classification approach:

- Minimises overfitting
- Increases performance
- Reducing training time

Classification Module

It is the framework for classifying a data collection into subcategories; vast data formats can be used. The key objective was to determine which category the data would belong to. Evaluation forecasting analysis conceptualizes the non-linear mapping from diverse input vectors to signal other predictable methods.

The images' essential elements are retrieved, and an ML model is developed to characterize the seriousness categories of an erythematous image.

- Characteristics such as feature map max-pooling are used to screen the images.
- This image analysis approach is utilized to analyze the images to retrieve information to obtain the outcome.
- KNN, Ensembles, SVM, Logistic Regression, and Decision Tree are examples of ML models. Grid-Dense layers may also be used to develop it with the assistance of Learning Algorithms.
- Therefore, to produce the optimum outcome, the results from various systems are integrated to generate efficient skin allergy intensity in classification findings.

```
[[ 41, 138, 131, ..., 123, 116,  38],
 [200, 119, 118, ..., 141, 150, 234],
 [224, 143, 126, ..., 173, 146, 240],
 ...,
 [224, 187, 171, ..., 165, 142, 213],
 [161,  97,  69, ..., 254, 253, 176],
 [136,  90,  92, ...,  91,  88, 123]]
```

Figure 9. Feature map of skin images.

Logistic Regression

Accuracy is: 59%

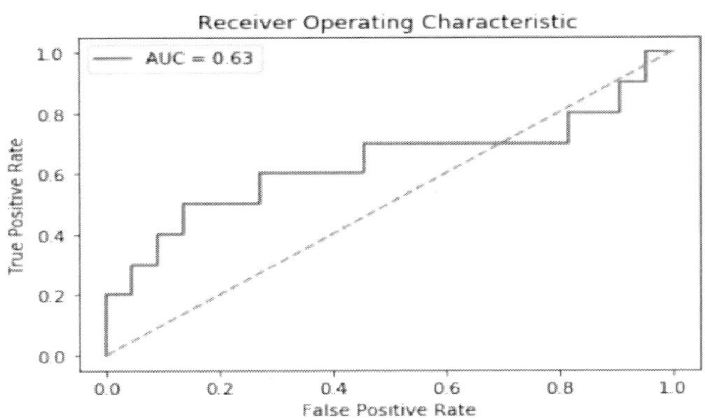

Figure 10. Roc curve for logistic regression.

Decision Tree

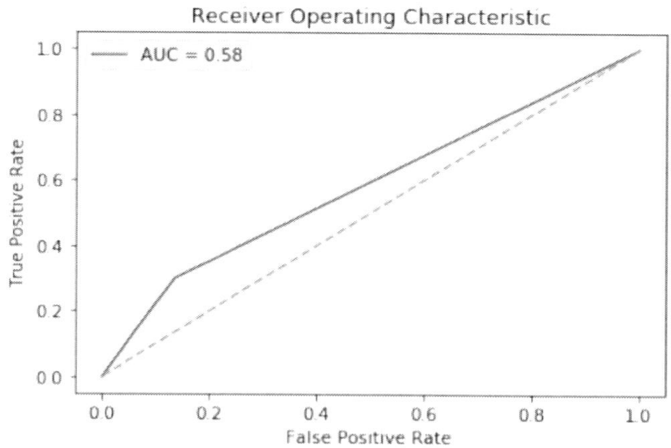

Figure 11. Roc curve for decision tree.

Gaussian NB

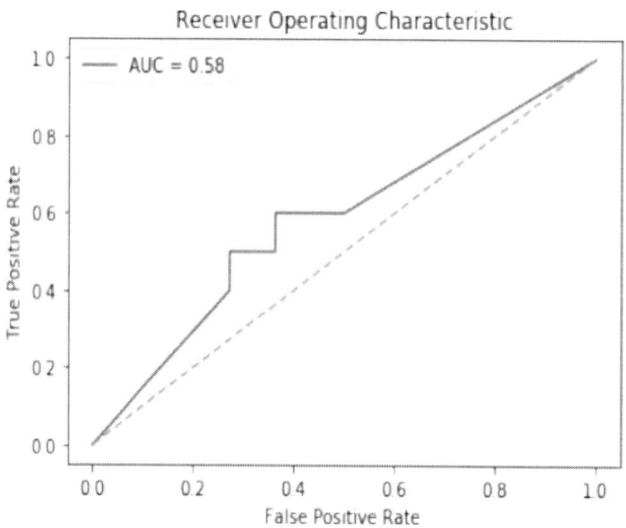

Figure 12. Roc curve for Gaussian Naive Bayes.

Neighbors Classifier

Accuracy is: 0.35%

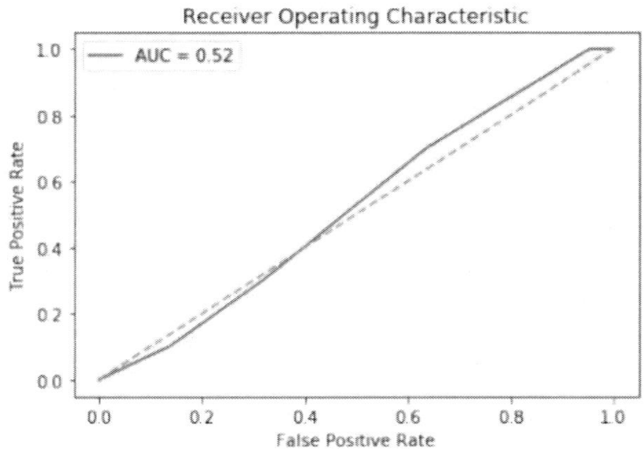

Figure 13. Roc curve for KNN classifier.

Random Forest Classifier

Accuracy is: 44%

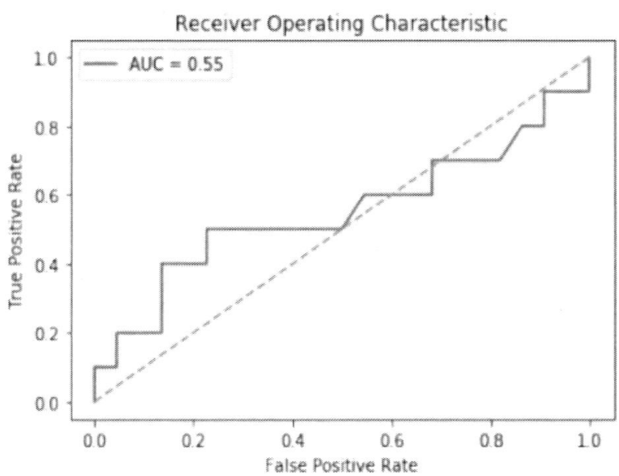

Figure 14. Roc curve for Random Forest classifier.

SVM

Accuracy: 34%

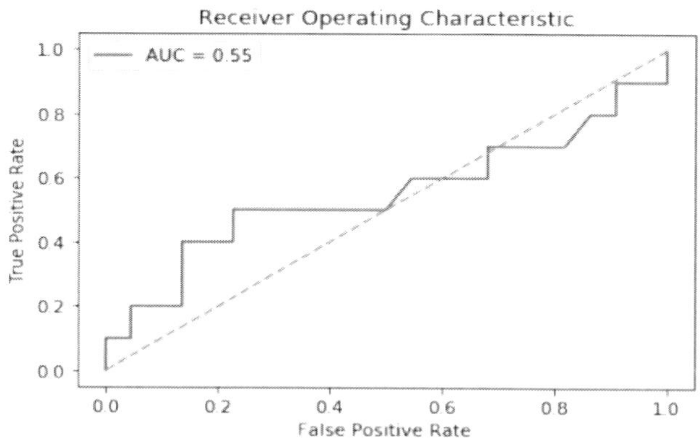

Figure 15. Roc curve for SVM.

Gradient Boosting Classifier

Accuracy: 0.47%

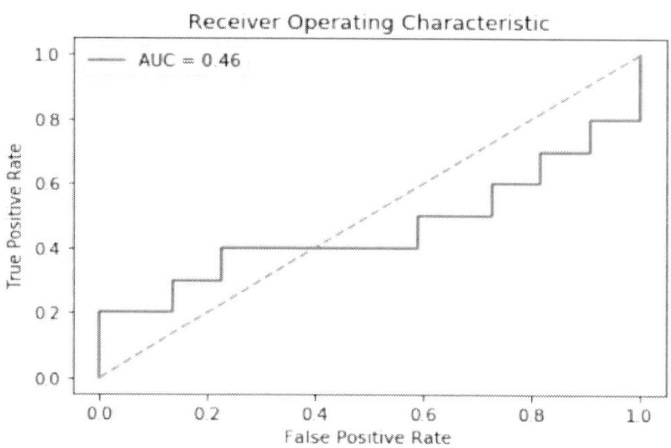

Figure 16. Roc curve for Gradient boosting.

XGB Classifier

Model accuracy is: 0.47%

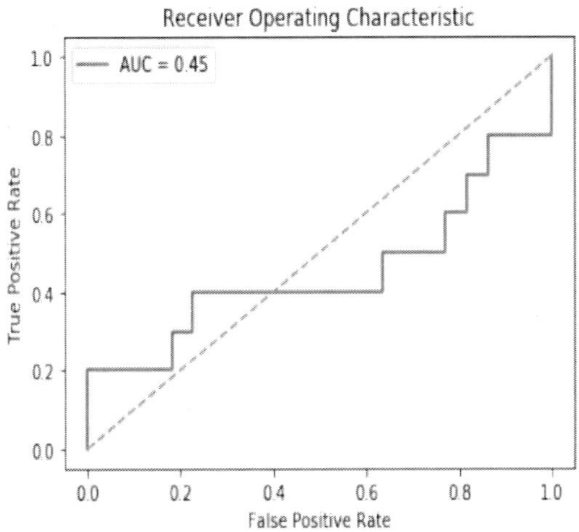

Figure 17. Roc curve for XGB.

SGD Classifier

Model accuracy is: 0.71%

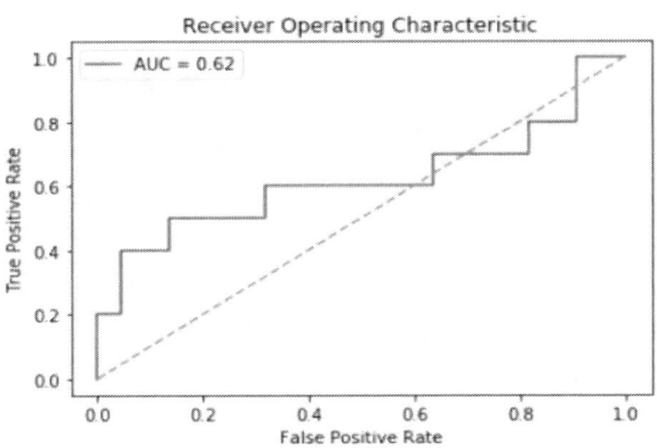

Figure 18. Roc curve for SGD.

Table 1. Classification report

	precision	recall	f1-score	support
1	0.60	0.60	0.60	10
0	0.80	0.73	0.76	11
micro avg	0.70	0.67	0.68	21
macro avg	0.70	0.66	0.68	21
weighted avg	0.70	0.67	0.68	21

Discussion

Knowing about COVID-19 dermatological symptoms might help with early identification and effective therapy for COVID-19 patients. This research analysis examines the vital cutaneous problems related to COVID-19 and the metabolic mechanism that may underpin them. The significance and pathophysiology of PPE-induced pressure ulcers are discussed, and alternative therapies are. For a thorough understanding of COVID-19, more research into its cutaneous symptoms is desperately needed. The SARS-CoV-2 outbreak has had far-reaching clinical, economic, and moral effects, affecting millions.

Furthermore, because of its long symptomless latent and pulmonary droplet transmission, this essential pathogenic illness is challenging to manage. There are still no experiments relating to irritation in the COVID19 global epidemic era, with most characterizing skin lesions indications in patients with SARSCoV2 inflammation. Irritation information is insufficient in many files, or more records will be obtainable in the forthcoming. Irritation about various factors of the global epidemic (for example, relevant to the area relating to COVID 19 virus, increased frequency of preceding skin irritation disabilities, allergic events to Personal protection equipment, mental tension irritation) has been valued highly.

Conclusion

Twenty months after the epidemic began spreading, cutaneous severe response signs have grown increasingly prevalent. These dermatological disorders must be addressed as soon as possible to avoid significant harm. In these extreme circumstances, the "wait and see" technique should not be used, as COVID-19 is causing numerous new diseases every day. This model aids in the early detection of skin allergies without the need for a visual examination by a dermatologist. This project is being developed to ensure that its primary goal is met and that the necessary assistance is offered at various levels to treat skin abnormalities. Because melanomas do not pose a life-threatening hazard, our research's primary purpose is to provide patients with high-quality therapy while also alleviating their discomfort. Patients diagnosed with clinical features of sickness may benefit from a specific therapy approach that helps symptoms and decreases pain.

Future Enhancement

There is a limited possibility that new viral variations associated with specific skin disorders will emerge. It's critical to create a model that can learn all of the current skin sensitivities, making it easier to treat the skin alterations brought on by these viruses. To maximize its performance utilizing deep neural networks, the built model should hold all of the anticipated training illnesses. With the help of OpenCV, this may be turned into more user-friendly and effective modelling that specialists can employ as automated systems in institutions.

References

[1] https://www.yourCOVIDrecovery.nhs.uk/managing-the-effects/effects-on-your-body/skindisorders/#:~:text=COVID%20can%20trigger%20a%20very,can%20last%20for%20months%20afterwards.

[2] https://consultqd.clevelandclinic.org/skin-rashes-an-emerging-symptom-of-COVID-19.

[3] Recalcati S. Cutaneous manifestations in COVID-19: a first perspective. *J Eur Acad Dermatol Venereol*. 2020. https://doi.org/10.1111/jdv.16387 [published online ahead of print, 2020 Mar 26.

[4] GBD 2017 Disease and Injury Incidence and Prevalence Collaborators. Global, regional, and national incidence, prevalence, and years lived with disability for 354 diseases and injuries for 195 countries and territories, 1990-2017: a systematic analysis for the Global Burden of Disease Study 2017. *Lancet*., 2018, 392(10159), 1789-1858. Doi:10.1016/S0140-6736(18)32279-7

[5] Chen, S. C., Pennie, M. L., Kolm, P., et al. (2006). Diagnosing and managing cutaneous pigmented lesions: primary care physicians versus dermatologists. *J Gen Intern Med*., 21(7), 678-682. Doi:10.1111/j.1525-1497.2006.00462.x

[6] Feldman, S. R., Fleischer, A. B. Jr, Williford, P. M., White, R., & Byington, R. (1997). Increasing utilization of dermatologists by managed care: an analysis of the National Ambulatory Medical Care Survey, 1990-1994. *J Am Acad Dermatol.*, 37(5, pt 1), 784-788. Doi:10.1016/S0190-9622(97)70118-X

[7] Kalwyna Rathod (2021), Skin Conditions to Watch Out for Post COVID-19 Infection", Jul 8, Femina.

[8] Harjas Singh, Harleen Kaur, Kanhaiya Singh, and Chandan K. Sen. *Advances in Wound Care*, Feb 2021.51-80.

[9] Zimmermann, P., & Curtis, N. (2020). COVID-19 in Children, Pregnancy, and Neonates: A Review of Epidemiologic and Clinical Features. *Pediatr Infect Dis J*, 39, 469.

[10] Chen, Yan, Hua Peng, Lin Wang, Yin Zhao, Lingkong Zeng, Hui Gao, and Yalan Liu. (2020). Infants Born to Mothers With a New Coronavirus (COVID-19). *Front Pediatr*, 8, 104.

[11] Mahé, A., Birckel, E., Krieger, S., Merklen, C., Bottlaender, L. A distinctive skin rash associated with coronavirus disease 2019? *J Eur Acad Dermatol Venereol*, 2020 Apr 15. doi:10.1111/jdv.16471.

[12] Joob, B., & Wiwanitkit, V. COVID-19 can present with a rash and be mistaken for Dengue. *J Am Acad Dermatol*, 2020 Mar 22. Doi: 10.1016/j.jaad.2020.03.036.

[13] Gary W. Cole, MD, FAAD, (2022), rash, Medically Reviewed on 11th Feb.

[14] Darlenski, R., & Tsankov, N. COVID-19 pandemic and the skin- What should dermatologists know? *Clin Dermatol*, 2020.

[15] https://www.livescience.com/skin-rashes-COVID-19-symptoms.html

[16] Bikdeli, B., Madhavan, M. V., Jimenez, D., et al. (2020). COVID-19, and thrombotic or thromboembolic disease: implications for prevention, antithrombotic therapy, and follow-up. *J Am Coll Cardiol.*, https://doi.org/10.1016/j.jacc.2020.04.031.

[17] Dong, E., Du, H., & Gardner, L. (2020). An interactive web-based dashboard to track COVID-19 in real-time. *Lancet Infect Dis.*, 20(5), 533–53.

[18] YourCOVIDrecovery.nhs.uk/managing-the-effects/effects-on-your-body/skin-disorders 24 June 2021.

[19] Osborne, N. J., Koplin, J. J., Martin, P. E., et al. (2011), HealthNuts Investigators. Prevalence of challenge-proven Ige-mediated food allergy using population-based sampling and predetermined challenge criteria in infants. *J Allergy Clin Immunol.*, 127(3), 668-76. e1, doi:10.1016/j.jaci.2011.01.039

[20] Blumenthal, K. G., Lai, K. H., Huang, M., Wallace, Z. S., Wickner, P. G., & Zhou, L. (2017). Adverse and hypersensitivity reactions to prescription nonsteroidal anti-inflammatory agents in a large health care system. *J Allergy Clin Immunol Pract.*, 5(3), 737-743.e3. Doi: 10.1016/j.jaip.2016.12.006

[21] Joob, B., & Wiwanitkit, V. (2020). COVID-19 can present with a rash and be mistaken for Dengue. *J Am Acad Dermatol.*, 82, e177 10.1016/j.jaad.2020.03.036.

[22] Jimenez-Cauhe J, Ortega-Quijano D, Prieto-Barrios M, Moreno-Arrones OM, Fernandez-Nieto D. Reply to "COVID-19 can present with a rash and be mistaken for dengue": petechial rash in a patient with COVID-19 infection. *J Am Acad Dermatol.*, 2020, [Epub ahead of print] 10.1016/j.jaad.2020.04.016.

[23] Thomas, E. A., John, M., & Bhatia, A. (2007). Cutaneous manifestations of Dengue viral infection in Punjab (North India). *Int J Dermatol.*, 46(7), 715-719. 10.1111/j.1365-4632.2007.03298. x.

[24] Yosipovitch, G., Ansari, N., Goon, A., Chan, Y. H., & Goh, C. L. (2002). Clinical characteristics of pruritus in chronic idiopathic urticaria. *Br J Dermatol.*, 147(1), 32-36. 10.1046/j.1365-2133.2002.04758. x.

[25] Huang, C., Wang, Y., Li, X., Ren, L., Zhao, J., Hu, Y., Zhang L., Fan G., Xu J., Gu X., Cheng Z., Yu T., Xia J., Wei Y., Wu W., Xie X., Yin W., Li H., Liu M., Xiao Y., Gao H., Guo L., Xie J., Wang G., Jiang R., Gao Z., Jin Q., Wang J., & Cao, B. (2020). Clinical features of patients infected with 2019 novel coronavirus in Wuhan, China. *The Lancet*, 395(10223), 497–506. 10.1016/S0140-6736(20)30183-5.

[26] Freeman, E. E. et al. (2020). The spectrum of COVID-19-associated dermatologic manifestations: an international registry of 716 patients from 31 countries. *J. Am. Acad. Dermatol.*, 83, 1118–1129

[27] Mirza, F. N., Malik, A. A., Omer, S. B. & Sethi, A. (2020). Dermatologic manifestations of COVID-19: a comprehensive systematic review. *Int. J. Dermatol.*, https://doi.org/10.1111/ijd.15168

[28] Genovese, G., Moltrasio, C., Berti, E. & Marzano, A. V. (2020). Skin manifestations associated with COVID-19: current knowledge and future perspectives. *Dermatology*, 237, 1–12.

[29] Genovese, G., Moltrasio, C., Berti, E., & Marzano, A, V. (2021). Skin Manifestations Associated with COVID-19: Current Knowledge and Future Perspectives. *Dermatology*, 237, 1-12. DOI: 10.1159/000512932.

[30] Marzano, A. V., Cassano, N., Genovese, G., Moltrasio, C., & Vena, G. A. (2020). Cutaneous manifestations in patients with COVID-19: a preliminary review of an emerging issue. *Br J Dermatol.*, Sep, 183(3), 431–42.

[31] Lin, P., Zhu, S., Huang, Y., et al. (2020). Adverse skin reactions among healthcare workers during the coronavirus disease 2019 outbreak: a survey in Wuhan and its surrounding regions. *Br J Dermatol*, 183, 190.

[32] Lan, J., Song, Z., Miao, X., et al. (2020). Skin damage among health care workers managing coronavirus disease-2019. *J Am Acad Dermatol*, 82, 1215.

[33] Jiang, Q., Song, S., Zhou, J., et al. (2020). The Prevalence, Characteristics, and Prevention Status of Skin Injury Caused by Personal Protective Equipment Among Medical Staff in Figurehting COVID-19: A Multicenter, Cross-Sectional Study. *Adv Wound Care (New Rochelle)*, 9, 357.

[34] Giavedoni, P., Podlipnik, S., Pericàs, J. M., Fuertes de Vega, I., García-Herrera, A., Alós L., et al. (2020). Skin manifestations in COVID-19: prevalence and relationship with disease severity. *J Clin Med.*, 9, 3261. Doi: 10.3390/jcm9103261

[35] Estébanez. A., Pérez-Santiago, L., Silva, E., Guillen-Climent, S., García-Vázquez, A., & Ramón, M. D. (2020). Cutaneous manifestations in COVID-19: a new contribution. *J Eur Acad Dermatol Venereol.*, 34, e250–1. Doi: 10.1111/jdv.16474

[36] Recalcati, S. (2020). Cutaneous manifestations in COVID-19: a first perspective. *J Eur Acad Dermatol Venereol.*, 34, e212–3. DOI: 10.1111/jdv.16387

[37] Diaz-Guimaraens, B., Dominguez-Santas, M., Suarez-Valle, A., Pindado-Ortega, C., Selda-Enriquez, G., Bea-Ardebol, S., et al. (2020). Petechial skin rash associated

with severe acute respiratory syndrome coronavirus 2 infection. *JAMA Dermatol.*, 156, 820–2. Doi: 10.1001/jamadermatol.2020.1741

[38] Piccolo, V., Neri, I., Filippeschi, C., Oranges, T., Argenziano, G., Battarra, V. C., et al. (2020). Chilblain-like lesions during COVID-19 epidemic: a preliminary study on 63 patients. *J Eur Acad Dermatol Venereol.*, 34, e291–3. DOI: 10.1111/jdv.16526.

[39] Kaya, G., Kaya, A., & Saurat, J.-H. (2020). "Clinical and histopathological features and potential pathological mechanisms of skin lesions in COVID-19: a review of the literature," *Dermatopathology*, vol. 7, no. 1, pp. 3–16,

[40] https://theconversation.com/8-ways-the-coronavirus-can-affect-your-skin-from-COVID-toes-to-rashes-and-hair-loss-144483.

[41] https://towardsdatascience.com/a-one-stop-shop-for-principal-component-analysis-5582 fb7e0a9c.

[42] Chiang, W. Y., Zhang, D., & Zhou, L. (2006). "Predicting and explaining patronage behavior toward web and traditional stores using neural networks: a comparative analysis with logistic regression," *Decision Support Systems*, Vol. 41, no.2, pp. 514-31.

[43] Elson, J., Tailor, A., Banerjee, S., Salim, R., Hillaby, K., & Jurkovic, D. (2006). "Expectant management of tubal ectopic pregnancy: prediction of successful outcome using decision tree analysis," *Ultrasound in Obstetrics and Gynecology: The Official Journal of the International Society of Ultrasound in Obstetrics and Gynecology*, Vol. 23, No.6, pp. 552-6.

[44] Schoslkopf, B., & Smola, A. (2002). "*Learning with Kernels*, Support Vector Machines," London: MIT Press.

[45] Ravikumar, G. Ramachandra, G. A., & Nagamani, K. (2014). "An Efficient Feature Selection System to Integrating SVM with Genetic Algorithm for Large Medical Datasets," *International Journal of Advanced Research in Computer Science and Software Engineering*, Vol. 4, N. 2, pp. 272-277.

[46] Altay, O., & Ulas, M. (2018 Mar). "Prediction of the autism spectrum disorder diagnosis with linear discriminant analysis classifier and K-nearest neighbor in children," In *2018 6th International Symposium on Digital Forensic and Security (ISDFS)*, 22, pp. 1-4. IEEE.

About the Editor

Dr. Vijayalakshmi Kakulapati

Professor

Department of Information Technology

Sreenidhi Institute of Science and Technology

Yamnampet, Ghatkesar, Hyderabad, Telangana-501301

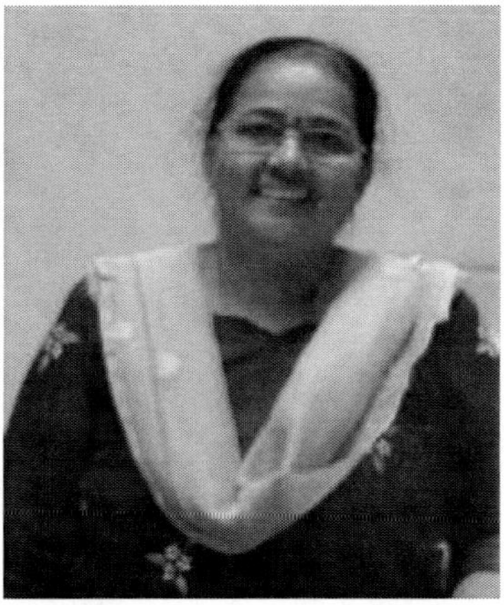

Prof. Vijayalakshmi Kakulapati received a PhD in Computer Science and Engineering from Jawaharlal Nehru Technological University (JNTU), Hyderabad. She is currently working as a professor in the Department of Information Technology, Sreenidhi Institute of Science and Technology, Hyderabad. She has twenty-six years of industry and teaching experience and is a member of various professional bodies, including the Institute of Electrical and Electronics Engineer (IEEE), Association for Computing Machinery (ACM), Computer Science Teachers Association (CSTA), LMISTE, LMCSI, International Association of Computer Science and Information Technology (IACSIT), FIETE, and more. She has more than 160 publications in national and international journals and conferences, 30 book chapters, and 4 books to her credit. She has received numerous awards, including Excellence in Research, Best Reviewer, appreciation awards, and more. Her areas of research include theoretical and practical information retrieval problems as well as machine learning applied to large-scale textual applications. Her research has focused on retrieval models, query/document representations, term weighting, term proximity models, and learning to rank (machine-learned ranking functions). She is also passionate about seeing research problems applied to real-world problems, especially those dealing with large, complex data sets. Along these lines, she is working with evaluating and designing novel search algorithms for web search and summarization. Currently, Dr. Kakulapati is working with big data analytics, health informatics, the Internet of Things, deep learning, artificial intelligence, and data sciences.

Index

D

E

F

Q

R

S